A Public Health Perspective on End of Life Care

A Public Health Perspective on End of Life Care

Edited by

Joachim Cohen
End-of-Life Care Research Group,
Ghent University & Vrije Universiteit Brussel,
Brussels, Belgium

Luc Deliens
End-of-Life Care Research Group,
Ghent University & Vrije Universiteit Brussel,
Brussels, Belgium, and VU University Medical Center,
Department of Public and Occupational Health, EMGO
Institute for Health and Care Research, Amsterdam, the Netherlands

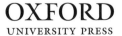

OXFORD
UNIVERSITY PRESS

OXFORD

UNIVERSITY PRESS

Great Clarendon Street, Oxford ox2 6DP

Oxford University Press is a department of the University of Oxford.
It furthers the University's objective of excellence in research, scholarship,
and education by publishing worldwide in

Oxford New York

Auckland Cape Town Dar es Salaam Hong Kong Karachi
Kuala Lumpur Madrid Melbourne Mexico City Nairobi
New Delhi Shanghai Taipei Toronto

With offices in

Argentina Austria Brazil Chile Czech Republic France Greece
Guatemala Hungary Italy Japan Poland Portugal Singapore
South Korea Switzerland Thailand Turkey Ukraine Vietnam

Oxford is a registered trade mark of Oxford University Press
in the UK and in certain other countries

Published in the United States
by Oxford University Press Inc., New York

British Library Cataloguing in Publication Data
Data available

Library of Congress Cataloging in Publication Data
Data available

Typeset in Minion by Cenveo, Bangalore, India
Printed and bound by
CPI Group (UK) Ltd,
Croydon, CR0 4YY

ISBN 978–0–19–959940–0

10 9 8 7 6 5 4 3 2 1

Oxford University Press makes no representation, express or implied, that the drug
dosages in this book are correct. Readers must therefore always check the product
information and clinical procedures with the most up-to-date published product
information and data sheets provided by the manufacturers and the most recent codes of
conduct and safety regulations. The authors and the publishers do not accept responsibility
or legal liability for any errors in the text or for the misuse or misapplication of material in
this work. Except where otherwise stated, drug dosages and recommendations are for the
non-pregnant adult who is not breastfeeding.

Foreword

Using the framework of 'new public health', this ambitious textbook argues convincingly for the concept that palliative care is a public health issue. This detailed seven part text describes the multidimensional aspects of public health and palliative care demonstrating how and why palliative care should be considered as an essential element in any national health strategy. This is the first such text devoted to identifying and codifying the elements of palliative care and public health and serves as an important reference book for the field demonstrating the depth and breadth of information and resources on public health palliative care policy and strategy. By clearly identifying the gaps and challenges in advancing palliative care within a public health agenda, this text stands as a robust resource for evidence-based information on the components required to advance palliative care in the scope of a public health perspective.

There is a rich and extensive history of palliative care advocacy for its public health priority. I write this from the perspective of a participant, an advocate, and a funder. From its earliest beginnings, it was a collaborative effort of several groups; the Modern Hospice Movement led by Drs Cicely Saunders and Robert Twycross, the efforts of the International Association for the Study of Pain to advance cancer pain management led by Drs John Bonica, Vittorio Ventafridda, Neil MacDonald, and myself, and the World Health Organization's Cancer Unit led by its director, Dr Jan Stjernsward. In fact, it was the seminal work of Dr Jan Stjernsward who, in 1982, as Director of the WHO Cancer Unit, created the framework for national cancer control programs and made palliative care one of the four essential elements of national and international cancer control policy discussions. Prevention, early diagnosis, curative therapy, and palliative care was the public health strategy he and his program championed. He advocated convincingly for the appropriate treatment of patients with cancer at all stages. Based on his WHO public health viewpoint, and with the knowledge that the majority of cancer cases lived in resource-poor settings and were patients with advanced incurable illness, he argued that quality of life and control of suffering were the key outcomes a cancer control policy must support.

From 1986 to 1997, with the publication of a series of widely translated and disseminated WHO monographs on international guidelines for pain management and palliative care for cancer patients, the concept of palliative care and pain relief as public health issues became an integral part of the agenda of the WHO Cancer Unit. Its name was subsequently changed to reflect its palliative care interest, to the WHO Cancer and Palliative Care Unit.

These ideas resonated with a growing number of international health care professionals and pain and palliative care experts and advocates and led to the creation of numerous international WHO Collaborating Centres, who took up the gauntlet to advocate for policy change, public and professional education, and drug availability. These centres' activities ranged from research in pain, patient–doctor communication, the development of assessment tools, and drug policy. International and national hospice and palliative care associations and palliative care professional organizations began to develop and grow with a common goal of advancing palliative care initially for cancer patients and eventually, now, for all patients with serious life-limiting illnesses.

Along with the three step ladder for analgesic dosing for cancer pain management, the WHO triangle became famous as the policy diagram schematically representing the three essential components necessary to institute palliative care at a national or country level: the development of national policies; professional and public education; and access to essential pain and palliative care medications. The WHO also strongly supported numerous advocacy efforts to make essential medicines available for palliative care. This policy work was grounded in the theory that palliative care programs at a country level needed to be context dependent and implementable.

In 1997 the WHO published its monograph on pain and palliative care in children and expanded the original definition of palliative care to emphasize the need for care for all children with life-limiting illnesses and that such care should begin at the time of diagnosis. By 2002, the WHO moved further in inclusiveness and published a broader definition of palliative care to demonstrate that palliative care was not just for cancer patients but for all with serious life-limiting illnesses like patients with HIV/AIDS, TB, and those with chronic illness from non-communicable diseases like cardiac, renal, and neurodegenerative diseases.

Palliative Care no longer was the domain of just the Cancer Unit. Palliative care language is now threaded through WHO's Aging program, its Stop TB program, its pediatric initiatives, and most recently into strategies with the Noncommunicable Diseases Program. There is now a WHO Office for Controlled Substances within the Access to Essential Medicines program to support efforts for access to pain medications and several new WHO Collaborating Centres in Palliative Care have been announced, some directed by chapter authors in this text like Irene Higginson and Xavier Gómez-Batiste giving further evidence to the public health status that palliative care now enjoys.

Palliative care is also now closely identified within the framework of the 'right to health'. Governments must be accountable to their citizens to provide such care and provide access to essential medicines for pain relief and palliative care. Human rights activists now work hand-in-hand with palliative care advocates asserting that it is the responsibility of governments to address the needs of those suffering and provide a system of care and appropriate government policies. Pain relief and palliative care are now clearly identified as human rights issues. Human Rights Watch has published four reports publicizing the lack of pain medications and palliative care services in India, Kenya, and the Ukraine. These reports call for regulatory reform to eliminate the barriers to effective palliative care policies. They have also presented examples of the lack of these services as documentation of human rights abuse before the Human Rights Council.

End of life care strategies like those recently developed in Britain point to progress on a public health framework. There are numerous countries, both resource-poor and resource-rich, who have developed model policies for palliative care in their national health strategies that give further credence to the fact that palliative care integration into public health agenda is now a reality.

Professor Clark's chapter, in Part VI, on the global aspects of palliative care, points to the important role of the Observatory on End of Life Care to serve as a public health resource tracking palliative care growth and development. More directories and data are needed and ongoing collaborations among WHO, IOELC, and the Worldwide Palliative Care Alliance to name only a few will lead to more evidence of the expansion of national and international palliative care efforts.

From the epidemiology of dying, to information on place of death, and the different trajectories of death to global issues, it is clear that the range of palliative care services needed is huge. This comprehensive text serves to organize and champion the field of palliative care as an important, growing, credible evidence-based public health concern. It provides an academic grounding to all of the components necessary for a public health strategy in palliative care. The editors, Joachim Cohen and Luc Deliens, are to be congratulated for providing such an expansive, thoughtful, and well-referenced text to encourage us to reflect, debate, grow, and plan for the future integration that will make palliative care available to all who need it.

Kathleen M. Foley, MD
Professor of Neurology, Neuroscience & Clinical Pharmacology
Weill Medical College of Cornell University
Attending Neurologist
Memorial Sloan-Kettering Cancer Center
Medical Director, International Palliative Care Initiative
Open Society Institute

Contents

Contributors

Julia Addington-Hall
Professor of End of Life Care,
Faculty of Health Sciences,
University of Southampton,
Southampton, UK

Elba Beas
Project Assistant,
WHO Collaborating Centre for Public
Health Palliative Care Programmes/The
'Qualy' End of Life Observatory,
Catalan Institute of Oncology,
L'Hospitalet de Llobregat, Spain

Lieve Van den Block
Professor, End-of-Life Care Research Group,
Ghent University & Vrije Universiteit
Brussel, Brussels, Belgium,
Professor of Communication and
Education in General Practice,
Department of Family Medicine,
Vrije Universiteit Brussel, Brussels, Belgium

Kevin Brazil
Professor, Department of Clinical
Epidemiology and Biostatistics,
Division of Palliative Care, Family Medicine,
Faculty of Health Science, McMaster
University, and
Director, St. Joseph's Health System
Research Network,
Ontario, Canada

Candela Calle
General Manager,
Catalan Institute of Oncology,
L'Hospitalet de Llobregat, Spain

David Clark
Professor of Medical Sociology, Director,
School of Interdisciplinary Studies,
University of Glasgow, Dumfries,
Scotland, UK

Chen-Hsiu Chen
Senior Lecturer,
Kang-Ning Junior College of Medical
Care and Management,
Taipei, Taiwan, Republic of China

Joachim Cohen
Postdoctoral Fellow of the Research
Foundation - Flanders (FWO), and
Senior Researcher, End-of-Life Care
Research Group,
Ghent University & Vrije Universiteit
Brussel, Brussels, Belgium

Leopold Curfs
Professor of Learning Disabilities,
Department of Clinical Genetics,
Maastricht University Medical Centre, and
Director of the Governor Kremers Centre
at the Academic Hospital Maastricht,
Maastricht University,
Maastricht, the Netherlands

Luc Deliens
Professor of Public Health and Palliative Care,
Director of the End-of-Life Care Research
Group,
Ghent University & Vrije Universiteit
Brussel, Brussels, Belgium, and
Palliative Care Centre of Expertise, EMGO
Institute for Health and Care Research,
VU University Medical Centre,
Amsterdam, the Netherlands

Julia Downing
Professor of Palliative Care,
Makerere University, Kampala, Uganda

Linda Emanuel
Buehler Professor of Medicine, and Director,
Buehler Center on Aging, Health &
Society, Feinberg School of Medicine, and
Adjunct Professor, Kellogg School of
Management,
Northwestern University, Chicago, USA

Jose Espinosa
Coordinator, WHO Collaborating Centre
for Public Health Palliative Care
Programmes/The 'Qualy' End of Life
Observatory,
Catalan Institute of Oncology,
L'Hospitalet de Llobregat, Spain

Konrad Fassbender
Assistant Professor, Division of Palliative
Care Medicine,
Adjunct Assistant Professor, School of
Public Health,
Fellow of the Institute of Public Economics,
University of Alberta, Edmonton, Canada

Chris Feudtner
Assistant Professor of Pediatrics,
Director, Department of Medical Ethics
Research Director, PACT,
Scientific Co-Director, PolicyLab,
The Children's Hospital of Philadelphia,
University of Pennsylvania School of
Medicine, Philadelphia, USA

Daniel J. Fischberg
Medical Director, Pain & Palliative Care
Department, The Queen's Medical
Center, and Associate Clinical Professor,
Department of Geriatric Medicine,
John A. Burns School of Medicine,
University of Hawaii, Honolulu, USA

Xavier Gómez-Batiste
Director, WHO Collaborating Centre for
Public Health Palliative Care Programmes/
The 'Qualy' End of Life Observatory,
Catalan Institute of Oncology,
L'Hospitalet de Llobregat, Spain

M. Pau González-Olmedo
Psychosocial Area Responsible, WHO
Collaborating Centre for Public Health
Palliative Care Programmes/The 'Qualy'
End of Life Observatory,
Catalan Institute of Oncology,
L'Hospitalet de Llobregat, Spain

Gunn Grande
Professor of Palliative Care,
School of Nursing, Midwifery & Social Work,
University of Manchester,
Manchester, UK

Richard Harding
Professor of Palliative Care, Department
of Family Medicine, Faculty of Health
Sciences, University of Cape Town,
South Africa

Agnes van der Heide
Senior Researcher,
Department of Public Health,
Erasmus University,
Rotterdam, the Netherlands

Margaret R. Helton
Professor,
Department of Family Medicine,
University of North Carolina,
Chapel Hill, USA

Irene J. Higginson
Professor of Palliative Care and Policy,
Department of Palliative Care, Policy and
Rehabilitation,
Cicely Saunders Institute, King's College
London, London, UK, and
Scientific Director, Cicely Saunders
International, London, UK and
WHO Collaborating Centre on
Palliative Care for Older People

Kari Hexem
Clinical Research Associate,
Department of General Pediatrics,
Children's Hospital of Philadelphia,
University of Pennsylvania School of
Medicine, Philadelphia, USA

Katherine Hunt
Senior Research Fellow,
Faculty of Health Sciences,
University of Southampton,
Southampton, UK

Amy S. Kelley
Assistant Professor,
Brookdale Department of Geriatrics and
Palliative Medicine,
Mount Sinai School of Medicine,
New York, USA

Allan Kellehear
Professor,
School of Health Administration,
Dalhousie University, Halifax,
Nova Scotia, Canada

Jonathan Koffman
Senior Lecturer in Palliative Care,
Department of Palliative Care,
Policy and Rehabilitation,
King's College London, London,
UK, and Scientific Director,
Cicely Saunders
International, London, UK and
WHO Collaborating Centre on
Palliative Care for Older People

Cristina Lasmarias
Training & Education Responsible,
WHO Collaborating Centre for Public
Health Palliative Care Programmes/
The 'Qualy' End of Life Observatory,
Catalan Institute of Oncology,
L'Hospitalet de Llobregat, Spain

Marisa Martínez-Muñoz
Research Area Responsible,
WHO Collaborating Centre for
Public Health Palliative Care
Programmes/The 'Qualy' End of
Life Observatory,
Catalan Institute of Oncology,
L'Hospitalet de Llobregat, Spain

Deepthi Mohankumar
Post-doctoral Fellow,
Faculty of Nursing,
University of Alberta,
Edmonton, Canada

R. Sean Morrison
Hermann Merkin Professor of Palliative
Care,
Brookdale Department of Geriatrics and
Palliative Medicine,
Mount Sinai School of Medicine,
New York, USA

Anna Novellas
Psychosocial Area Assistant,
WHO Collaborating Centre for Public
Health Palliative Care Programmes/The
'Qualy' End of Life Observatory,
Catalan Institute of Oncology,
L'Hospitalet de Llobregat, Spain

Josep Porta-Sales
Chair, Palliative Care Service,
Catalan Institute of Oncology,
L'Hospitalet de Llobregat, Spain

Miel W. Ribbe
Professor in Nursing Home Medicine,
Department of Nursing Home Medicine,
EMGO Institute for Health and Care
Research,
VU University Medical Center,
Amsterdam, the Netherlands

Judith Rietjens
Assistant Professor,
Department of Public Health,
Erasmus MC, Rotterdam, the
Netherlands, and
Professor, End-of-Life Care Research Group,
Ghent University & Vrije Universiteit
Brussel, Brussels, Belgium

Philip D. Sloane
Goodwin Distinguished Professor of
Family Medicine,
Co-Director, Program on Aging,
Disability and Long-Term Care,
Cecil G. Sheps Center for Health Services
Research,
University of North Carolina,
Chapel Hill, USA

Jenny van der Steen
Senior Researcher,
Department of Nursing Home Medicine,
and Department of Public and
Occupational Health,
EMGO Institute for Health and Care
Research, VU University Medical Center,
Amsterdam, the Netherlands

Jan Stjernsward
Senior Consultant,
WHO Collaborating Centre for Public
Health Palliative Care Programmes/The
'Qualy' End of Life Observatory,
Catalan Institute of Oncology,
L'Hospitalet de Llobregat, Spain

Lindsey Sutherland
Research Assistant,
Department of Oncology,
University of Alberta, Edmonton, Canada

Jordi Trelis
Medical Director,
Catalan Institute of Oncology,
L'Hospitalet de Llobregat, Spain

Irene Tuffrey-Wijne
Senior Research Fellow,
Division of Population Health Sciences
and Education,
St George's University of London,
London, UK

Siew Tzuh Tang
Professor,
School of Nursing,
Chang Gung University, Tao-Yuan,
Taiwan, Republic of China

Annemieke Wagemans
ID Physician, Maasveld, Koraalgroep, and
Research Fellow, Department of General
Practice-Governor Kremers Centre,
Maastricht University, Maastricht,
the Netherlands

Kirsten Wentlandt
Research Fellow,
Department of Psychosocial Oncology and
Palliative Care, Princess Margaret Hospital,
University Health Network, Toronto,
Canada

Donna M. Wilson
Professor,
Faculty of Nursing,
University of Alberta, Edmonton, Canada

Camilla Zimmermann
Head, Palliative Care Program, University
Health Network, and
Associate Professor of Medicine, Division
of Medical Oncology and Haematology,
University of Toronto, Toronto, Canada

Acknowledgement

The authors would like to thank Jane Ruthven for her work editing each chapter of the
book.

Part I

Introduction

Chapter 1

Applying a public health perspective to end-of-life care

Joachim Cohen and Luc Deliens

Introduction

Guaranteeing a good ending to life for people with life-threatening illnesses requires impeccable assessment and evaluation of their own and their family's needs and preferences and the consequent delivery of adequate and patient-centred care. Traditionally, this aim has been approached primarily from the perspective of the carer–patient relationship, or at best as the interaction between patient, family, and caregivers. This is reflected in most textbooks on palliative care (e.g. the *Oxford Textbook on Palliative Nursing* (1) and the *Oxford Textbook on Palliative Medicine* (2)) which are mostly aimed at optimizing individual care relationships, improving the understanding and honouring of the patient's and family's experiences near the end of life, and addressing the physical, psychological, social, and moral distress that impedes a peaceful dying. The needs of the dying person are the primary concern, but responsibilities towards the family and the support network, such as bereavement support, grief counselling, and social support, are also considered. Patients are viewed as individuals with their own stories and histories.

Such an individual approach to the end of life may be sufficient, and in fact most appropriate, to meet the needs of the dying person and all other actors involved, but it may be inadequate to address the problems on a population level. This book will argue for, and illustrate the need of, a public health approach to organizing and safeguarding good end of life through impeccable assessment and evaluation of the needs and preferences of dying people and their families, and through the delivery of patient-centred care.

In this introductory chapter we will first describe the essential features of palliative care and of public health. By indicating how demographic, epidemiological, and societal changes are affecting the circumstances of death and dying and creating societal challenges to its organization, we will illustrate how—from a societal perspective—the quality of dying is an issue of health promotion that a society should increasingly consider as a crucial aspect of population health, and will provide a sociological justification for adopting a public health approach to end-of-life issues. Next, we will elaborate on what we think this means by describing the concept of the 'new public health' and applying it to the end of life. As such we want to narrow down the definition of a public health approach in end-of-life care and explain why areas that are rather clinically oriented, that pertain to traditional laboratory science, or that focus on individual instead of population health, will not be covered by the book. Subsequently we will try to identify the core end-of-life care domains as approached from a new public health perspective.

Palliative care and public health: definitions

The World Health Organization (WHO) has defined palliative care as *an approach that improves the quality of life of patients and their families facing the problems associated with life-threatening illness, through the prevention and relief of suffering by means of early identification and impeccable assessment and treatment of pain and other problems, physical, psychosocial, and spiritual* (3). The WHO definition further states that palliative care:

- provides relief from pain and other distressing symptoms
- affirms life and regards dying as a normal process
- intends neither to hasten nor postpone death
- integrates the psychological and spiritual aspects of patient care
- offers a support system to help patients live as actively as possible until death
- offers a support system to help the family cope during the patient's illness and in their own bereavement
- uses a team approach to address the needs of patients and their families, including bereavement counselling, if indicated
- will enhance quality of life, and may also positively influence the course of illness; is applicable early in the course of illness, in conjunction with other therapies that are intended to prolong life such as chemotherapy or radiation therapy, and includes those investigations needed to better understand and manage distressing clinical complications.

The WHO definition of palliative care applies not only to individual carer–patient–family relationships but also implies that public health systems need to monitor the problems people with life-threatening illnesses are experiencing and create circumstances favourable to tackling them in the best possible ways. While the WHO has recognized palliative care as a major public health priority for all countries (4;5), it remains a theme only sporadically dealt with within public health. The focus of public health has traditionally been on preventing illness and premature death; preventing suffering and optimizing the quality of dying has not been part of this paradigm. Conversely, a population health approach is rarely deliberately applied within the end-of-life care field, where the individualistic approach persists.

Public health can be broadly defined as one of the tools used by society to protect, promote, and restore people's health. It is the combination of sciences, skills, and beliefs that is directed to the maintenance and improvement of health through collective or social actions (6). The 'promotion and restoration' of health does not have to be seen only as a curative approach illness; health can also be defined in a positive way as energy and vitality, the ability to do things, a general feeling of well-being, being able to maintain social relationships, or as psychosocial well-being (7). As such, health and well-being will be influenced by circumstances such as tiredness, fear, anxiety, stress, and burdensome symptoms, and also by the physical and social environment. Hence, health promotion also includes improving those circumstances for dying people.

The reference to 'collective or social actions' suggests that public health could be regarded as a collective counterpart of individual patient care (6); rather than the health of an individual patient and their family it is focused on the health of the population.

Applying a public health perspective to end-of-life care

Important demographic and social changes have occurred, and continue to occur, in most developed countries, progressively increasing the importance of good supportive and end-of-life care, increasingly confronting societies with the challenges of the care needs of old age and death, and of dying as part of societal life.

Increase in life expectancy

As a result of public health measures, most developed countries have experienced a strong increase in life expectancy over the previous century. Figure 1.1 shows that in Sweden (a country with very early mortality data) a rise in life expectancy at birth occurred particularly in the twentieth century, largely as a result of the public health policy approach towards population health in that period. After the Second World War life expectancy rose almost linearly with around one season increase per year.

Not all countries have mortality data going back as far as Sweden does, but it can safely be assumed that most countries which industrialized early experienced similar shifts in

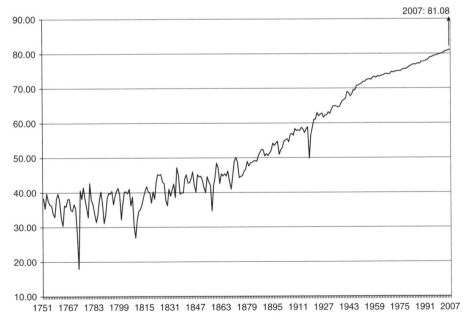

Fig. 1.1 Change in life expectancy in Sweden 1751–2007.
Source: graph made by the authors based on data obtained through the Human Mortality Database, www.mortality.org (8).

life expectancy. In most of these countries a sharp increase in life expectancy at birth can be observed from 1950 onwards, and several counties now have an average life expectancy (men and women together) of over 80 (8). Moreover, life expectancy keeps increasing, and it should be borne in mind that the life expectancy at birth in a particular year (e.g. 2007) is actually based on observed mortality and hence mostly on that of people born several decades previously. With a progressively increasing life expectancy, the cohorts that are young now or even middle-aged, and the very large baby-boom generation (i.e. the generation born in the years after the Second World War) can be expected to die at an even older age.

An aging population

This increase in life expectancy contributes to an aging population, especially as it coincides with a dramatic drop in the fertility rate after the generation born in the years after the Second World War. The implications for the structure of the population are obvious in Figure 1.2. At the end of the nineteenth century (see the example of the Netherlands) or even shortly before the Second World War (see the example of the USA) the population structure in most developed countries had was shaped like a pyramid, with every generation, generally, more numerous than the previous one. The period roughly between 1946 and the early 1960s was characterized by a high birth rate, giving life to the so-called baby-boom generation. In the age pyramids of around 1955 this large generation can already be observed in the bottom age categories. Today this generation is aged around 50–65, and we can see how its size, the aging of the population, and the low birth rate has impacted on population structure.

With this situation, it can be expected that the number and proportion of older people will increase sharply in the coming years. In the European Union (27 member states) the proportion of people aged 65 years or over in the total population is projected to increase from 17.1% in 2008 to 30.0% in 2060 with the number rising from 84.6 million to 151.5 million. Similarly, the number of people aged 80 years or over is projected almost to triple from 21.8 million (4.4%) in 2008 to 61.4 million (12.1%) by 2060 (9). According to projections by the UN, the number of people aged 80 years and over worldwide will rise from 102 million in 2009 to 395 million in 2050 (10). Needless to say, this will increasingly confront societies with the challenge of taking care of frail and older people and guaranteeing them a good quality of life. Moreover, even if the life expectancy free of disabilities or health problems increases, the period people will live with disabilities or health problems will still increase as the total lifespan increases (6). This will also increase the period in which people will need care.

Increasing the informal care burden

This expected and increasing burden will moreover have to be borne by a relatively, and increasingly, smaller group. The old age dependency ratio, expressed as the level of support of those aged 65 years or over by those aged between 15 and 64, may be indicative of the care burden within society. The old age dependency ratio is expected to rise substantially

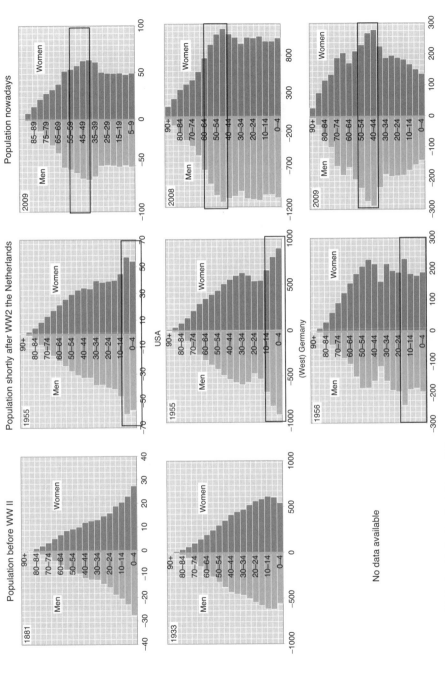

Fig. 1.2 Age pyramids in the Netherlands, USA, and Germany.
Source: graphs made by the authors based on data obtained through the Human Mortality Database, www.mortality.org (8)
Population numbers* 10000 dark grey squares roughly represent the baby-boom generation.

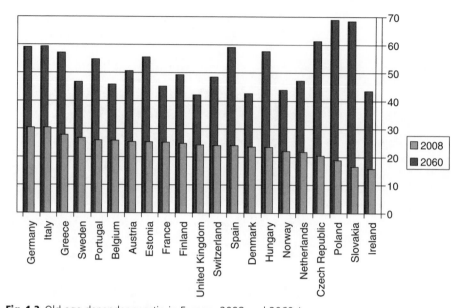

Fig. 1.3 Old age dependency ratio in Europe, 2008 and 2060.*
*Old age dependency ratio = population aged 65 and over/population aged 15–64. Figures for 2060 based on population projections (graph made by the authors based on data obtained through Eurostat).

in the European Union from its current levels of 25.4% to 53.5% in 2060, with variable figures for the different member states (Figure 1.3) (9).

Increasing death rates

As a result of this population ageing, the number of deaths has also begun to increase (Figure 1.4). While most developed countries still have higher birth than death rates (e.g. USA), some (e.g. Germany, Japan) have already entered the stage of higher death than birth rates, sometimes referred to as the fifth stage in the demographic transition (11;12). From 2015 onwards deaths are expected to outnumber births within the European Union. Most developed countries will at some point experience similar shifts. Projections made by Statistics Canada for instance show that, depending on how optimistic a scenario for the evolution in life expectancy is assumed, that the number of deaths in 2055 will be about double, or more, that of deaths currently taking place (13).

Moreover, it has been estimated that each death potentially affects the lives of on average five other people in terms of caregiving and grieving; it is estimated that currently about 290 million people worldwide are affected each year by death and dying and that this number will increase sharply in the near future (14). By 2030 there will be an estimated 74 million deaths per year, which will increase the number of people affected by death and dying per year to 370 million (14). Obviously death and dying will become a major issue for the health of populations.

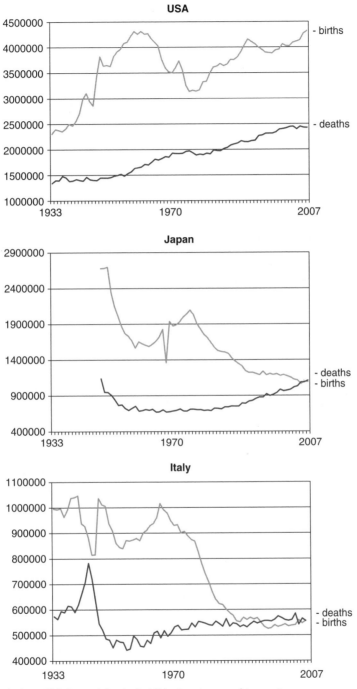

Fig. 1.4 Evolution of births and deaths in USA, Germany, and Japan.*
*Graphs made by the authors based on data obtained through the Human Mortality Database, www.mortality.org (8).

Epidemiological transition

Along with the ageing of the population and the subsequent increase in the number of deaths, there is also an ongoing shift in the predominant causes of death (15;16;17). People increasingly die from chronic diseases like cancer and chronic heart disease and growing old is increasingly typified by a slow degenerative dying process rather than by a sudden or quick death. Even among those dying at an old age the causes have changed dramatically, and dying is increasingly related to circulatory diseases such as congestive heart failure, neurological diseases like dementia, or cancer in old age.

Currently it is estimated on the basis of the conditions leading to death in developed countries that at least about 40% of all deaths could benefit from some form of palliative care or care with an end-of-life focus (5;18). With the ongoing changes in the predominant causes of death this proportion can be expected to increase in the future.

Cultural changes in society

Apart from these demographic and epidemiological changes, a number of cultural and attitudinal changes have occurred (e.g. increased intolerance of pain and suffering, increasing value put on personal autonomy, individualism, and right to self-determination, and changed medical aspirations) which have changed our concerns about and expectations of the circumstances in which death and dying take place (19–21). One could say that gaining some form of planning over one's death and achieving a 'good death' have become more important in the minds of people in many developed countries. With the 'empowered' post-war generation reaching old age it can be expected that even stronger demands regarding the circumstances of and care at the end of life will be made in the near future.

In short, there have been and will continue to be a number of demographic, epidemiological, and societal changes that increasingly confront societies with challenges regarding the organization of end-of-life care and of death and dying. Rising life expectancy and dropping birth rates have, in developed countries, contributed to aged populations and are soon to result in a relatively large group of older people. As this shift is also associated with an increase in older people living with certain health problems or care needs, it will confront societies with the public health challenge of organizing long term and end-of-life care for older patients. With a much smaller group of younger people to take care of older relatives the burden on informal caregivers will have an important influence on population health and will need to be balanced against the costs of organizing formal care to support end-of-life care needs. The number of deaths is on the rise and is, as a result of the large generation born in the years after the Second World War, expected to increase in the coming decades. Additionally, the proportion dying from or with conditions for which some type of palliative care is beneficial also increases, which means that palliative care or care with an end-of-life focus will need to become public health priorities in order to guarantee a good quality of end of life. The so-called 'baby-boom generation', culturally different from its predecessors, may pose stronger demands as to the quality of end-of-life care and even increase the public health demand for a 'good enough' death. If we also take into account that several other people are affected by each death in terms of informal caregiving and grieving the public health challenge to protect the health and well-being of the population directly or indirectly involved with death and dying is even more obvious.

A 'new public health' approach to end-of-life care

The term 'public health' has described different things over time and its field of application has periodically changed. Wile there is variation between different countries (for instance also between the United Kingdom and the European continent), we could conveniently date the origins of public health to the beginning of the nineteenth century, when governments were putting considerable public effort into controlling disease and creating healthier living environments, mainly as a response to health problems (in particular cholera and typhoid) emanating from industrialization and urbanization (7). Public health legislation and sanitary reforms were the main spheres of action. Some of the most important population health successes were made in this period, mainly through non-medical intervention. The economic affluence of the 1950s to 1970s inspired a strong public health focus on improving the quality of life and on developments in clinical medicine, driven by the mounting Enlightenment belief that medicine would be able to conquer disease and premature death. This led to an individualistic approach to public health with a strong focus on clinically-oriented health care interventions. From the 1970s onwards a focus developed on the effects of affluence on chronic diseases, focusing strongly on individual behaviour and lifestyle, and the first large-scale post-war economic crisis led to a rationing of health care spending. This era paved the way for the 'new public health' which from the mid-1980s developed as a reaction to the public health approach that had been dominant since the 1950s, in which too much focus had been placed on the medical profession or on the prevention and cure of disease. The new public health criticized this approach and formulated a number of new directions in public health. It put less emphasis on the biomedical approach and more on social and economic aspects and aimed to focus more on equity and on attempting to break down barriers between professional groups and lay people. It essentially put population health in the foreground instead of individual health such as clinical interventions. Regarding methodology, the new public health recognized the usefulness of methodologies other than epidemiological research.

For this book on end-of-life care from a public health perspective, we use the concept of 'the new public health' as the most useful approach in narrowing the scope of the book (7). In applying it we want to make a distinction between the public health approach, primarily concerned with population health and hence the quality of end-of-life care on a population level, and the medical patient–caregiver approach that focuses on clinical interventions or other aspects of individual quality of end-of-life care and quality of the end of life. As such, we could describe the field of public health at the end of life as the efforts organized by society to optimize the circumstances of the dying and all those involved through collective or social actions. From a public health perspective, we are concerned with the quality of end-of-life care of populations, not just the individuals within them. This implies a much wider view than the strictly medical or paramedical, and in fact requires input and insights from different scientific disciplines (e.g. medical, paramedical, sociological, psychological, anthropological, health economics) acquired through different research methodologies. The reader will notice this variation in scientific disciplines in the selection of the authors of the separate chapters discussing findings based on various research methodologies.

End-of-life care foci from a new public health approach (outline of the book)

Good end-of-life care is amenable to population-based and public sector interventions and has the potential to improve the circumstances of dying on a population scale (22). Hence, end of life care is an important public health issue. Applying a new public health approach to end-of-life care may make little difference to the quality of care for individual patients, but the relevance is that with the growing proportion of people benefiting from it, these small differences can make a big difference on a population level.

In the next paragraph we delineate possible issues of concern with a new public health for the end of life approach, both from a public health policy perspective and a public health research perspective. These issues will be dealt with in the subsequent chapters.

In order to inform a public health policy debate, it is first necessary to gather population-based data on the manner and circumstances in which people die; before public policies try to impact on these circumstances, and improve the quality of the end of life, it is first necessary to be aware of existing problems and concerns. While the causes of mortality and morbidity have been extensively described, there has not been a systematic public health interest in the other circumstances of death and dying. Part II of the book will describe the clinical and social context of death and dying in our societies.

First, Chapter 2 by Tang and Chen will describe where people die in various European, Asian, and North-American countries, and which factors influence place of death. Generally, terminal patients and their informal caregivers prefer death to occur at home (23), and there is ample evidence that dying at home can contribute to a better death compared with dying in an institution (24;25). In reality, however, only a minority of people eventually die at home (26). Knowing which people die where and which factors influence this is essential in developing rational and appropriate public health policies that support the preference of many to die at home. The systematic description and cross-national comparison in the chapter by Tang and Chen is instructive in this context as it allows the identification of factors (e.g. the organization of care provision) facilitating home death.

Chapter 3, by Irene Higginson, will look beyond where people die to the circumstances in which they die, including symptoms, physical, psychological, social and spiritual concerns, the quality of life and of dying, and the experiences of caregivers. Hitherto little has been known about the circumstances of dying and death on a population level, with most studies being limited to patients with certain terminal diagnoses or those making use of certain forms of care. The few population-based studies that do provide important information in this respect unequivocally suggest unmet care needs for many of the dying and a rather unattractive picture of the care of dying people, with many experiencing severe pain, a high number of transitions among health care settings in the last weeks before death, a high average number of days spent in an ICU, and many unmet care needs (27–34). The chapter by Higginson discusses the findings of some of those and other studies regarding the experiences of patients and families towards the end of life and the circumstances of death and dying.

Within the context of an ageing population and a growing tension between medical-therapeutic possibilities on the one hand, and demands for more patient-centred and comfort-oriented approaches at the end of life on the other, end-of-life care decisions are also becoming an increasingly important issue in medicine and public health (21;34–37). Chapter 4 by Agnes van der Heide and Judith Rietjens describes the empirical population-based evidence worldwide on how often and in which ways these decisions are made and thereby provides important information to facilitate interventions to improve the quality of end-of-life care and to safeguard good end-of-life practice.

Another way in which the type of care one receives influences circumstances at the end of life is through its financial implications, both for society and for patients and families. The costs of medical care seem increasingly to be a burden on society and therefore are becoming an economic health policy issue. The costs of medical care sharply increase towards the end of life (38). Studies in the USA indicate that about 80% of medical care expenditure occurs in the last year of life, 40% in the last month (38). In the UK, about 12% of total health care costs (39) and in the USA about a quarter of total Medicare expenditure (40) is spent on the end of life (40). Hence end-of-life is a major public health concern, leading to the need to look for efficient distribution of means and rational and cost-effective ways of providing good end-of-life care. In Chapter 5, Konrad Fassbender and Lindsey Sutherland present evidence of the costs of the final stage of life and particularly of the economic implications for families providing care for their dying relatives themselves and the costs of this for society as a whole.

Public health is essentially concerned with good access to appropriate health care and equity in that access. In terms of end-of-life care this implies that public health policy needs to be concerned with what type of health care people are accessing or receiving at the end of life and why they are or are not accessing or receiving it. It also implies that people with equal needs at the end of life should have the same access to the same end-of-life care. Part III of the book deals with the issues of access and use of end-of-life care services, and the barriers thereto. The first chapter of this section (Chapter 6), by Kirsten Wentlandt and Camilla Zimmermann, addresses the issue of how the end of life is characterized for a majority of patients by an aggressive care approach, with an overuse of certain aggressive treatments and acute care services (eg chemotherapy, emergency department visits, intensive care unit admission) very near to death, and by an under-utilization of palliative care/hospice. Reasons for this pattern of health service use are discussed, as are implications for the quality of life of patients and their families.

Such overly aggressive treatment and under-use of palliative care services may be the consequence of patients accessing palliative care too late or not at all (36). Gunn Grande, in Chapter 7, presents empirical data on which patients access palliative care and which do not, and indicates a number of barriers to access and a number of reasons why access is often missed or happens rather late in the dying process.

One major public health policy option through which undesired over-treatment at the end of life can be avoided, access to palliative care stimulated, and a good quality of end-of-life care safeguarded is through the stimulation of good communication between professional caregivers, patients, and families. In Chapter 8 Linda Emanuel documents some of the difficulties with communication at the end of life, identifies communication issues of importance, and reviews some of the mechanisms involved in processing and managing them. The chapter outlines a number of approaches for health policy-makers, for professional caregivers, and for patients and families to consider which may optimize communication near the end of life.

Public health end-of-life policy should always focus on care at the end of life and the proper evaluation of existing and new care models is crucial. Part IV of the book describes palliative care services developed in different care settings. Three chapters on, respectively, palliative care in primary care, in nursing homes, and in hospitals, will address the organization of services, different models emerging in different countries, benefits and disadvantages of the models, and challenges in the organization of care; home, hospital, and increasingly nursing homes will continue to be important settings of end-of-life care (41), and the setting also influences the organizational characteristics and caregiving provided (42). In Chapter 9 Lieve Van den Block focuses on palliative care delivered in the home, outlines different models of primary palliative care organization, and in particular focuses on the Gold Standard Framework used as a means of referral to palliative care in primary care in the UK.

In Chapter 10 the challenges and needs in the development of new care models for long-term care settings are addressed by Jenny van der Steen et al. These settings are likely to become the most important places for end-of-life care in the near future. The specific models developed in the USA and the Netherlands (with its unique and specific nursing home physicians and a relatively high proportion of deaths occurring in care homes (43)) are discussed and serve as illustrations of how to address important challenges.

Chapter 11, by Amy Kelley, Daniel Fischberg, and Sean Morrison, discusses hospital-based palliative care programmes. There are rapid advances in medical therapies and, partly as a result, meeting the care needs of patients in palliative care is becoming increasingly complex and technical. Palliative care (or palliative medicine) is increasingly becoming a medical specialty and hospital-based palliative care programmes have, as a result, become more important. The organization of palliative care services in hospitals, with a particular focus on the USA, and its impact on patient outcomes and health care costs, is discussed, as are the challenges hospital palliative care programmes may face in the future.

The pursuit of equity is a core feature of a new public health approach. The public health focus on the pursuit of equity was particularly stimulated by the publication in 1980 of the Black Report in the UK and similar reports in other countries, which clearly demonstrated that, despite universal access to health care and progressive social security systems, in many European countries considerable differences in health and access to health care persist between different social groups (44;45). Substantial social inequalities in prevalence of and mortality from cancer, cardiovascular diseases, and other diseases exist (46;47), and are also partly the result of social inequalities in secondary prevention (i.e. screening and early detection) (47). Social inequalities also exist in the use of and access to various treatments and health care services in general (48) as well as in the quality of care received (47).

While social inequalities have been a major research issue within public health and medicine in general (49), much less attention has been paid to social inequalities in the way people die and are cared for at the end of life. A number of publications, however, have drawn attention to the 'disadvantaged dying' (50;51) and the WHO has also demanded better palliative care and better access to palliative care for all (4). To provide effective end-of-life care for all, inequalities in the access of high-quality care need to be identified. This book aims to make a contribution in that respect and tries to put social inequalities in end-of-life care on the public health agenda. Several chapters address different social groups and discuss how these groups are locked out of access to the best possible care or circumstances at the end of life by virtue of their primary disease, their age, their intellectual abilities, where they live, or some related form of discrimination, prejudice, or social exclusion. Julia Addington-Hall and Katherine Hunt describe in Chapter 12 how and why palliative care has predominantly been modelled on the relatively younger cancer patient. Kevin Brazil in Chapter 13 and Karin Hexem and Chris Feudtner in Chapter 14 describe the problems and disadvantages with respect to end-of-life care in older people and in children. In Chapter 15 Irene Tuffrey-Wijne et al. discuss inequalities at the end of life for patients with intellectual disabilities. Donna Wilson and Deepthi Mohankumar address in Chapter 16 how people living in urban and rural/remote areas differ in the manner in which they die and the type of care they access. In Chapter 17 Jonathan Koffman appraises the evidence, principally from the UK and the USA, to determine in which ways socially excluded groups–the poor, black and minority ethnic groups, asylum seekers and refugees, the homeless, those within the penal system, and drug users—are disadvantaged in terms of accessing specialist palliative care and related services. He also makes a number of suggestions for how to develop a socially inclusive public health policy for the end of life.

As mentioned earlier, the end of life has some characteristics in common with other public health priority issues, such as a major impact with respect to health consequences or costs for families, and the potential for preventing the suffering associated with illness (52). In order to impact effectively on the quality of end-of-life care and on equality of access on a population level, effective public health policies must be developed. Part VI of the book contains three chapters describing past policies with regard to end-of-life and palliative care and future challenges in the development of an end-of-life public health policy. Chapter 18 by Gomez-Battiste et al. considers the development of public health policy with regard to the end of life on a supra-national level by explaining the principles, aims, and elements of the WHO Palliative Care Public Health Programmes. Chapter 19 on sub-Saharan Africa by Julia Downing and Richard Harding serves as an illustration of how policies have been set out in developing countries and what specific challenges these regions face. In Chapter 20 David Clark illustrates how palliative care has been developed internationally and explains how and why the progress in integrating palliative care within global, regional and national policy-making remains limited.

In the delivery of end-of-life care, from a public health perspective, families, and relatives of dying patients must not be overlooked. Dying is essentially a family affair (53) as is the quality of dying. When someone is diagnosed with a life-threatening illness this impacts the whole family; the characteristics and circumstances of dying will also impact on the quality of life of family members, and—essentially—a large part of the care for a dying person (e.g. personal care, administration, but also things such as monitoring pain medication) is provided by family carers (53). In Chapter 21, Allan Kellehear argues for the enhancement and support of family care as a major focus of attention for a public health policy of the end of life. This attention, so he argues, should go beyond direct service provision and involve health promotion, community development and service partnerships.

This book, in describing these end-of-life care issues and themes in its different sections and chapters, hopes to sketch an empiricism-based image of the end of life of populations, to evaluate how 'healthy' the end of life of populations is, to suggest how the end of life can be improved, and to map out the agenda of a new public health policy for the end of life. A summary of these findings is presented in the concluding Chapter 22.

References

(1) *Oxford Textbook of Palliative Nursing*, 3rd edn. New York: Oxford University Press; 2010.

(2) Hanks G, Cherny NI, Christakis NA, Fallon M, Kaasa S, Portenoy RK. *Oxford Textbook of Palliative Medicine*, 4th edn. Oxford: Oxford University Press; 2009.

(3) National cancer control programmes: Policies and managerial guidelines. Geneva: World Health Organization; 2002.

(4) Davies E, Higginson IJ. Better palliative care for older people. World Health Organisation Europe; 2004.

(5) Davies E, Higginson I. Palliative care: The solid facts. Copenhagen: World Health Organization Europe; 2004.

(6) Public health and health care [in Dutch: Volksgezondheid en gezondheidszorg], 2nd edn. Maarssen: Elsevier/Bunge; 1999.

(7) Baum F. *The New Public Health*. 3rd edn. Oxford: Oxford University Press; 2011.

(8) University of California Berkeley (USA) and Max Planck Institute for Demographic Research (Germany). Human Mortality Database. 2010. Available at www.mortality.org or www.human-mortality.de (data downloaded on 01/12/2010). Ref Type: Data File.

(9) Giannakouris K. Ageing characterises the demographic perspectives of the European societies. Eurostat; 2008.

(10) United Nations Department of Economic and Social Affairs/Population Division. World Population Ageing 2009. 2009 Dec. Report No. ESA/P/WP/212.

(11) Caldwell JC, Caldwell BK, Caldwell P, McDonald PF, Schindlmayr T. *Demographic Transition Theory*. Dordrecht, The Netherlands: Springer; 2006.

(12) Population Division USCB. International Data base. 2009. Population Division, US Census Bureau. 24-2-2010. Ref Type: Online Source.

(13) Statistics Canada. Population Projections for Canada, Provinces and Territories 2005–2031. Retrieved online 15 June 2010 from http://www.statcan.gc.ca/pub/91-520-x/91-520-x2005001-eng.pdf. 2005. Ref Type: Data File.

(14) Gomes B, Higginson IJ, Davies E. Hospice and palliative care: Public health aspects. In: Heggenhougen K, Quah S (eds), *International Encyclopedia of Public Health*, first edn. San Diego: Academic Press; 2008, 460–9.

(15) Mackenbach JP. [The epidemiological transition in The Netherlands]. *Ned Tijdschr Geneeskd* 1993 Jan 16; **137** (3): 132–8.

(16) Wolleswinkel-van Den Bosch JH, Looman CW, Van Poppel FW, Mackenbach JP. Cause-specific mortality trends in The Netherlands, 1875–1992: A formal analysis of the epidemiologic transition. *Int J Epidemiol* 1997 Aug; **26** (4): 772–81.

(17) Wilson DM, Cohen J, Birch S, Macleod R, Mohankumar D, Armstrong P, et al. 'No One Dies of Old Age': Implications for research, practice, and policy. *Journal of Palliative Care.* 2011; **27** (2): 148–56.

(18) Rosenwax LK, McNamara B, Blackmore AM, Holman CD. Estimating the size of a potential palliative care population. *Palliat Med* 2005 Oct; **19** (7): 556–62.

(19) Illich I. *Medical Nemesis. The Expropriation of Health.* New York: Bantam Books; 1979.

(20) Baker ME. Economic, political and ethnic influences on end-of-life decision-making: A decade in review. *J Health Soc Policy* 2002; **14** (3): 27–39.

(21) Seale C. Changing patterns of death and dying. *Soc Sci Med* 2000 Sep; **51** (6): 917–30.

(22) O'Neill JF, Wolf RC. Palliative care as a public health issue. In: Bruera E, Higginson I, von Gunten C, Ripamonti C (eds), *Textbook of Palliative Medicine.* London: Edward Arnold; 2005, 68–76.

(23) Higginson IJ, Sen-Gupta GJ. Place of care in advanced cancer: A qualitative systematic literature review of patient preferences. *J Palliat Med* 2000; **3** (3): 287–300.

(24) Barbera L, Paszat L, Chartier C. Death in hospital for cancer patients: An indicator of quality of end-of-life care. *Palliat Med* 2005 Jul; **19** (5): 435–6.

(25) Yao CA, Hu WY, Lai YF, Cheng SY, Chen CY, Chiu TY. Does dying at home influence the good death of terminal cancer patients? *J Pain Symptom Manage* 2007 Nov; **34** (5): 497–504.

(26) Cohen J, Houttekier D, Onwuteaka-Philipsen B, Miccinesi G, Addington-Hall J, Kaasa S, et al. Which patients with cancer die at home? A study of six European countries using death certificate data. *J Clin Oncol* 2010 May 1; **28** (13): 2267–73.

(27) Addington-Hall J, McCarthy M. Regional Study of Care for the Dying: Methods and sample characteristics. *Palliat Med* 1995 Jan; **9** (1): 27–35.

(28) Addington-Hall JM, O'Callaghan AC. A comparison of the quality of care provided to cancer patients in the UK in the last three months of life in in-patient hospices compared with hospitals, from the perspective of bereaved relatives: Results from a survey using the VOICES questionnaire. *Palliat Med* 2009 Apr; **23** (3): 190–7.

(29) Cartwright A, Hockey J, Anderson J. *Life Before Death.* London: Routledge & Kegan Paul; 1973.

(30) Seale C, Cartwright A. *The Year Before Death.* Avebury: Aldershot; 1994.

(31) Costantini M, Beccaro M, Merlo F. The last three months of life of Italian cancer patients. Methods, sample characteristics and response rate of the Italian Survey of the Dying of Cancer (ISDOC). *Palliat Med* 2005 Dec; **19** (8): 628–38.

(32) Lentzner HR, Pamuk ER, Rhodenhiser EP, Rothenberg R, Powell-Griner E. The quality of life in the year before death. *Am J Public Health* 1992 Aug; **82** (8): 1093–8.

(33) Brock DB, Foley DJ, Salive ME. Hospital and nursing home use in the last three months of life. *J Aging Health* 1996 Aug; **8** (3): 307–19.

(34) A controlled trial to improve care for seriously ill hospitalized patients. The study to understand prognoses and preferences for outcomes and risks of treatments (SUPPORT). The SUPPORT Principal Investigators. *JAMA* 1995 Nov 22; **274** (20): 1591–8.

(35) Danis M, Mutran E, Garrett JM, Stearns SC, Slifkin RT, Hanson L, et al. A prospective study of the impact of patient preferences on life-sustaining treatment and hospital cost. *Crit Care Med* 1996 Nov; **24** (11): 1811–17.

(36) Earle CC, Neville BA, Landrum MB, Ayanian JZ, Block SD, Weeks JC. Trends in the aggressiveness of cancer care near the end of life. *J Clin Oncol* 2004 Jan 15; **22** (2): 315–21.

(37) Prendergast TJ, Claessens MT, Luce JM. A national survey of end-of-life care for critically ill patients. *Am J Respir Crit Care Med* 1998 Oct; **158** (4): 1163–7.

(38) Luce JM, Rubenfeld GD. Can health care costs be reduced by limiting intensive care at the end of life? *Am J Respir Crit Care Med* 2002 Mar 15; **165** (6): 750–4.

(39) Higginson IJ, Koffman J. Public health and palliative care. *Clin Geriatr Med* 2005 Feb; **21** (1): 45–55, viii.

(40) Miller SC, Intrator O, Gozalo P, Roy J, Barber J, Mor V. Government expenditures at the end of life for short- and long-stay nursing home residents: Differences by hospice enrollment status. *J Am Geriatr Soc* 2004 Aug; **52** (8):1284–92.

(41) Houttekier D, Cohen J, Surkyn J, Deliens L. Study of recent and future trends in place of death in Belgium using death certificate data: A shift from hospitals to care homes. *BMC Public Health* 2011 Apr 13; **11** (1): 228.

(42) Cohen J, Bilsen J, Fischer S, Lofmark R, Norup M, van der HA, et al. End-of-life decision-making in Belgium, Denmark, Sweden and Switzerland: Does place of death make a difference? *J Epidemiol Community Health* 2007 Dec; **61** (12): 1062–8.

(43) Cohen J, Bilsen J, Addington-Hall J, Lofmark R, Miccinesi G, Kaasa S, et al. Population-based study of dying in hospital in six European countries. *Palliat Med* 2008 Sep; **22** (6): 702–10.

(44) Navarro V. The 'Black Report' of Spain—The Commission on Social Inequalities in Health. *Am J Public Health* 1997 Mar; **87** (3): 334–5.

(45) Macintyre S. The Black Report and beyond: What are the issues? *Soc Sci Med* 1997 Mar; **44** (6): 723–45.

(46) Huisman M, Kunst AE, Bopp M, Borgan JK, Borrell C, Costa G, et al. Educational inequalities in cause-specific mortality in middle-aged and older men and women in eight western European populations. *Lancet* 2005 Feb 5; **365** (9458): 493–500.

(47) Ward E, Jemal A, Cokkinides V, Singh GK, Cardinez C, Ghafoor A, et al. Cancer disparities by race/ethnicity and socioeconomic status. *CA Cancer J Clin* 2004 Mar; **54** (2): 78–93.

(48) Pappas G, Hadden WC, Kozak LJ, Fisher GF. Potentially avoidable hospitalizations: Inequalities in rates between US socioeconomic groups. *Am J Public Health* 1997 May; **87** (5): 811–16.

(49) Macintyre S. The Black Report and beyond: What are the issues? *Soc Sci Med* 1997 Mar; **44** (6): 723–45.

(50) Oliviere D, Monroe B. *Death, Dying and Social Differences.* Oxford: Oxford University Press; 2004.

(51) Exley C. Review article: The sociology of dying, death and bereavement. *Sociol Health Illn* 2004 Jan; **26** (1): 110–22.

(52) Rao JK, Anderson LA, Smith SM. End of life is a public health issue. *Am J Prev Med* 2002 Oct; **23** (3): 215–20.

(53) *Family Carers in Palliative Care. A guide for health and social care professionals,* first edn. Oxford: Oxford University Press; 2009.

Part II

Clinical and social context of death and dying

Chapter 2

Place of death and end-of-life care

Siew Tzuh Tang and Chen-Hsiu Chen

Place of death: a convergence of humanitarian and cost containment concerns in end-of-life care

The basic tenets of end-of-life care are philosophically rooted in an acknowledgement of the individual's inherent dignity and are directed toward helping the patient to die with dignity intact (1,2). To maintain their dignity, patients must have a sense of control over the circumstances of their dying and must be able to make their own decisions and to preside over their own dying (1,2). One specific need of these patients is to decide where they prefer to die (2). Setting affects the philosophy of care as well as the types and intensity of services that can be delivered to the dying. Therefore, setting has a tangible, direct, and immediate impact on a patient's quality of life at the end of life (3). Correspondingly, one domain of quality of dying and death has been specifically defined as dying in the place of one's choice (2). Having a sense of control over selecting the place of death can alleviate concerns about the unknown process of dying, reduce anxieties about both the present and the future, enhance quality of life, and even the quality of death itself (2). Therefore, place of death has been suggested as an important indicator of human development and public health (4–6). Achieving a patient's preferred place of death is a marker of all efforts to enable a 'good' death, one in accordance with the wishes of the patient and their family, as suggested by the Institute of Medicine (7).

Cancer patients worldwide have a strong preference for dying at home (Table 2.1). The choice of home as a terminally ill patient's preferred place of death has been motivated by quality of life considerations (16,20,21); the principal reasons given by patients who prefer to die at home are being with their families, enjoying a more 'normal' life, having greater autonomy, and being surrounded by a familiar and comfortable home environment. Dying at home—while almost a universal aspiration across different cultures—may be particularly important in some cultures such as the Chinese (18).

In contrast, a preference for dying in an institution may indicate a resigned acceptance of the inevitability of in-patient care. This acceptance may result from limited informal care resources for providing end-of-life care at home, the intention not to burden family caregivers, a sense of security gained from the concept of professionals better managing symptoms and maximizing personal dignity once bodily functions are lost, and practical considerations in managing a dead body at home (4,15,16,20,21–25). Although dying at home may not be feasible for all terminally ill patients, reasons for preferring *not* to die at

Table 2.1 Preferences for dying at home among cancer patients

Authors(Ref #)	Published year	Country	Preference of dying at home (%)
Tang & McCorkle (8)	2003	USA	87.4
Agar et al. (9)	2008	USA	35.0
Brazil et al. (10)	2005	Canada	63.1
Stajduhar et al. (11)	2008	Canada	50.0
Koffman & Higginson (12)	2004	UK	81.0
Wood et al. (13)	2007	UK	73.0
Gyllenhammar et al. (14)	2003	Sweden	77.0
Beccaro et al. (4)	2006	Italy	93.5
Foreman et al. (15)	2006	Australia	58.1
Sanjo et al. (16)	2007	Japan	73.0
Choi et al. (17)	2010	Japan	68.0
Tang et al. (18)	2005	Taiwan	61.0
Hsieh et al. (19)	2007	Taiwan	74.0

home may highlight directions for clinical interventions and public health policy. Thus, resources could be allocated to improving the availability of homecare services and effectively coordinating end-of-life care between hospital and community to ensure that it responds to patient choice of place of death.

The current interest in place of death and the de-hospitalization of death also arises from the fiscal pressure of the high costs of end-of-life care (see Chapter 6 in this book). The primary driver of end-of-life care spending in the US (26,27), Canada (28), the Netherlands (29), and Taiwan (30) is the use of in-patient services. However, intense in-patient end-of-life care patterns not only fail to increase survival, but also do not enhance patient quality of life, satisfaction with care quality, or family bereavement adjustment (31–33). An attractive alternative to in-patient end-of-life care is hospice home care, which shifts end-of-life care from hospital to home. Given that the preference of the majority of terminally ill patients is to die at home and the potential cost saving for the society at large, contemporary health care policy is directed at facilitating death at home when desired and preventing crisis admissions in the last few days of life (34).

Actual place of death

All causes of death

Contemporary population-based studies indicate that the most common place of death around the world, for all causes of death, is hospital (Table 2.2). Furthermore, a substantial and continuing decline in hospital deaths was only found for the US (40,41) and Canada (6). Correspondingly, deaths occurring at home increased in the US and Canada, a highly notable trend because it is the opposite of that in England and Wales (43), Japan (42), and Korea (37).

Table 2.2 Proportions of death in a hospital for all causes of death from population-based study

Country	All causes of death			Cancer		
	Authors (Ref #)	Published year	Proportions of death in a hospital	Authors (Ref #)	Published year	Proportions of death in a hospital
Australia	McNamara et al. (39)	2007	48.6			
Australia	Currow et al. (46)	2008	60.0	Currow et al. (46)	2008	60.0
Belgium	Cohen et al. (35,36,53)	2007, 2008, 2010	48.9–51.6	Cohen et al. (35,53)	2008, 2010	59.5–61.4
Canada	Wilson et al. (6)	2009	60.6–77.7	Wilson et al. (6)	2009	68.5
Denmark	Cohen et al. (36)	2007	39.8			
England	Cohen et al. (35)	2008, 2010	58.1–61.0	Cohen et al. (35,53)	2008, 2010	49.5–49.9
Greece				Mystakidou. (45)	2009	56.0–59.8
Italy	Costantini et al. (40)	2000	52.6	Beccaro et al. (4)	2006	34.6
Japan	Yang et al. (42)	2006	87.0			
Korea	Yun et al. (38)	2006	39.9	Yun et al. (48)	2007	66.2
Netherlands	Cohen et al. (35,53)	2008, 2010	33.9–35.1	Cohen et al. (35,53)	2008	30.8–31.0
Scotland	Cohen et al. (35)	2008	58.5	Cohen et al. (35)	2008	57.4
Sweden	Cohen et al. (35,36)	2007, 2008	43.9–62.5	Cohen et al. (35)	2008	85.1
Switzerland	Cohen et al. (36)	2007	37.3			
Taiwan	Lin et al. (37)	2007	34.2	Tang et al. (47)	2010	66.1
USA	Gruneir et al. (41)	2007	52.8	Gruneir et al. (41)	2007	41.9
USA	Flory et al. (42)	2004	54.0	Flory et al. (42)	2004	37.0
Wales	Cohen et al. (35,53)	2008, 2010	62.8–63.6	Cohen et al. (35)	2008	59.8–60.1

Cancer death

The majority of cancer patients also died in hospital (Table 2.2). Furthermore, home deaths for cancer patients show decreasing trends in the UK (44), Italy (40), Greece (45), Korea (38), and Taiwan (47). Increasing trends for home deaths were reported in the US (42) and Canada (6).

A great discrepancy between preferred and actual place of death

One can conclude from the above review of epidemiologic studies on preferred and actual place of death for patients with all diseases, and specifically for cancer patients, that despite the predominant preference for dying at home, the reality is that few patients achieve their preference. Indeed, a recent systematic review reported that overall congruence between preferred and actual place of death ranged from 30% to 90%, with kappa statistics ranging from 0.11 to 0.68 (49). No study achieved better than moderate agreement, indicating that there is a great discrepancy between preferred and actual place of death. Most importantly, terminally ill patients who preferred to die at home had a lower probability of dying in their preferred place than those who preferred to die in hospital or in-patient hospice (4,8,50).

Reversing the trend toward institutional place of death will be an enormous task (5,44). The first step in this task should be to identify the factors predisposing terminally ill patients to die in a specific place; understanding these factors would lead to better organization of end-of-life care and ultimately to a better death, regardless of place. Factors associated with place of death could serve as focal points for policies facilitating patients dying in their place of choice.

Determinants of place of death

Where a person dies is influenced by greatly differing circumstances, implying that place of death is a multi-factorial phenomenon (41,44). Place of death has been most extensively investigated among cancer populations, therefore, the following section on determinants of place of death will be based on the cancer literature. A systematic review (44) concluded that where cancer patients died was influenced by a complicated network of 17 factors that could be categorized into six groups: individual factors, factors related to illness, personal attitudinal variables, social support, environmental factors, and macro-social factors (historical trends). This categorization will be used to organize the following review and is supplemented by evidence from the most current literature. The review will also include recent findings on how place of death is influenced by services received at the end of life to illustrate an area that has been under-investigated (Figure 2.1).

Individual factors: socio-demographic characteristics of the dying person

Age, gender, and socio-economic status (SES) are the most commonly investigated socio-demographic characteristics. However, the impact of those variables on place of death was found to be inconsistent (44). More recent studies have shown that the proportion of home deaths decreased significantly with increasing age in the UK (51,52), Belgium, Norway, and the Netherlands (53) but increased significantly with age in Italy (53) and Taiwan (47).

The greater likelihood of *elderly cancer patients dying at home compared with younger patients* in some countries, such as Italy or Taiwan, *may be due to cultural considerations.* Death in older age is more likely to be accepted in these countries as 'nature taking its course'. Aggressive life-sustaining treatments, which can only be administered in hospitals, are commonly avoided for terminally ill elderly cancer patients, in contrast to an expectation that 'everything' should be done for children or young adults nearing the end of life. Consequently, the propensity for elderly cancer patients to die in an acute hospital is low. Furthermore, Taiwanese culture highly values *shou zhong zheng qin* (dying naturally of

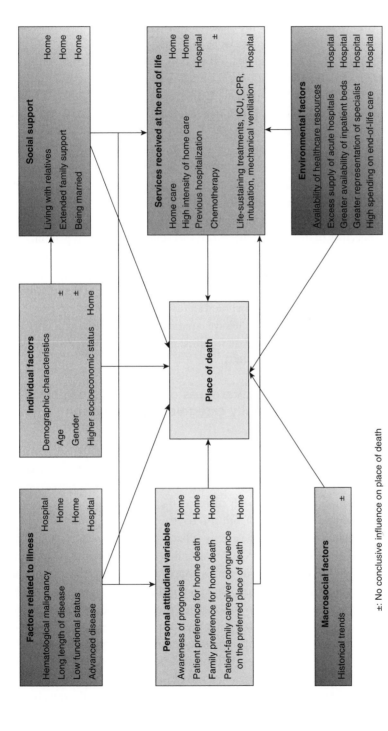

Fig. 2.1. Factors influencing place of death for cancer patients.

old age at home in one's bed). Such a death is the most glorious and fortunate way of dying. Taiwanese people are highly motivated to fulfil their older family member's wish of *shou zhong zheng qin* as one aspect of the important virtue of filial piety (54). Therefore, elderly Taiwanese cancer patients are more likely to die at home.

The effect of gender on the place of death is equivocal and differs from country to country (35,43,47,53,55). Social conditions such as education, social class, and urbanization were shown to influence dying at home (53,56). Furthermore, higher SES, both individual and area, has been consistently reported in recent studies as positively associated with increased chances of a home death (51,53).

Factors related to illness

Death at home was consistently associated with three factors related to illness: non-solid tumors, length of disease, and functional status (56). Patients with non-solid tumours (leukaemia, lymphoma, or haematological malignancies) were the most likely to die in hospital, whereas a long trajectory of disease and low functional status that enabled planning and discussions about preferences were associated with home death. These last two observations have been repeatedly confirmed, i.e. a diagnosis of haematological malignancy (35,47,53) and longer survival (47,55) increase the propensity to die in a hospital and at home respectively. The association between functional status and place of death has not been reported since Gomes and Higginson's (56) systematic review. However, patients with advanced cancer, as manifested by a disease with distant metastasis, have recently been reported as more likely to die in hospital (47).

Personal attitudinal variables: awareness of prognosis, preferred place of death, and patient-family caregiver agreement on preferred place of death

Home death was associated in Gomes and Higginson's (56) review not only with patients' increasing awareness of dying and a preference for home death, but also with family caregivers' clear recognition and endorsement of patients' preferences. Patient-family caregiver congruence on the preferred place of death not only increases the likelihood of patients dying in the preferred place, home or hospice (57), but also contributes significantly to terminally ill cancer patients' quality of life (58). The extent of patient-family caregiver congruence on preferred place of death was found to increase with higher patient-rated importance for dying at a preferred place, and patient-family concordance on preferred end-of-life care options (59). In contrast, the extent of patient-family caregiver congruence influence on preferred place of death decreased when patients understood their prognosis and when their family caregivers reported higher negative impact of caregiving on their life. This study highlights the importance of open patient-family communication about prognosis and end-of-life care options, not only to promote end-of-life care decisions that are consistent with the values and wishes of terminally ill cancer patients, but also to facilitate family caregivers' understanding of patients' actual preferences for end-of-life care, including place of death. Health policy and commitment by health care professionals should also ensure that supporting patients dying at home does not create an intolerable burden for family caregivers.

Social support: marital status, living arrangements, the extent of family support

The feasibility of maintaining terminally ill cancer patients at home and facilitating home deaths depends heavily on whether family caregivers are available, willing, and capable of supporting patients at home. The likelihood of dying at home was found to increase for patients living with relatives and having extended family support (56). Married people have better chances of dying at home because of the potential social support (47,52,53,55).

Environmental factors: available health care resources

Where cancer patients died was found to heavily and consistently depend on the formal health care services available in their local area and on contextual characteristics (56). A higher probability of death in a hospital setting was associated with structural variations in acute health care supply variables, including excess supply of acute hospitals, greater availability of in-patient beds, and greater representation of specialist rather than primary care physicians at both the primary hospital and regional levels (47,53,60).

Services received by patients and their family caregivers

Home death has been associated with use and intensity of home care at the end of life (55,56,61) whereas dying in an acute hospital has been associated with hospitalization at the end of life (47,56). Except for hospitalization and home care received at the end of life, the association between other services received at the end of life and place of death has rarely been examined. This gap in knowledge is due to previous population-based research relying heavily on death certificates to examine the determinants of place of death (35,45,53,55). Such research is limited by focusing largely on individual-level factors and to a lesser extent on health care resources at both the primary hospital and regional levels (35,41,53,56), without input from patients' clinical needs and services provided at the end of life. Evidence indicates wide variations in home death across regions with different levels of health care intensity or expenditures. Patients residing in high-intensity hospital service areas (62) or regions with greater spending on end-of-life care (63) have a lower probability of dying at home. Nevertheless, the association between aggressive care received by cancer patients at the end of life and place of death has only been examined in a handful of studies.

US Medicare patients treated with chemotherapy at the end of life were reported to be more likely than those not receiving chemotherapy to die in hospital (64), but this observation was not confirmed in Taiwanese cancer decedents 2001–6 (47). Elderly patients who chose cardiopulmonary resuscitation (CPR) were 70% more likely to die in a hospital and 11% less likely to die at home ($P <0.001$) than those who completed a do-not-resuscitate order (65). Similarly, the likelihood of home death of Taiwanese cancer patients was significantly decreased by receiving life-sustaining treatments (ICU care, CPR, intubation, and mechanical ventilation) in their last month of life (47).

Aggressive life-sustaining treatments can only be administered in hospitals. Therefore, if cancer patients receive such care in their last month of life, their propensity to die at home would be decreased. Furthermore, receiving life-sustaining treatments in the last month of life suggests that a patient or his/her family preferred aggressive care. In such a case, hospice care might be refused or delayed by them. Since receiving hospice or palliative care facilitates home death (55,56,61) the likelihood of home death decreases significantly for patients who receive life-sustaining treatments in the last month of life.

Determinants of congruence between preferred and actual place of death

Factors influencing the extent of congruence between preferred and actual place of death were recently examined in a systematic review (50). This review led to several conclusions: (1) no specific individual factor was consistently related to extent of congruence, (2) poor symptom control was the only illness-related factor consistently related to decreased congruence, (3) among personal attitudinal variables, those wishing to die at home were less likely to have their preference met than those wishing to die elsewhere, (4) among social support factors, lack of family support and of family caregiving ability consistently decreased the extent of congruence, and (5) environmental factors, including physician support, hospice enrolment, and when patients are given additional skilled care and support in navigating the health care system, consistently improved the extent of congruence, whereas rehospitalization decreased the likelihood of congruence between preferred and actual place of death (50).

Impact of dying at home for family caregivers

Patients' preferred place of death was suggested to be contingent on their understanding of informal care resources and the security offered. A major barrier to patients' preference for dying at home is their concern at being a burden to family caregivers (4,20,21,24,25) because death at home presents significant challenges and consequences for them. Caregiving responsibilities generate competing demands that make family caregivers vulnerable to *physical disease,* psychological distress, and economic hardship, which hinder social engagement (66,67) and extend into the bereavement stage with increased morbidity and mortality (68).

The evidence on the impact of death at home on family caregivers' post-bereavement experience appears to be conflicting. In earlier studies, bereaved families of the home-death group were found to experience greater sleeping disturbance (69) and higher levels of psychological distress, to be more likely to dwell on thoughts regarding the deceased and to withdraw from social contacts and responsibilities, and to be less likely to look forward to the future or come to terms with the death of their relative (70,71). Families of patients who died at home or in hospital have been reported not to differ in bereavement outcomes (19,57,72). However, a recent study showed that hospital deaths were associated with a heightened risk of prolonged grief disorder for bereaved family caregivers (73).

The decision to provide end-of-life caregiving at home most commonly derives from a family caregiver's promise to grant the patient's wish to die at home (22). As time goes by, however, family caregivers may re-evaluate this promise in light of important contextual factors and their own caregiving experiences. The final months of life can be overwhelming and devastatingly expensive for families (67); however, many health care systems have no formal compensation for the substantial time, effort, and financial costs that family members devote to caring for terminally ill patients at home. Therefore, one might speculate that some patients who die in an institutional setting, against their own preferences and the original preferences of their caregivers, had family caregivers who could no longer cope physically or mentally with home care, and/or became exhausted.

This hypothesis was confirmed by a recent longitudinal study on the caregiving impact of home death in Taiwan (74). Family caregivers were more likely and willing to shoulder the 'care burden' and keep their promise to let the patient die at home under certain conditions: (1) they found meaning and rewards in caregiving, (2) they received adequate resources for fulfilling caregiving demands, and (3) they judged that caregiving would not *interfere* with their daily schedule and risk their own health or quality of life beyond a level that they could tolerate. When family caregivers can fulfil their promise to let their relative die at home, they may feel a sense of achievement and may cope better in bereavement. In contrast, failure to keep the promise to grant the dying relative's wish to die at home may predispose family caregivers to suffer a worse bereavement outcome (75).

Therefore, home deaths should not be advocated without recognizing that the well-being of family members both before and after the patient dies may be compromised by the dynamic and complex interaction between pre-existing family relationships and available resources for end-of-life caregiving at home (22). Family caregivers *perform an important service for society and their relatives, and they do so at considerable costs to their own well-being.* For the good of both patients and society, policy-makers and health care professionals need to commit to increasing *support for* family caregivers *in providing* end-of-life care at home. *This support is vital not only to offset the effects of caregiving stress, but also to allow families to keep their promise to* fulfil the patient's wish to die at home.

Conclusion and future directions for research and clinical care

The large documented discrepancy between patients' preferred and actual place of death highlights the challenge inherent in achieving patient preferences for place of death. Decisions about preferred place of death are not made in isolation but are embedded within individual social settings and relationships and are mediated by a range of complex clinical, interpersonal, social, and pragmatic considerations. Health care professionals have not fully understood how preferences for place of death change as illness advances and in responses to the demands imposed by deterioration of patient physical health and probable exhaustion of family resources. Knowledge accumulated about the factors determining place of death includes the roles played by functional status, personal preferences, use of formal home care, and the availability of informal and social support in determining place of death. However, other factors that can contribute to explaining within-country and cross-national differences in place of death are under-investigated; these include clinical needs and services other than home care or palliative care received at the end of life. Most importantly, research efforts should go beyond the long-standing interest of investigating place of death per se to identifying factors that will facilitate the extent of congruence between terminally ill patients' preferred and actual place of death.

If one of the primary goals of end-of-life care is to enhance the quality of life of dying patients and their family caregivers, policies must be prioritized to ensure that patients die in their location of choice. The preference for home deaths cannot be optimally realized unless health care professionals and policy-makers better understand and value the importance of family caregiving and make an increased policy commitment to provide end-of-life care at home, thus raising levels of funding for home care services to support family caregivers. The interface between in-patient and community care of terminally ill patients should be improved to facilitate a move towards home death. With these efforts, these patients' sense of control over end-of-life care decisions may be improved, thus preserving their integrity. Their confidence that their preferred place of death can be honoured without imposing an intolerable burden on their loved ones may be enhanced, lifting the feeling of being a burden to others. Furthermore, rigorous research is urgently needed on the quality of dying at home and to evaluate the cost-effectiveness of providing end-of-life care at home, for which very little evidence is available.

Since death and dying cannot be, nor should be, entirely shifted out of hospital, and the major improvements in end-of-life care are likely to be in hospital, resources should be allocated to promoting the development of excellent care within hospitals. Because death is inevitable and everyone dies, achieving a good death in any setting is of paramount interest. A clear understanding of the insufficiencies of current health care systems in providing end-of-life care for patients might help policy-makers and health care professionals identify opportunities to improve end-of-life care, develop innovations for advancing the quality of end-of-life care, evaluate the impact of interventions, and hold institutions accountable for the quality of end-of-life care they provide. Eventually, knowledge built around place of death will be instrumental in the better organization of end-of-life care, effectively removing barriers to dying in one's preferred place and leading ultimately to a better death for everyone no matter where they die.

References

(1) Chochinov HM, Hack T, McClement S, Kristjanson L, Harlos M. Dignity in the terminally ill: A developing empirical model. *Soc Sci Med*. 2002; **54**: 433–43.

(2) Patrick DL, Engelberg RA, Curtis JR. Evaluating the quality of dying and death. *J Pain Symptom Manage*. 2001; **22**: 717–26.

(3) Mezey M, Dubler NN, Mitty E, Brody AA. What impact do setting and transitions have on the quality of life at the end of life and the quality of the dying process? *Gerontologist*. 2002; **42** (Supp III): 54–67.

(4) Beccaro M, Costantini M, Rossi PG, Miccinesi G, Grimaldi M, Bruzzi P. Actual and preferred place of death of cancer patients. *J Epidemiol Commun H*. 2006; **60**: 412–16.

(5) Mpinga EK, Pennec S, Gomes B, Cohen J, Higginson IJ, Wilson D, et al. First international symposium on places of death: An agenda for the 21st century. *J Palliat Care*. 2006; **22**: 293–6.

(6) Wilson DM, Truman CD, Thomas R, Fainsinger R, Kovacs-Burns K, Froggatt K, et al. The rapidly changing location of death in Canada, 1994–2004. *Soc Sci Med*. 2009; **68**: 1752–8.

(7) Field MJ, Cassel C (eds). *Approaching Death: Improving Care at the End of Life*. Washington, DC: National Academy Press, 1997.

(8) Tang ST, McCorkle R. Determinants of congruence between the preferred and actual place of death for terminally ill cancer patients. *J Palliat Care*. 2003; **19**: 230–7.

(9) Agar M, Currow DC, Shelby-James TM, Plummer J, Sanderson C, Abernethy AP. Preference for place of care and place of death in palliative care: Are these different questions? *Palliat Med*. 2008; **22**: 787–95.

(10) Brazil K, Howell D, Bedard M, Krueger P, Heidebrecht C. Preferences for place of care and place of death among informal caregivers of the terminally ill. *Palliat Med*. 2005; **19**: 492–9.

(11) Stajduhar KI, Allan DE, Cohen SR, Heyland DK. Preferences for location of death of seriously ill hospitalized patients: Perspectives from Canadian patients and their family caregivers. *Palliat Med*. 2008; **22**: 85–8.

(12) Koffman J, Higginson IJ. Dying to be home? Preferred location of death of first-generation black Caribbean and native-born white patients in the United Kingdom. *J Palliat Med*. 2004; **7**: 628–36.

(13) Wood J, Storey L, Clark D. Letter to the editor: Preferred place of care: An analysis of the 'first 100' patient assessments. *Palliat Med*. 2007; **21**: 449–50.

(14) Gyllenhammar E, Thoren-Todoulos E, Strang P, Strom G, Eriksson E, Kinch M. Predictive factors for home deaths among cancer patients in Swedish palliative home care. *Support Care Cancer*. 2003; **11**: 560–7.

(15) Foreman LM, Hunt RW, Luke CG, Roder DM. Factors predictive of preferred place of death in the general population of South Australia. *Palliat Med*. 2006; **20**: 447–53.

(16) Sanjo M, Miyashita M, Morita T, Hirai K, Kawa M, Akechi T, et al. Preferences regarding end-of-life cancer care and associations with good-death concepts: A population-based survey in Japan. *Ann Oncol*. 2007; **18**: 1539–47.

(17) Choi J, Miyashita M, Hirai K, Sato K, Morita T, Tsuneto S, et al. Preference of place for end-of-life cancer care and death among bereaved Japanese families who experienced home hospice care and death of a loved one. *Support Care Cancer*. 2010; **18**: 1445–53.

(18) Tang ST, Liu TW, Lai MS, McCorkle R. Discrepancy in the preferences of place of death between terminally ill cancer patients and their primary family caregivers in Taiwan. *Soc Sci Med*. 2005; **61**: 1560–6.

(19) Hsieh MC, Huang MC, Lai YL, Lin CC. Grief reactions in family caregivers of advanced cancer patients in Taiwan. *Cancer Nurs*. 2007; **30**: 278–84.

(20) Seymour J, Payne S, Chapman A, Holloway M. Hospice or home? Expectations of end-of-life care among white and Chinese older people in the UK. *Sociol Health Illn*. 2007; **29**: 872–90.

(21) Tang ST. When death is imminent, where terminally ill cancer patients prefer to die and why. *Cancer Nurs*. 2003; **26**: 245–51.

(22) Exley C, Allen D. A critical examination of home care: End of life care as an illustrative case. *Soc Sci Med*. 2007; **65**: 2317–27.

(23) Evans WG, Cutson TM, Steinhauser KE, Tulsky JA. Is there no place like home? Caregivers recall reasons for and experience upon transfer from home hospice to inpatient facilities. *J Palliat Med*. 2006; **9**: 100–10.

(24) Higginson IJ, Sen-Gupta GJA. Place of care in advanced cancer: A qualitative systematic literature review of patient preferences. *J Palliat Med*. 2000; **3**: 287–300.

(25) Thomas C, Clark MD. Place of death: Preferences among cancer patients and their carers. *Soc Sci Med*. 2004; **58**: 2431–44.

(26) Levinsky NG, Yu W, Ash A. Moskowitz M, Gazelle G, Saynina O, et al. Influence of age on Medicare expenditures and medical care in the last year of life. *JAMA*. 2001; **286**: 1349–55.

(27) Wennberg JE, Fisher ES, Goodman DC, Skinner JS. Tracking the care of patients with severe chronic illness: The Dartmouth atlas of health care. 2008. Available at: http://www.dartmouthatlas.org/at lases/2008_Chronic_Care_Atlas.pdf. Accessed 7 April 2010.

(28) Fassbender K, Fainsinger RL, Carson M, Finegan BA. Cost trajectories at the end of life: The Canadian experience. *J Pain Symptom Manage*. 2009; **38**: 75–80.

(29) Polder JJ, Barendregt JJ, van Oers H. Health care costs in the last year of life: The Dutch experience. *Soc Sci Med*. 2006; **63**, 1720–31.

(30) Liu CN, Yang MC. National health insurance expenditure for adult beneficiaries in Taiwan in their last year of life. *J Formosa Med Ass*. 2002; **101**: 552–9.

(31) Barnato AE, Chang CC, Farrell MH, Lave JR, Roberts MS, Angus DC. Is survival better at hospitals with higher 'end-of-life' treatment intensity? *Med Care* 2010; **48**: 125–32.

(32) Wennberg JE, Bronner K, Skinner JS, Fisher ES, Goodman DC. Inpatient care intensity and patients' ratings of their hospital experiences. *Health Aff* 2009; **28**: 103–12.

(33) Wright AA, Zhang B, Ray A, Mark JW, Trice E, Balboni T, et al. Associations between end-of-life discussions, patient mental health, medical care near death, and caregiver bereavement adjustment. *JAMA*. 2008; **300**: 1665–73.

(34) World Health Organization. Palliative care: The solid facts. World Health Organization, Geneva. 2004. Available at: www.who.int/entity/cancer/palliative/en/. Accessed 29 March 2010.

(35) Cohen J, Bilsen J, Addington-Hall J, Löfmark R, Miccinesi G, Kaasa S, et al. Population-based study of dying in hospital in six European countries. *Palliat Med*. 2008; **22**: 702–10.

(36) Cohen J, Bilsen J, Fischer S, Löfmark R, Norup M, van der Heide A, et al. End-of-life decision-making in Belgium, Denmark, Sweden and Switzerland: Does place of death make a difference? *J Epidemiol Community Health*. 2007; **61**: 1062–8.

(37) Lin HC, Lin YJ, Liu TC, Chen CS, Lin CC. Urbanization and place of death for the elderly. *Palliat Med*. 2007; **21**, 705–11.

(38) Yun YH, Lim MK, Choi KS, Rhee YS. Predictors associated with the place of death in a country with increasing hospital deaths. *Palliat Med*. 2006; 20, 455–61.

(39) McNamara B, Rosenwax L. Factors affecting place of death in Western Australia. *Health Place*. 2007; **13**: 356–67.

(40) Costantini M, Balzi D, Garronec E, Orlandini C, Parodi S, Vercelli M, et al. Geographical variations of place of death among Italian communities suggest an inappropriate hospital use in the terminal phase of cancer disease. *Public Health*. 2000; **114**: 15–20.

(41) Gruneir A, Mor V, Weitzen S, Truchil R, Teno J, Roy J. Where people die—A multilevel approach to understanding influences on site of death in America. *Med Care*. 2007; **64**: 351–78.

(42) Flory J, Young-Xu Y, Gurol I, Levinsky N, Ash A, Emanuel E. Place of death: U.S. trends since 1980. *Health Aff*. 2004; **23**: 194–200.

(43) Yang L, Sakamoto N, Marui E. A study of home deaths in Japan from 1951 to 2002. *BMC Palliat Care*. 2006; 5: 1–9.

(44) Gomes B, Higginson IJ. Where people die (1974–2030): Past trends, future projections and implications for care. *Palliat Med*. 2008; **22**: 33–41.

(45) Mystakidou K, Parpa E, Tsilika E, Galanos A, Patiraki E, Tsiatas M, et al. Where do cancer patients die in Greece? A population-based study on the place of death in 1993 and 2003. *J Pain Symptom Manage*. 2009; **38**: 309–14.

(46) Currow DC, Burns CM, Abernethy AP. Place of death for people with noncancer and cancer illness in South Australia. *J Palliat Care*. 2008; **24**: 144–50.

(47) Tang ST, Huang EW, Liu TW, Rau KM, Hung YN, Wu SC. Propensity for home death among Taiwanese cancer decedents, 2001–2006 determined by services received at end of life. *J Pain Symptom Manage.* 2010; **40**, 566–74.

(48) Yun YH, Kwak M, Park SM, Kim S, Choi JS, Lim HY, et al. Chemotherapy use and associated factors among cancer patients near the end of life. *Oncol.* 2007; **72**: 164–71.

(49) Bell CL, Somogyi-Zalud E, Masaki KH. Methodological review: measured and reported congruence between preferred and actual place of death. *Palliat Med.* 2009; **23**: 482–90.

(50) Bell CL, Somogyi-Zalud E, Masaki KH. Factors associated with congruence between preferred and actual place of death. *J Pain Symptom Manage.* 2010; **39**: 591–604.

(51) Davies,E, Linklater KM, Jack RH, Clark L, Møller H. How is place of death from cancer changing and what affects it? *Br J Cancer.* 2006; **95**: 593–600.

(52) Grundy E, Mayer D, Young H, Sloggett A. Living arrangements and place of death of older people with cancer in England and Wales. *Br J Cancer.* 2004; **91**, 907–12.

(53) Cohen J, Houttekier D, Onwuteaka-Philipsen B, Miccinesi G, Addington-Hall J, Kaasa S, et al. Which patients with cancer die at home? A study of six European countries using death certificate data. *J Clin Oncol.* 2010; **28**: 2267–73.

(54) Dai YT, Dimond MF. Filial piety: A cross-cultural comparison and its implications for the well-being of older parents. *J Gerontol Nurs.* 1998; **24**: 13–18.

(55) Aabom B, Kragstrup J, Vondeling H, Bakketeig LS, Stovring H. Population-based study of place of death of patients with cancer. *Br J General Practice.* 2005; **55**: 684–9.

(56) Gomes B, Higginson IJ. Factors influencing death at home in terminally ill patients with cancer: Systematic review. *BMJ.* 2006; **332**: 515–21.

(57) Grande GE, Ewing G. Informal carer bereavement outcome: Relation to quality of end of life support and achievement of preferred place of death. *Palliat Med.* 2009; **23**: 248–56.

(58) Tang ST, Liu TW, Tsai CM, Wang CH, Chang GC, Liu LN. Patient awareness of prognosis, patient-family caregiver congruence on the preferred place of death, and caregiving burden of families contribute to the quality of life for terminally ill cancer patients in Taiwan. *Psycho-Oncol.* 2008; **17**: 1202–9.

(59) Tang ST, Chen CCH, Tang WR, Liu TW. Determinants of patient-family caregiver congruence on preferred place of death in Taiwan. *J Pain Symptom Manage.* 2010; **40**: 235–45.

(60) Lackan NA, Eschbach K, Stimpson JP, Freeman JL, Goodwin JS. Ethnic differences in in-hospital place of death among older adults in California: effects of individual and contextual characteristics and medical resource supply. *Med Care.* 2009; **47**: 138–45.

(61) Back AL, LiYF, Sales AE. Impact of palliative care case management on resource use by patients dying of cancer at a Veterans Affairs Medical Center. *J Palliat Med.* 2005; **8**: 26–35.

(62) Teno JM, Mor V, Ward N, Roy J, Clarridge B, Wennberg JE, et al. Bereaved family member perceptions of quality of end-of-life care in U.S. regions with high and low usage of intensive care unit care. *J Am Geriatr Soc.* 2005; **53**: 1905–11.

(63) Barnato AE, Herndon MB, Anthony DL, Gallagher PM, Skinner JS, Bynum JPW, et al. Are regional variations in end-of-life intensity explained by patient preferences? A study of the US Medicare population. *Med Care.* 2007; **45**: 386–93.

(64) Earle CC, Neville BA, Landrum MB, Ayanian JZ, Block SD, Weeks JC. Trends in the aggressiveness of cancer care near the end of life. *J Clin Oncol.* 2004; **22**: 315–21.

(65) Temkin-Greener H, Mukamel DB. Predicting place of death in the program of All-Inclusive Care for the Elderly (PACE): Participant versus program characteristics. *J Am Geriatr Soc.* 2002; **50**: 125–35.

(66) Covinsky KE, Goldman L, Cook EF, Oye R, Desbiens N, Reding D, et al. The impact of serious illness on patients' families. *JAMA.* 1994; **272**: 1839–44.

(67) Emanuel EJ, Fairclough DL, Slutsman J, Emanuel LL. Understanding economic and other burdens of terminal illness: The experience of patients and their caregivers. *Ann Intern Med.* 2000; **132**: 451–9.

(68) Christakis NA, Allison PD. Mortality after the hospitalization of a spouse. *New Eng J Med.* 2006; **354**: 719–30.

(69) Carlsson ME, Rollison B. A comparison of patients dying at home and patients dying at a hospice: Sociodemographic factors and caregivers' experiences. *Palliat Suppor Care.* 2003; **1**: 33–9.

(70) Addington-Hall J, Karlsen S. Do home deaths increase distress in bereavement? *Palliat Med.* 2000; **14**: 161–2.

(71) Steele LL. The death surround: Factors influencing the grief experience of survivors. *Oncol Nurs Forum.* 1990; **17**: 235–41.

(72) Grande GE, Farquhar MC, Barclay SIG, Todd CJ. Caregiver bereavement outcome: relationship with hospice at home, satisfaction with care, and home death. *J Palliat Care.* 2004; **20**: 69–77.

(73) Wright AA, Keating NL, Balboni TA, Matulonis UA, Block SD, Prigerson HG. Place of death: Correlations with quality of life of patients with cancer and predictors of bereaved caregivers' mental health. *J Clin Oncol.* 2010; **28**: 4457–64.

(74) Tang ST Supporting terminally ill cancer patients dying at home or at a hospital for Taiwanese family caregivers. *Cancer Nurs.* 2009; **32**: 151–7.

(75) McNamara B, Rosenwax L. Which carers of family members at the end of life need more support from health services and why? *Soc Sci Med.* 2010; **70**: 1035–41.

Chapter 3

Circumstances of death and dying

Irene J. Higginson

From a public health perspective it is important to understand and map the circumstances in which people die, including symptoms, physical, psychological, social and spiritual concerns, the quality of life and of dying, and the experiences of caregivers. Such information is critical for planning interventions and services to improve palliative and end-of-life care. This chapter appraises research and other evidence about the experiences of patients and families towards the end of life, and the circumstances of death and dying. Public health takes a population perspective, concerned with the health and health care for individuals needing palliative and end-of-life care. This chapter considers five aspects—who is affected, the patient and family (lay caregiver) reports of the circumstances of death and dying, when are we concerned, inequities in care, and (briefly) models to improve care.

Who is concerned with death and dying: the population affected

Each year 58 million people die in the world, 85% in developing countries (1). Each death potentially affects the lives of on average five other people in terms of caregiving and grieving. It is therefore estimated that the total number of people affected each year by death and dying currently stands at 290 million (2).

As chapter one has shown, age specific death rates have been falling and people are living longer in most parts of the world. This, coupled with the baby boom years, means that soon there will be a considerable increase in the annual number of deaths (3). By 2030 there will be an estimated 74 million deaths per year, which will increase the number of people affected by death and dying per year to 370 million (2;4). After reaching the age of 65, people now live on average another 12–22 years (5). If more people live to older ages and with increasing chronic disease (see below), then larger numbers will be living with the effects, for longer, and dying from them.

Improvements in public health and the control of infectious diseases, industrialization, and consumerism have resulted in great changes in the way people live and the diseases they suffer and die from (5;6). Chronic diseases and cancers are now the leading causes of death. Chronic diseases currently account for 35 million deaths annually, 60% of all world deaths (1;2). Table 3.1 shows the predictions for 2030—rising numbers of people dying from heart disease, cerebrovascular disease including stroke, chronic respiratory disease and respiratory infections, and cancers.

Table 3.1 World deaths (millions) by leading causes, 2005 and 2030

	2005			2030		
	Rank	Deaths	%	Rank	Deaths	%
Ischaemic heart disease	1	7.6m	13.0%	1	9.7m	13.1%
Cerebrovascular disease	2	5.7m	9.9%	2	7.7m	10.3%
Lower respiratory infections	3	3.7m	6.3%	5	2.6m	3.5%
Chronic obstructive pulmonary disease	4	3.0m	5.2%	3	6.5m	8.7%
HIV/AIDS	5	2.8m	4.9%	4	5.9m	7.9%
Perinatal conditions	6	2.3m	4.0%	10	1.6m	2.1%
Diarrhoeal diseases	7	1.7m	2.9%	16	0.9m	1.2%
Tuberculosis	8	1.6m	2.8%	9	1.8m	2.4%
Trachea, bronchus, lung cancers	9	1.3m	2.3%	7	2.2m	3.0%
Road traffic accidents	10	1.3m	2.3%	8	2.1m	2.8%
Diabetes mellitus	11	1.1m	1.9%	6	2.3m	3.1%
Stomach cancer	15	0.9m	1.6%	11	1.4m	1.8%

Source: *Global Burden of Disease*, 2005.

In 2005 24.6 million people were living with cancer and 7.5 million died from it (1;2). Although cancer deaths are expected to reach 11.4 million by 2030, these will account for only 15.3% of all world deaths. Cardiovascular diseases will cause twice as many deaths (23 million) as cancer. The pandemic of HIV/AIDS, which killed 2.8 million in 2005, is expected to become the third leading cause of death in the world by 2030. In Africa, the scale of palliative care needs for HIV disease and AIDS already outweighs by up to 10 times the needs for cancer care. In Uganda, for example, 20,000 cancer patients need palliative care, while 200,000 AIDS patients need these services (1;2).

Patient and family reports of the experience of death and dying

Information in this section is drawn from surveys and longitudinal studies among patients and families on the experiences in death and dying during the last 50 years.

For a long time now, we have known that people reaching the end of life experience complex symptoms, emotional, social and spiritual concerns, along with physical and functional limitations (7). Their families and lay caregivers too have pressures in providing care, as well as the emotional effects of the illness on themselves (7). In 1963, in a prospective study of patients with terminal diseases in the area of King's College Hospital, London, Hinton described the physical and mental distress of dying (8) . In retrospective studies of bereaved relatives, Parkes first described the problems experienced by patients and families, and then showed the positive benefits for individuals who received hospice care from St Christopher's Hospice (9–12).

Cartwright conducted the first population based research, using mortality follow-back interviews (interviews with bereaved relatives) in 1969, based on a random sample of deaths from death registrations (13;14). Informal caregivers reported high prevalence of symptoms in the last year of life, for people with cancer and non cancer, with around 80% reporting pain, and a multitude of symptoms including breathlessness, constipation, nausea, vomiting, weakness or fatigue, depression, and especially among older people dizziness, confusion, incontinence, hearing and sight problems. The survey was repeated in 1987 (15–19). The repeated study found that the proportion of people living alone in the year before they died had doubled (32% compared with 15 per cent in the 1969). There had also been an increase in the proportions living in institutions and being admitted to hospital in the 12 months before death. Home visiting by general practitioners had fallen, although more of those dying in 1987 than in 1969 had had a home help. There was an increased age at which people were dying in the later study: longer life was sometimes associated with the prolongation of unpleasant symptoms.

McCarthy and Addington-Hall repeated the survey methods in 1990 (20–3), and then Addington-Hall developed a postal version. Their first study was carried out in twenty health districts in the UK. Although self-selected, districts were nationally representative in terms of social characteristics. Interviews were obtained for 3,696 patients (response rate of 69%) dying from all causes (2,074 were cancer deaths). They analysed the results for different diagnoses, including cancer, heart failure, neurological disease, stroke, and dementia. There was a high level of symptoms for all patients, and of emotional, social, information, and communication needs. At some stage in the last year of life, 88% of cancer patients were reported to have been in pain, 66% were said to have found it to be 'very distressing', and 61% to have experienced it in their last week. Treatment that only partially controlled the pain, if at all, was said to have been received by 47% of those treated for pain by their GPs and by 35% of hospital patients. Other common symptoms experienced by more than half the sample in their last year were loss of appetite, constipation, dry mouth or thirst, vomiting or nausea, breathlessness, low mood, and sleeplessness. Half of the respondents (51%) were unable to get all the information they wanted about the patient's medical condition when they wanted it. Relatives bore the brunt of caring for 81% of the sample. More help with activities of daily living was reportedly needed by 31% (20–4). For example, in the dementia group, the symptoms most commonly reported in the last year were mental confusion (83%), urinary incontinence (72%), pain (64%), low mood (61%), constipation (59%), and loss of appetite (57%). Dementia patients saw their GP less often than cancer patients and their respondents rated GP assistance less highly. Dementia patients needed more help at home compared with cancer patients, and received more social services (22;23).

Solano et al. undertook research to determine any similarities or differences in the prevalence of symptoms across diseases. They found that the prevalence of 11 symptoms was often widely but homogeneously spread across the five diseases (Table 3.2). Three symptoms—pain, breathlessness, and fatigue—were found among more than 50% of patients for all five diseases. Most striking was the pattern of similarity of symptoms and problems across diseases in the face of palliative care services being available only to cancer patients. Thus there appeared to be a common pathway toward death for malignant and non-malignant diseases (25). This has important implications for planning and developing services, as

Table 3.2 Palliative Symptom Grid of symptom prevalence in far advanced disease

Symptoms	Cancer	AIDS	Heart disease	COPD	Renal disease
Pain	35–96%	63–80%	41–77%	34–77%	47–50%
Depression	3–77%	10–82%	9–36%	37–71%	5–60%
Anxiety	13–79%	8–34%	49%	51–75%	39–70%
Confusion	6–93%	30–65%	18–32%	18–33%	—
Fatigue	32–90%	54–85%	69–82%	68–80%	73–87%
Breathlessness	10–70%	11–62%	60–88%	90–95%	11–62%
Insomnia	9–69%	74%	36–48%	55–65%	31–71%
Nausea	6–68%	43–49%	17–48%	—	30–43%
Constipation	23–65%	34–35%	38–42%	27–44%	29–70%
Diarrhoea	3–29%	30–90%	12%	—	21%
Anorexia	30–92%	51%	21–41%	35–67%	25–64%

Source: Solano, Gomes, & Higginson, *JPSM*, 2006.

Notes:

1. *Minimum–maximum prevalence ranges were extracted from 64 original studies, identified through a systematic search of medical databases (Medline, Embase and Psycinfo) and 12 textbooks of palliative care, internal medicine, and oncology.*

2. *COPD = chronic obstructive pulmonary disease.*

3. *On two occasions, a single study reported a prevalence range rather than a single point prevalence—anxiety for COPD and constipation for renal failure. '—' was displayed when no data were found for a specific symptom and condition (e.g. confusion for renal failure).*

it implies that palliative care can and should be developed for many diseases together. This would also fit with the needs of the future ageing population, who will have multiple conditions (5;6). Here palliative care needs to be provided for the problems that one individual might have e.g. cancer, heart failure and respiratory or neurological diseases.

In 1990, Higginson et al. investigated the current problems and needs of terminally ill cancer patients and their family members and discovered their views of hospital, community, and palliative care support team services in a prospective study of patients and families by questionnaire interviews in the patients' homes. They found that symptom control and family/carer anxiety were rated as the most severe current problems by both patients and families. Palliative care support teams received the most praise, being rated by 58 (89%) patients and 59 (91%) of family members as good as excellent. General practitioners and district nurses were rated good or excellent by 46 (71%) patients and 46 (71%) family members, but 6 (9%) in each group rated the service as poor or very bad. Hospital doctors and nurses had the poorest ratings—they were rated good or excellent by only a third of patients and family members, and 14 (22%) patients and 15 (23%) family members rated this service as poor or very bad. Negative comments referred to communication (especially at diagnosis), coordination of services, the attitude of the doctor, delays in diagnosis, and difficulties in getting doctors to visit at home (26).

In the US the Study to Understand Prognoses and Preferences for Outcomes and Risks of Treatments (SUPPORT) provided insights into the experiences of end-of-life care in the US in the late 1990s. Although this study was actually a randomized trial to test nurses counselling patients in advance directives (which incidentally showed no effect), it provided useful descriptive information about the end-of-life care in hospitals in the USA (27;28).

SUPPORT comprised a two year prospective observational study (phase I) with 4,301 patients followed by a two year controlled clinical trial (phase II) with 4,804 patients and their physicians randomized by specialty group to the intervention group (n = 2652) or control group (n = 2152). All patients were recruited from five teaching hospitals in the United States and had one or more of nine life-threatening diagnoses. The six-month mortality rate was 47%. The phase I observation documented shortcomings in communication, frequency of aggressive treatment, and the characteristics of hospital death: only 47% of physicians knew when their patients preferred to avoid Cardio-Pulmonary Resuscitation (CPR); 46% of do-not-resuscitate (DNR) orders were written within two days of death; 38% of patients who died spent at least 10 days in an intensive care unit (ICU), and for 50% of conscious patients who died in the hospital, family members reported moderate to severe pain at least half the time (27;28). Looking specifically at the last three days of life, SUPPORT found that 55% of patients were conscious. Among these patients, pain, dyspnoea, and fatigue were prevalent. Four in 10 patients had severe pain most of the time. Severe fatigue affected almost eight in 10 patients. Overall, 11% of patients had a final resuscitation attempt. A ventilator was used in one-quarter of patients, and a feeding tube was used in almost half (4/10). Most patients (59%) were reported to prefer a treatment plan that focused on comfort, but care was reported to be contrary to the preferred approach in 10% of cases (27).

Using the methods of Cartwright, McCarthy and Addington-Hall, in Italy Costantini et al. translated and adapted Addington-Hall's postal questionnaire the Views of Informal Carers—Evaluation of Services (VOICES) to conduct the Italian Survey of the Dying of Cancer (ISDOC)(29–31). The study used a two-stage probability sample to estimate end-of-life outcomes of about 160,000 Italian cancer deaths, interviewing a sample of 1,900 lay caregivers or family members. According to their reports, 82.3% [95% confidence interval (CI) 79.9% to 84.4%] patients experienced pain, and 61.0% (95% CI 57.9% to 64.0%) very distressing pain. Only 59.5% (95% CI 3.7% to 65.0%) received analgesic treatment with opioids for moderate to severe pain; pain was 'only partially relieved' or 'not relieved at all' in 54% of the patients with very distressing pain(32). In a sub-analysis of those dying in hospital, ISDOC found that most Italian cancer patients suffered from many untreated or poorly treated symptoms, and only a few reported acceptable control over physical suffering. Moreover, only two-thirds of patients and one-third of caregivers received basic information on therapies and care. About one-third of the caregivers expressed dissatisfaction with the health care received (30;32).

ISDOC quantified some of the major effects on caregivers and the financial effects. During the last three months of the patient's life, 44% of caregivers reported difficulties in their regular employment. Of the 68% of families who had to pay for some of the care, 37% had to pay for drugs, 36% for nursing and assistance and 22% for physicians. Paying for care was more frequent in the south of Italy (OR 2.5; 95% CI 1.0 to 6.3) and when the patient was a housewife (OR for unit increase 2.7; 95% CI 1.6 to 6.1). To cover the costs of patient care, 26% of families used all or most of their savings. Economic difficulties were greater in the south of Italy (OR 3; 95% CI 1.8 to 5.1), for female caregivers (OR 1.4; 95% CI 1.0 to 1.9) and for disadvantaged patients (33).

Overall, the global picture of the circumstances of death and dying of patients with cancer and other progressive is of multiple symptoms, coupled with physical, emotional, and social problems experienced by patients and families. There are also concerns about the information given and communication, and the adequacy of, and (especially from the US SUPPORT study) appropriateness of treatment. Good face-to-face communication is highly valued, and failings in communication can leave individuals traumatized for long periods (34). Patients want services to be of high quality and to be well co-ordinated. They want to be offered optimal symptom control and psychological, social and spiritual support (35;36). Studies have consistently shown that, in addition to receiving the best treatments, patients want and expect to be treated as individuals, with dignity and respect, to have their voices heard in relation to decisions about treatment and care, and to receive the best symptom management and holistic care (37).

The need for care, support, and optimal symptom management is intensified when the illness progresses, as patients become more ill and are less able to actively demand services. There are concerns that death is over medicalized and depersonalized. In some situations there is over-treatment with high technological care, while simple nursing care and symptom management is neglected (27;28;38). There is, however, no reason why more appropriate technologies and patient-centred interventions should not be used.

Although some patients report positively on their experience of care, there are still too many who do not receive adequate symptom management, information, care, and support, particularly in advanced illness, across a range of illnesses including cancer, heart failure, respiratory conditions, stroke, HIV/AIDS, neurological conditions, and dementia (5;20; 24;25;34;39–44). Even when effective treatments are available, patients often miss out on these, particularly those in nursing and residential homes, those of minority ethnic groups, and those belonging to deprived populations (45). Their families and caregivers also have unresolved needs and problems continuing during bereavement which are often as severe and sometimes more so than those of patients, and yet often go unresolved (46). All who observe, participate in and survive the care of individuals with progressive illness experience personal effects such as a sense of loss and grief. The quality of care effects their capacity to live their lives and make future choices. Poor quality bereavement leads to caregiver depression, despair and unresolved grief. Improving care and bereavement therefore has an important role in prevention.

When are we concerned with death and dying: trajectories of experience?

To understand the circumstances experienced by patients and families it is important to consider these in a longitudinal way, to map how long people were experiencing their symptoms and problems, and how these affected them.

The problems experienced by patients and families at the end of life have many simi-larities. But the timing before death may vary by condition, and here some distinctions by diagnosis or other categories are useful.

In the United States, McCusker conducted early work on trajectories, attempting to define the incidence, prevalence and duration of terminal cancer, and examined patient characteristics and patterns of care during the terminal care period (TCP). She estimated that 90% of all cancer deaths had a TCP of average duration of 94 days.

Lynn and colleagues modelled the trajectory of functional decline in cancer and other conditions (47). As Figure 3.1 shows, they proposed three different trajectories. For mostly cancer they suggest there is a period of stable (good) function, followed by a period of rapid decline. For organ failure they suggest there is a varied spiky trajectory, and for frailty they suggest slow dwindling. Work has replicated the cancer trajectories, and shows these apply even among older patients (48;49).

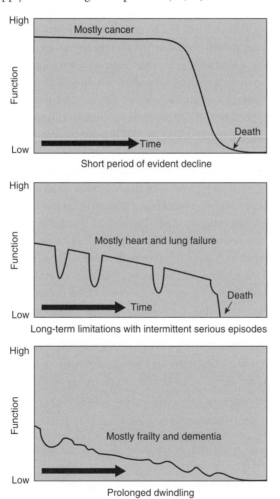

Fig. 3.1 Illness trajectory for serious chronic diseases: original hypotheses.
Source: Adapted from J Lynn and DM Adamson, Living Well at the End of Life: Adapting Health Care to Serious Chronic Illness in Old Age, White Paper; WP-137 (2003) with permission of Rand Health.

Murray and colleagues have identified that the trajectories beyond function, however, are more complex than this. In a qualitative study they mapped the trajectories of patient circumstances, including social, psychological, and spiritual well-being and the distress of family caregivers. They found that family members or carers followed clear patterns of social, psychological, and spiritual well-being and distress that mirrored the experiences of those for whom they were caring, with some carers also experiencing deterioration in physical health that impacted on their ability to care. However, psychological and spiritual distress were particularly dynamic and commonly experienced. In addition to the 'why us?' response, witnessing suffering triggered personal reflections in carers on the meaning and purpose of life. Certain key points in the illness tended to be particularly problematic for both carers and patients: at diagnosis, at home after initial treatment, at recurrence, and during the terminal stage (50).

The data on which many of these models are validated are cross-sectionally collected on different patients at different times before death (51). Therefore, we cannot be sure that these trajectories reflect the longitudinal trajectory of individual patients. Recent research has questioned the 'mean' or average trajectory, as this is not reproduced in individual patients. Bausewein et al. compared summary and individual trajectories of breathlessness and overall symptom burden over time and towards the end of life in two groups of patients: those with advanced cancer and those with severe chronic obstructive pulmonary disease (COPD). In the summary trajectories in cancer patients, breathlessness increased towards death. In COPD patients, breathlessness increased over time.

However, individual breathlessness and symptom burden trajectories revealed wide individual variations which were missed in the summary trajectories. Individual patients (both cancer and CODP) fell into one of four different main patterns: fluctuation, increasing, stable, and decreasing breathlessness (Figure 3.2). The authors concluded that symptom trajectories on the population level mask individual variation, which is reflected in distinct symptom trajectories with different patterns (52). Similarly Murtagh et al., studying patients dying from renal failure (an increasingly common group), found great individual variation (53). For planning services it is the individual trajectories, rather than the 'average', which is vital. The summary trajectories indicate a slow decline for many conditions. But in fact, many more individual patients have markedly fluctuating trajectories, meaning that they need services which can respond rapidly to their rapidly changing needs. Planning using summary trajectories will seriously underestimate the need for rapid response services. In the future planning services should allow for the individual trajectories of patients and families, and the inclusion of aspects beyond functional status.

Inequities in care

Epidemiology and Public Health have always paid particular attention to those groups who draw the poorest lot in society, through poor access to care, social exclusion, or deprivation. There are three main groups that are relevant here.

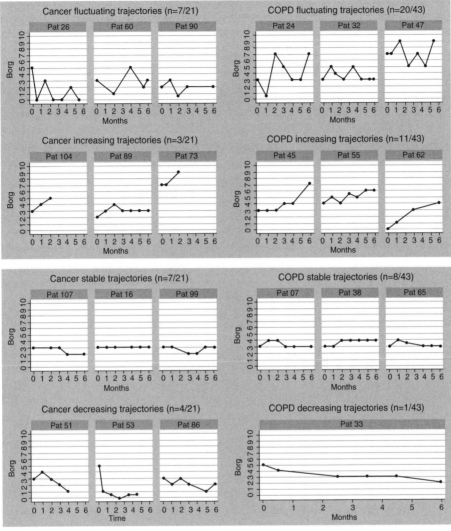

Fig. 3.2 Evidence of different trajectories even within diseases from research data: the main symptom trajectories being fluctuating, increasing, decreasing and stable. Higher scores or increasing indicates more severe symptoms. (COPD = chronic obstructive pulmonary disease.) Republished from Claudia Bausewein et al., *Individual breathlessness trajectories do not match summary trajectories in advanced cancer and chronic obstructive pulmonary disease: Results from a longitudinal study*, Palliative Medicine, Volume 24, Number 8, pp. 777–786 (2010), with permission of SAGE Publications.

Economic

Despite preferences to the contrary, in areas of high socioeconomic deprivation fewer people die at home (see Figure 3.3) (54;55). They also die at younger ages (56), often with a poorer quality of life (57). Furthermore, services tend to require more resources to achieve the same level of care (45). An inverse law of hospice care is thus present, where provision is in indirect ratio to need. McCusker's USA-based study showed a trend of

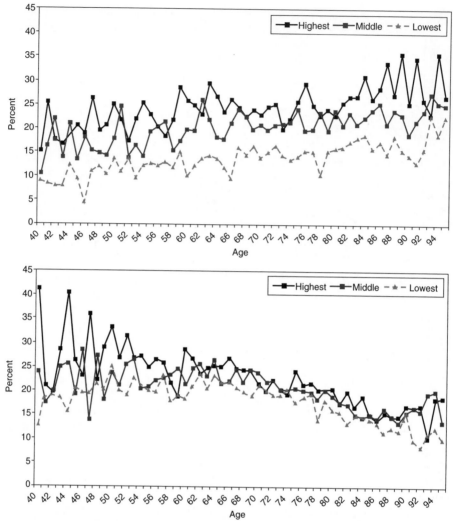

Fig. 3.3 Proportion of cancer deaths at home by socio-economic status and age in New York (top) and London (bottom). Data from 1995–8.
Republished from Sandra L. Decker, Irene J. Higginson, *A tale of two cities: Factors affecting place of cancer death in London and New York*, The European Journal of Public Health, Volume 17, Issue 3 (2007), with permission of Oxford University Press.

less well-educated people dying away from home, to be reversed only for people in areas sufficiently deprived to warrant reimbursement of home care services (58).

Older people

In many countries older people and their carers have experienced age-based discrimination in access to and availability of services (59). In general terms, older people are less likely to be cared for at home, and more likely to be in nursing and residential homes, where staff are often ill-equipped to manage the symptoms associated with advanced disease (60–3).

In recent years dementia has become a major concern for all developed countries and greatly affects the use of health and social care services (64;65). Mental confusion, urinary incontinence, pain, low mood, constipation, and loss of appetite were frequently reported, and many of these were experienced for longer periods of time than in patients with a cancer diagnosis (23). Models of, or processes similar to, palliative care services have demonstrated some benefits among people with dementia (66).

People from black and minority ethnic groups

Minority ethnic groups are more likely than the rest of the population to be poor. Minority ethnic communities thus experience a double disadvantage—they are disproportionately concentrated in deprived areas and suffer all the problems that affect other people in these areas and may also suffer overt and inadvertent racial discrimination inadequate understanding of their cultures, and additional barriers like language, cultural and religious differences.

A study in an inner London health authority demonstrated that black Caribbean patients with advanced disease experienced restricted access to some specialist palliative care services compared with white patients (34). This supports other research among minority ethnic communities (67;68).

Are there models of care that improve the circumstances?

It is beyond the scope of this chapter to provide a detailed analysis of models of care that improve the circumstances of people at the end of life and their families. A meta-analysis found that multi-professional palliative care for patients and families produced better outcomes at the end of life than conventional care (70;71). Palliative care in hospitals is associated with significant reductions in per diem costs and total costs, and can generate substantial savings to the health system by 'cost avoidance' (67;72). A recent randomized trial of palliative care among patients with lung cancer found that patients assigned to early palliative care had a better subsequent quality of life than did patients assigned to standard care (mean score on the FACT-L scale [in which scores range from 0 to 136, with higher scores indicating better quality of life], 98.0 vs. 91.5; P = 0.03). In addition, fewer patients in the palliative care group had subsequent depressive symptoms (16% vs. 38%, P = 0.01) and although fewer received aggressive end-of-life care (33% vs. 54%, P = 0.05), median survival was longer (11.6 months vs. 8.9 months, P = 0.02) (73). Thus although the circumstances of patients and families indicate the severity of problems which they face, it is important to remember that these circumstances are not inevitable, and that access to palliative care and other interventions that improve symptoms, emotional, social, and spiritual concerns is needed.

Conclusions

Populations are aging, and increasing numbers of people are reaching the end of life. The overall picture of the circumstances of death and dying is one of common complex and multiple symptoms, emotional, spiritual and social concerns, with more similarities than differences in the experience between patients of different conditions. There are often gaps in the provision of services providing support and symptom relief, but equally examples of inappropriate or over-treatment in some hospitals (although the latter is based mainly on US data). Family members and caregivers often carry a great burden and their health suffers. Older people, those from low socio-economic groups and black and minority ethnic groups often experience disadvantage in access to services despite similar levels of problems. The trajectory of illness is more complex that the early models of functional decline showed, and can be different within–as well as across–diseases. Indeed there can be similar trajectories in cancer and non-cancer patients. Fluctuating and increasing trajectories of problems are most common. The trajectory is also different for aspects beyond function, and is especially varied for emotional, social and spiritual concerns. Models of care—especially palliative care—can improve the experiences of patients and families.

References

(1) World Health Organization (2005) *Preventing Chronic Diseases: A Vital Investment*. Geneva: World Health Organization.

(2) Gomes, B, Higginson, IJ, and Davies E (2008) Hospice and palliative care: Public health aspects. In: K Heggenhougen and S. Quah (eds), *International Encyclopedia of Public Health*, first edn. San Diego: Academic Press.

(3) Gomes, B, and Higginson, IJ (2008) Where people die (1974—2030): Past trends, future projections and implications for care. *Palliat Med*, **22** (1): 33–41.

(4) Mathers, CD, and Loncar, D (2005) Updated projections of global mortality and burden of disease, 2002–2030: Data sources, methods and results. Geneva: World Health Organisation.

(5) Davies, E, and Higginson, IJ (2004) *Better Palliative Care for Older People*. Geneva: World Health Organization.

(6) Davies, E, and Higginson, IJ (2004) *Palliative Care: The Solid Facts*. Denmark: World Health Organisation.

(7) Higginson, IJ (1993) Palliative care: A review of past changes and future trends. *J Public Health Med*, **15** (1): 3–8.

(8) Hinton, J (1963) The physical and mental distress of the dying. *Quarterly Journal of Medicine*, **125:** 1–20.

(9) Parkes, CM (1975) The emotional impact of cancer of ear, nose and throat on patients and their families. *Journal of Laryngology and Otology*, **89:** 1271–9.

(10) Parkes, CM (1979) Terminal care: Evaluation of in-patient services at St Christopher's Hospice: Part 2—Self assessment of effects of the service on surviving spouses. *Postgraduate Medical Journal*, **55:** 523–7.

(11) Parkes, CM (1979) Terminal care evaluation of in-patient service at St Christopher's Hospice: Part 1—Views of surviving spouse on effects of the service on the patient. *Postgrad Med J*, **55:** 517–25.

(12) Parkes, CM (1985) Bereavement. *British Journal of Psychiatry*, **146:** 11–17.

(13) Bowling, A, and Cartwright, A. (1982) *Life After Death: A Study of the Elderly Widowed*. London: Tavistock.

(14) Cartwright, A, Hockey, J, and Anderson JL (1973) *Life Before Death*. London: Routledge & Kegan Paul.

(15) Cartwright, A (1991) The relationship between general practitioners, hospital consultants and community nurses when caring for people in the last year of their lives. *Fam Pract*, **8** (4): 350–5.

(16) Cartwright, A (1991) Changes in life and care in the year before death 1969–1987. *J Public Health Med*, **13** (2): 81–7.

(17) Cartwright, A (1991) The role of hospitals in caring for people in the last year of life. *Age & Ageing*, **20:** 271–4.

(18) Cartwright, A. The role of residential and nursing homes in the last year of people's lives. *British Journal of Social Work*, **21:** 627–45.

(19) Seale, C, and Cartwright, A (1994) *The Year Before Death*. Aldershot: Avebury.

(20) Addington-Hall, J, Lay, M, Altmann, D, and McCarthy, M (1998) Community care for stroke patients in the last year of life: Results of a national retrospective survey of surviving family, friends and officials. *Health Soc Care Community*, **6** (2): 112–19.

(21) Addington-Hall, JM, and McCarthy, M (1995) Dying from cancer: Results of a national population-based investigation. *Palliat Med*, **9:** 295–305.

(22) McCarthy, M, Lay, M, and Addington-Hall, JM (1996) Dying from heart disease. *J Royal College of Physicians of London*, **30:** 325–8.

(23) McCarthy, M, Addington-Hall, J, and Altmann, D (1997) The experience of dying with dementia: A retrospective study. *Int J Geriatr Psychiatry*, **12** (3): 404–9.

(24) Addington-Hall, J, Lay, M, Altmann, D, and McCarthy, M (1995) Symptom control, communication with health professionals, and hospital care of stroke patients in the last year of life as reported by surviving family, friends, and officials. *Stroke*, **26** (12): 2242–8.

(25) Solano, JP, Gomes, B, and Higginson, IJ (2006) A comparison of symptom prevalence in far advanced cancer, AIDS, heart disease, chronic obstructive pulmonary disease and renal disease. *Journal of Pain & Symptom Management*, **31:** 58–69.

(26) Higginson, I, Wade, A, and McCarthy, M (1990) Palliative care: Views of patients and their families. *BMJ*, **301:** 277–81.

(27) Lynn, J, Teno, JM, Phillips, RS, Wu, AW, Desbiens, N, Harrold, J, et al. (1997) Perceptions by family members of the dying experience of older and seriously ill patients. *Ann Intern Med*, **126** (2): 97–106.

(28) Teno, J, Lynn, J, Wenger, N, Phillips, RS, Murphy, D, Connors, AF Jr., et al. (1997) Advance directives for seriously-ill hospitalized patients: Effectiveness with the Patient Self-Determination Act and the SUPPORT intervention. *J Am Geriatr Soc*, **45** (4): 500–7.

(29) Beccaro, M, Costantini, M, and Merlo, DF (2007) Inequity in the provision of and access to palliative care for cancer patients. Results from the Italian survey of the dying of cancer (ISDOC). *BMC Public Health*, **7:** 66.

(30) Beccaro, M, Caraceni, A, and Costantini, M (2010) End-of-life care in Italian hospitals: Quality of and satisfaction with care from the caregivers' point of view—Results from the Italian Survey of the Dying of Cancer. *J Pain Symptom Manage*, **39** (6): 1003–15.

(31) Costantini, M, Beccaro, M, and Merlo, F (2005) The last three months of life of Italian cancer patients. Methods, sample characteristics and response rate of the Italian Survey of the Dying of Cancer (ISDOC). *Palliat Med*, **19** (8): 628–38.

(32) Costantini, M, Ripamonti, C, Beccaro, M, Montella, M, Borgia, P, Casella, C, et al. (2009) Prevalence, distress, management, and relief of pain during the last 3 months of cancer patients' life. Results of an Italian mortality follow-back survey. *Ann Oncol* **20** (4): 729–35.

(33) Giorgi, RP, Beccaro, M, Miccinesi, G, Borgia, P, Costantini, M, Chini, F, et al. (2007) Dying of cancer in Italy: Impact on family and caregiver. The Italian Survey of Dying of Cancer. *J Epidemiol Community Health*, **61** (6): 547–54.

(34) Koffman, J, and Higginson, IJ (2001) Accounts of carers' satisfaction with health care at the end of life: A comparison of first generation black Caribbeans and white patients with advanced disease. *Palliat Med*, **15:** 337–45.

(35) Selman, L, Harding, R, Speck, P, Robinson, V, Aguma, A, Rhys, A, et al. (2010) Spiritual care recommendations for people from black and minority ethnic (BME) groups receiving palliative care in the UK. Palliative Care, Policy & Rehabilitation, King's College London.

(36) Steinhauser, KE, Christakis, NA, Clipp, EC, McNeilly, M, Grambow, S, Parker, J, et al. (2001) Preparing for the end of life: Preferences of patients, families, physicians, and other care providers. *J Pain and Symptom Management*, **22:** 727–37.

(37) National Institute of Clinical Excellence (NICE) (2004) *Improving Supportive and Palliative Care for Adults with Cancer—The Manual*. London: National Institute of Clinical Excellence.

(38) Mills, M, Davies, TO, and Macrae, WA (1994) Care of dying patients in hospital. *BMJ*, **309:** 583–6.

(39) Addington-Hall, JM, MacDonald, L, Anderson, H, and Freeling, P (1991) Dying from cancer: The views of bereaved family and the friends about the experiences of terminally ill patients. *Palliat Med*, **5:** 207–14.

(40) Bausewein, C, Booth, S, Gysels, M, Kuhnbach, R, Haberland, B, and Higginson, IJ (2010) Understanding breathlessness: Cross-sectional comparison of symptom burden and palliative care needs in chronic obstructive pulmonary disease and cancer. *J Palliat Med*, **13** (9): 1109–18.

(41) Edmonds, P, Vivat, B, Burman, R, Silber, E, and Higginson, IJ (2007) 'Fighting for everything': Service experiences of people severely affected by multiple sclerosis. *Mult Scler*, **13** (5): 660–7.

(42) Gysels, M, Richardson, A, and Higginson, IJ (2004) Communication training for health professionals who care for patients with cancer: A systematic review of effectiveness. *Support Care Cancer*, **12** (10): 692–700.

(43) Higginson, IJ, Astin, P, and Dolan, S (1998) Where do cancer patients die? Ten-year trends in the place of death of cancer patients in England. *Palliat Med*, **12** (5): 353–63.

(44) Murtagh, FE, Addington-Hall, JM, Donohoe, P, and Higginson, IJ (2006) Symptom management in patients with established renal failure managed without dialysis. *EDTNA ERCA J*, **32** (2): 93–8.

(45) Higginson, IJ, and Koffman, J (2005) Public health and palliative care. *Clinics in Geriatric Medicine*, **21:** 45–55.

(46) Harding, R, and Higginson, IJ (2003) What is the best way to help caregivers in cancer and palliative care? A systematic literature review of interventions and their effectiveness. *Palliative Medicine*, **17** (1): 63–71.

(47) Lynn, J, and Adamson, DM (2003) *Living Well at the End of Life: Adapting Health Care to Serious Chronic Illness in Old Age*. Arlington, VA: Rand Health.

(48) Costantini, M, Beccaro, M, and Higginson, IJ (2008) Cancer trajectories at the end of life: Is there an effect of age and gender? *BMC Cancer*, **8:** 127.

(49) Teno, JM, Weitzen, S, Fennell, ML, and Mor, V (2001) Dying trajectory in the last year of life: Does cancer trajectory fit other diseases? *J Palliat Med*, **4** (4): 457–64.

(50) Murray, SA, Kendall, M, Boyd, K, Grant, L, Highet, G, and Sheikh, A (2010) Archetypal trajectories of social, psychological, and spiritual wellbeing and distress in family care givers of patients with lung cancer: Secondary analysis of serial qualitative interviews. *BMJ*, **340:** c2581.

(51) Lunney, JR, Lynn, J, Foley, DJ, Lipson, S, and Guralnik, JM (2003) Patterns of functional decline at the end of life. *Journal of the American Medical Association*, **289:** 2387–92.

(52) Bausewein, C, Booth, S, Gysels, M, Kuhnbach, R, Haberland, B, and Higginson, IJ (2010) Individual breathlessness trajectories do not match summary trajectories in advanced cancer and chronic obstructive pulmonary disease: Results from a longitudinal study. *Palliat Med*, Sep 16.

(53) Murtagh, FE, Addington-Hall, J, Edmonds, P, Donohoe, P, Carey, I, Jenkins, K, et al. (2010) Symptoms in the month before death for stage 5 chronic kidney disease patients managed without dialysis. *J Pain Symptom Manage*, **40** (3): 342–52.

(54) Decker, SL, and Higginson, IJ (2007) A tale of two cities: Factors affecting place of cancer death in London and New York. *Eur J Public Health*, **17** (3): 285–90.

(55) Higginson, IJ, Jarman, B, Astin, P, and Dolan, S (1999) Do social factors affect where patients die: An analysis of 10 years of cancer deaths in England. *Journal of Public Health Medicine*, **21:** 22–8.

(56) Raleigh, SV, and Kiri A (1997) Life expectancy in England: Variations and trends by gender, health authority and level of deprivation. *Journal of Epidemiology and Community Health*, **51:** 649–58.

(57) Cartwright, A (1992) Social class differences in health and care in the year before death. *J Epidemiol Comm Hlth*, **46:** 54–7.

(58) McCusker, J (1983) Where cancer patients die: An epidemiologic study. *Public Health Rep*, **98:** 170–6.

(59) Age Concern (1999) *Turning Your Back On Us. Older People and the NHS*. London: Age Concern.

(60) Bernabei, R, Gambassi, G, Lapane, K, Landi, F, Gatsonis, C, Dunlop, R, et al. (1998) Management of pain in elderly patients with cancer. SAGE Study Group. Systematic Assessment of Geriatric Drug Use via Epidemiology. *JAMA*, **279** (23): 1877–82.

(61) Eve, A, and Higginson, IJ (2000) Minimum dataset activity for hospice and hospital palliative care services in the UK 1997/98. *Palliat Med*, **14:** 395–404.

(62) Katz, J, Komaromy, C, and Sidell, M (1999) Understanding palliative care in residential and nursing homes. *International Journal of Palliative Nursing*, **5:** 58–64.

(63) Komaromy, C, Sidell, M, and Katz, J (2000) Dying in care: Factors which influence the quality of terminal care given to older people in residential and nursing homes. *International Journal of Palliative Nursing*, **6:** 192–205.

(64) Koffman, J, Fulop, NJ, Pashley, D, and Coleman, K (1996) No way out: The delayed discharge of elderly mentally ill acute and assessment patients in north and south Thames regions. *Age Ageing*, **25** (4): 268–72.

(65) Koffman, J, and Taylor, S (1997) The needs of caregivers. *Elder Care*, **9** (6): 16–19.

(66) Woods, RT, Wills, W, Higginson, IJ, Hobbins, J, and Whitby, M (2003) Support in the community for people with dementia and their carers: A comparative outcome study of specialist mental health service interventions. *International Journal of Geriatric Psychiatry*, **18:** 298–307.

(67) Farrell, J (2000) *Do Disadvantaged and Minority Ethnic Groups Receive Adequate Access to Palliative Care Services?* Glasgow: Glasgow University.

(68) Skilbeck, J, Corner, J, Beech, N, Clark, D, Hughes, P, Douglas, H-R, et al. (2002) Clinical nurse specialists in palliative care. Part 1. A description of a Macmillan Nurse caseload. *Palliative Medicine*, **16:** 285–96.

(69) Gomes, B, and Higginson, IJ (2006) Factors influencing death at home in terminally ill patients with cancer: Systematic review. *BMJ*, **332** (7540): 515–21.

(70) Higginson, IJ, Finlay, I, Goodwin, DM, Cook, AM, Hood, K, Edwards, AGK, et al. (2002) Do hospital-based palliative teams improve care for patients or families at the end of life? *J Pain Symptom Manage*, **23:** 96–106.

(71) Higginson, IJ, Finlay, IG, Goodwin, DM, Hood, K, Edwards, AGK, Cook, A, et al. (2003) Is there evidence that palliative care teams alter end-of-life experiences of patients and their caregivers? *J Pain Symptom Manage*, **25:** 150–68.

(72) Smith, TJ, and Cassel, JB (2009) Cost and non-clinical outcomes of palliative care. *J Pain Symptom Manage*, **38** (1): 32–44.

(73) Temel, JS, Greer, JA, Muzikansky, A, Gallagher, ER, Admane, S, Jackson, VA, et al. (2010) Early palliative care for patients with metastatic non-small-cell lung cancer. *N Engl J Med*, **363** (8): 733–42.

Chapter 4

End-of-life decisions

Agnes van der Heide and Judith Rietjens

Introduction

During the second half of the twentieth century, medical progress has contributed significantly to the increase in life expectancy (1). Improvements in clinical management have increased survival for many types of cancer (2,3) and the risk of cardiac death has decreased significantly due to effective drug management, technical devices and sophisticated intensive care (4,5). Neonatal and paediatric intensive care have also enormously increased medicine's capabilities to sustain and prolong vulnerable life in its earliest stages. However, the growing number of life-prolonging options also complicates decision-making at the end of life. People increasingly wish to have some control over the last phase of their lives (6–10) and end-of-life care frequently involves questions about when the application of burdensome or costly life-prolonging interventions is appropriate, when refraining from such treatment is appropriate, and when the need to alleviate suffering is more important than the risk of hastening death.

Empirical data about end-of-life decision-making practices are scarce. The broadly accepted notion within palliative care that continued 'aggressive' care might not always be beneficial has not yet been translated into end-of-life decision-making as an accepted field of research. This is probably due to the sensitive nature of the issue: conscious abandonment of the paradigmatic medical goal of postponing death is not easily addressed empirically without evoking debate about what is right and what is wrong.

In this chapter, we will give a brief overview of the legal regulation of physician assistance in dying in the Netherlands and elsewhere. Further, we will present research data on the frequency of end-of-life decisions and their main characteristics in different countries. Finally, we will briefly discuss the possible consequences of legalizing euthanasia for the practice of end-of-life decision-making.

Regulation of physician-assisted dying

The Netherlands was the first country worldwide where euthanasia and assisted suicide were officially accepted and regulated. The debate was triggered in 1973 by the so-called 'Postma case'. A physician helped her dying mother end her own life following repeated and explicit requests for euthanasia. The physician eventually received a short suspended sentence. While the court upheld that she did indeed commit murder, it offered an opening for regulating euthanasia by acknowledging that a physician does not always have to keep a patient alive against his or her will when faced with pointless suffering. As the first euthanasia test case, it broke social taboos in a country with strong Christian traditions. It also reflected a wave of awareness among many young medical professionals of the limits of medical care and of self-determination of patients. In the 1980s, the debate about euthanasia progressed and formalized. In 1980, the Committee of Attorneys General took a special interest in physicians' end-of-life decisions. To achieve uniformity in policy, they decided that every case of euthanasia should be scrutinized and that it should be decided whether or not the attending physician should be prosecuted. In 1982, the Health Council advised that a State Commission should be installed to address the definition of euthanasia as well as the criteria under which it should be allowed. In 1985, the Commission produced its report. The Commission defined euthanasia as 'intentionally terminating another person's life at the person's request'. This definition has been used ever since. The Commission also drew up a series of criteria for due care to be met in every case of euthanasia.

After the start of the debate on euthanasia, some physicians were willing to report euthanasia cases and thus to be held accountable. However, until the mid-1980s only a very small number of cases were reported. In 1990 the Ministry of Justice—together with the Royal Dutch Medical Association—agreed a formal and uniform notification procedure, aiming at transparency, accountability, and the harmonizing of regional prosecution policies. Physicians who had complied with the criteria for due care for euthanasia, as determined by the Association, would not be prosecuted. As a next step, in 1998, a national reporting procedure was developed through the establishing of multidisciplinary review committees consisting of a lawyer, a physician, and an ethicist. These committees examined the cases reported and advised the public prosecutor about whether or not the criteria for due care had been met. The reporting procedure was endorsed by many physicians and the review committees only rarely found serious violations of the requirements.

In 2001, after two decades of policy interventions in which public acceptance of euthanasia had further increased (from almost 50% in 1966 up to 90% in 1988 (11)), parliament decided that euthanasia should be legalized and the Euthanasia Act came into effect to regulate the ending of life by a physician at the request of a patient who was suffering unbearably without hope of relief. The criteria for due care, originally formulated by the State Commission, had meanwhile been further developed, partly through case law (12). They require a physician to assess that:

1. the patient's request is voluntary and well-considered

2. the patient's suffering is unbearable and without hope of improvement

3. the patient is informed about his or her situation and prospects

4. there are no reasonable alternative treatment options.

Further,

5. another independent physician should be consulted and

6. the termination of life should be performed with due medical care.

The Act officially legalized euthanasia, but in effect it largely legalized existing practice. The only major change was that, under the Act, the review committees needed to forward to the public prosecutor only those cases in which the due care criteria are not met. As such, the Act has diminished legal interference with physicians' medical end-of-life practices. In the period 2003–9, the review committees gave a verdict of non-compliance in 38 out of a total of 14,500 reported cases. The main reason for a verdict of non-compliance was a failure to fulfil the requirement of consultation of a second independent physician. None of the physicians involved was prosecuted. Most physicians think that the Act has improved their legal certainty and contributes to the care with which euthanasia and physician-assisted suicide are practised.

Legalization of euthanasia and assisted suicide in the Netherlands was followed by comparable laws in Belgium in 2002 and Luxembourg in 2009. Physician-assisted suicide is currently legal in the US states of Oregon and Washington, and has been discussed in Montana. Under the Oregon and Washington laws an adult state resident who has been diagnosed with a terminal illness that will end their life within six months may request from their physician a prescription for a lethal dose of medication to end their life. The request must be countersigned by two witnesses. A second physician must examine the patient's medical records and confirm the diagnosis. The patient must be competent. If the request is authorized, the patient must wait at least fifteen days and make a second oral request before the prescription may be written.

In Switzerland, physician-assisted suicide is allowed if it is done without any self-interest on the part of the physician or any other person. In 1995 the world's first euthanasia legislation, the Rights of the Terminally Ill Act, was passed in the Northern Territory of Australia, but was overturned in 1997 by Australia's Federal Parliament. Currently, the legalization of euthanasia or assisted dying is under discussion in many countries such as the UK, France, Canada, Columbia, and Australia.

Frequencies of end-of-life decisions

The first study to provide large-scale representative data on frequencies of end-of-life decisions was a Dutch nationwide study on the practice of euthanasia and other end-of-life decisions performed in 1990 (13,14). In this study, end-of-life decisions were characterized by the nature of the act involved (e.g. administering drugs or forgoing treatment), the intention of the physician (death was intended or accepted as an unintended effect of treatment aimed at alleviation of symptoms), patient involvement, and the life-shortening effect. The study introduced the following classification of end-of-life decisions (13):

1. physician-assisted dying, which is defined as intentionally providing a patient with lethal drugs. Physician-assisted dying is euthanasia if a physician administers the drug upon the explicit request of the patient; it is assisted suicide if the patient self-administers the lethal drugs.

2. alleviation of symptoms while taking into account or appreciating the hastening of death as a possible side effect.

3. limitation of treatment by withholding or withdrawing potentially life-prolonging interventions.

The study was repeated in 1995, 2001, and 2005 (15–17). Continuous deep sedation until death was introduced as a specific type of decision in 2001. Continuous deep sedation is often seen as an intervention that should not be used to hasten death, although it may have such an effect depending on how and when it is used. As such, decisions about continuous deep sedation may or may not be included in the classification of end-of-life decisions.

The Dutch questionnaire and classification system were used in several studies in other countries. In 1998, a Belgian study assessed end-of-life decision-making practices in Flanders, using a study design that was similar to the Dutch studies (18). Studies in Australia (1996) and the United Kingdom (UK) (2006) used a similar questionnaire, but a different study design (19,20). The 2001 study in the Netherlands was conducted in conjunction with the EURELD project that, using identical study designs, simultaneously studied end-of-life practices in six different European countries: Belgium, Denmark, Italy, the Netherlands, Sweden and Switzerland (21). Table 4.1 gives an overview of the frequency of end-of-life decisions as found in the studies using the Dutch questionnaire and classification. The rates of euthanasia and assisted suicide are clearly higher in the Netherlands than elsewhere, although the 2005 study found a significant decline compared with 2001. The Australian study was conducted during a short period in which euthanasia was legally allowed in the state of Northern Territory. Physician-assisted dying is sometimes provided in the absence of an explicit patient request. This practice is rare in most countries studied, but the rates are relatively high in Belgium and Australia (see Table 4.1).

The frequency of assisted suicide has also regularly been studied in the state of Oregon, USA, where assistance in suicide is allowed and where this practice is involved in about 0.1% of all deaths (22) Other studies on end-of-life decision-making practices mainly concerned intensive care units (ICUs), e.g. the ETHICUS study, a comparative study conducted in 1999/2000 in 37 ICUs in 17 European countries (23). This study asked physicians if they had actively shortened the dying process in patients who died at ICUs. This was found to be the case in 0–19% of all deaths at ICUs in the different countries (23). With many patients in the ICU being non-competent patients, this practice is largely

Table 4.1 Most important decision concerning the end of life, as percentage of all deaths*

	BE	NL	NL	BE	CH	DK	SW	IT	AU	UK
	2007	2005	EURELD study, 2001						1996	2006
Euthanasia + physician-assisted suicide	2.0	1.8	2.8	0.3	0.6	0.1	0.0	0.0	1.8	0.2
Ending of life without explicit patient request	1.8	0.4	0.6	1.5	0.4	0.7	0.2	0.1	3.5	0.3
Intensified alleviation of symptoms	27	25	20	22	22	26	21	19	31	33
Limiting life-prolonging treatment	17	16	20	15	28	14	14	4	29	30
Total	48	43	44	38	51	41	36	23	65	64

NL, Netherlands; BE, Belgium; CH, Switzerland; DK, Denmark; SW, Sweden; IT, Italy; AU, Australia; UK, United Kingdom.

*Studies in the NL, BE, CH, DK, SW, and IT used death certificates as the sampling unit, whereas the AU and UK studies asked samples of physicians to provide information on their most recent death case.

Sources: NL 2005 ref. 17; EURELD study 2001 ref. 21; AU 1996 ref. 19; UK 2006 ref. 20; BE 2007 ref. 24.

similar to ending of life without an explicit patient request or intensified alleviation of symptoms with shortening of life as a welcomed side effect.

Intensified alleviation of symptoms with shortening of life as an expected side effect is a practice that occurs frequently and at rather similar rates in most countries (25). It is most frequently found in Australia and the UK (see Table 4.1). The 2001 EURELD study also yielded comparative data about the use of continuous deep sedation until death and found it to be most common in Belgium (8.2%) and Italy (8.5%) (26). More recent studies found frequencies of 8.2% in the Netherlands in 2005 and 14.5% in Belgium in 2007 (17,24). Most other studies found higher rates, from 15% of deaths to more than 60%, but these studies often involved specialized end-of-life settings and broader definitions, so that higher frequencies are to be expected (27–30)

Wide variations between and within countries and between care settings have been found for the rates of withdrawing and withholding treatments and the proportion of deaths preceded by do-not-resuscitate (DNR) orders (21,31–33). Decisions to limit life-prolonging treatment are rare in Italy, more common in Denmark, Sweden, Belgium, and the Netherlands, and they are rather frequently made in Switzerland, Australia and the UK (see Table 4.1). In the EURELD study a DNR order had preceded death in about half of all cases in Switzerland, the Netherlands and Sweden, in about 40% in Belgium and Denmark, and in a quarter in Italy (33). It has been suggested that the variation in the frequency of decisions to limit treatment reflects differences in the attitudes of physicians towards the importance of aiming at the prolongation of life and applying aggressive interventions to achieve that goal in all cases (31). However, different concepts of futility may also affect perceptions of whether the non-application of a therapeutic option is standard care or the result of an explicit decision. Death at an ICU is even more frequently preceded by treatment limitations. The ETHICUS study found that 73% of all deceased patients in ICUs had received limitations of treatment (23). Percentages of deceased ICU patients for whom life-sustaining treatment had been withheld varied between 16% and 70% per country; for withdrawing treatment the range was 5–69% (23).

Patient involvement in end-of-life decisions

Large variations between countries have been found in the extent to which physicians consider the patients for whom they make end-of-life decisions as competent and able to participate in the decision-making process. Further, high frequencies of end-of-life decisions seem to be associated with high levels of patient involvement in decision-making. In the EURELD study, Dutch and Swiss physicians reported that one third of their deceased patients had been competent, and these rates were significantly even lower in Denmark, Belgium, Sweden, and especially Italy, where only 9% were considered competent (21). The rates at which physicians discussed their decisions with competent patients were rather low in Sweden (38%) and Italy (42%), but much higher in Switzerland (78%) and the Netherlands (92%) (21). These figures were comparable but somewhat less remark-able for discussing decisions with family in cases of non-competent patients. A decision-making model in which self-determination plays an important role may involve higher rates of end-of-life decision-making than a more paternalistic model. This hypothesis is in accordance with the frequently-reported patient disapproval of continued aggressive care at the end of life, and with the finding that the dying process typically involves less than optimal communication between caregivers and patients (34,35).

End-of-life decisions in clinical practice

Physician-assisted dying

Euthanasia and physician-assistance with suicide are mainly provided at the request of patients with cancer who die under the age of 80 (17,21,22) whose estimated life expectancy is usually limited to one month or less. Typical reasons why patients ask their physician to provide assistance in dying are the absence of any prospect of improvement, loss of dignity, and suffering from severe symptoms.

In the Netherlands, over 80% of all cases of euthanasia and physician-assistance in suicide are performed by general practitioners, at the patient's home. In Belgium and Oregon, assistance in dying is also often provided in hospitals by clinical specialists (17,21,22).

Ending of life without an explicit patient request mostly involves the use of opioids in patients with an estimated life expectancy of less than one week often with cancer, and who have lost competence in the terminal stage of their disease (36).

Alleviation of symptoms

Intensive alleviation of symptoms, mostly with opioids or sedatives, is typically used for patients with a very limited life expectancy, who are approaching death while suffering from severe symptoms such as pain, dyspnoea or anxiety. Cancer patients are also over-represented in this group. Patients dying in hospitals and patients dying at home more often receive opioids or sedatives as compared with those dying in nursing homes (25,37).

Continuous deep sedation

In a few countries national or local guidelines have been developed for the use of sedatives in the last phase of life. In the Netherlands the Royal Dutch Medical Association launched a nationwide guideline in 2006. Recently, the European Association for Palliative Care (EAPC) published a framework of recommendations for the use of sedation in palliative care comparable with earlier published international recommendations (38); the bottom-line of all these recommendations is that sedation can be considered when the patient is suffering unbearably from refractory symptoms. The disease should be advanced and without prospect of improvement, with death expected within hours or days. When possible, the patient and/or their family should be actively involved in the decision-making and benzodiazepines should be the drugs of first choice. The purpose of continuous sedation until death should be symptom relief and not the hastening of death.

The 2001 EURELD study showed that patients who received continuous deep sedation until death were more often male, younger than 80 years, more likely to have had cancer, and died more often in a hospital compared to non-sudden deaths without continuous deep sedation (26). Furthermore, several studies have shown that use of sedation until death is increasing. In the Netherlands, the use of continuous deep sedation in conjunction with an end-of-life decision increased from 5.6% of deaths in 2001 to 7.1% in 2005, mostly in patients treated by general practitioners and in those with cancer (17). In Belgium, its use increased from 8.2% in 2001 to 14.5% in 2007 (24).

A review of the use of sedation in end-of-life care showed that sedation is most often used to alleviate severe delirium, dyspnoea and pain. Benzodiazepines such as midazolam are most often used to induce sedation, sometimes in combination with opioids. In almost all instances, consent to use sedation is obtained from competent patient; in case of lack of competence, consent was almost always obtained from family members (39).

Limitation of treatment

Limitation of treatment more often than other decisions involves elderly patients (21). Further, these decisions are often made earlier in the disease process and involve more shortening of life than intensive alleviation of symptoms (31). Decisions to refrain from potentially life-prolonging treatment and DNR agreements are most often made by clinical specialists and nursing home physicians (33).

Legalizing euthanasia: a slippery slope?

The studies from the Netherlands and Belgium discussed in this chapter strongly suggest that public control and transparency of the practice of euthanasia is to a large extent possible, and that the legalization of euthanasia and physician-assisted suicide in several countries has not resulted in a slippery slope for medical end-of-life practices. Besides religious or principle-based arguments, the slippery slope argument is the mainstay of opponents of the legalization of euthanasia. Briefly, the argument states that: if we allow A (the use euthanasia at the request of terminally ill patients) then B (abuse of euthanasia, that is, ending the life of vulnerable patient groups without their consent) will necessarily or very likely follow. B is morally not acceptable; therefore, we must not allow A. Until now, studies show no clear evidence of a slippery slope (17,24). The frequency of the ending of life without explicit patient request did not increase over the studied years. Also, there is no evidence of a higher frequency of euthanasia among the elderly, people with low educational status, the poor, the physically disabled or chronically ill, minors, people with psychiatric illnesses including depression, or racial or ethnic minorities, compared with background populations (40).

Conclusions

End-of-life decision-making practices vary within and between industrialized Western countries. The differences between them may have a significant impact on patterns of death and dying. End-of-life decision-making is related to patient characteristics such as age, diagnosis and prognosis, but cross-national differences in the distribution of age at death and causes of death are limited. The variations in end-of-life decision-making and their impact on experiences around death and dying require further study.

An important lesson that can already be drawn from the past two decades of research on end-of-life decision-making is that it is feasible to study this subject. Most studies show that quite large proportions of physicians in several countries were willing to share their experiences.

Research further shows that end-of-life decision-making is a significant aspect of end-of-life care. In approximately 4 out of every 10 patients, death is preceded by a decision that possibly or certainly hastens the dying process, and this percentage seems to be increasing. This points to the growing awareness that high quality end-of-life care is not always aimed at prolonging the patient's life at all costs but is also aimed at improving the quality of life through the prevention and relief of symptoms, sometimes to the extent that patients request and receive euthanasia.

Medical end-of-life decision-making is a crucial part of end-of-life care in which fundamental human values are at stake. It should therefore be given continuous attention in public health policy and medical training. High quality, widely accessible, rational and transparent end-of-life care is indispensable to a just and equitable practice of end-of-life decision-making that contributes to the quality of death and dying, both for the individual and at the population level. Systematic periodic research is crucial to enhancing our understanding of end-of-life care in modern medicine, in which the pursuit of a good quality of dying is now widely recognized as an important goal, in addition to traditional goals such as curing disease and prolonging life.

References

(1) Wilmoth JR. Demography of longevity: Past, present, and future trends. *Exp Gerontol* 2000; **35**: 1111–29.

(2) Gondos A, Bray F, Brewster DH, Coebergh JW, Hakulinen T, Janssen-Heijnen ML, Kurtinaitis J, Brenner H. The EUNICE Survival Working Group. Recent trends in cancer survival across Europe between 2000 and 2004: A model-based period analysis from 12 cancer registries. *Eur J Cancer* 2008; **44**: 1463–75.

(3) Den Dulk M, Krijnen P, Marijnen CA, Rutten HJ, van de Poll-Franse LV, Putter H, Meershoek-Klein Kranenbarg E, Jansen-Landheer ML, Coebergh JW, van de Velde CJ. Improved overall survival for patients with rectal cancer since 1990: The effects of TME surgery and pre-operative radiotherapy. *Eur J Cancer* 2008; doi: 10.1016/j.ejca.2008.05.004.

(4) Turakhia M, Tseng ZH. Sudden cardiac death: Epidemiology, mechanisms and therapy. *Curr Probl Cardiol* 2007; **32**: 501–46.

(5) Thompson BT, Cox PN, Antonelli M, Carlet J, Cassell J, Hill NS, Hinds CJ, Pimentel JM, Reinhart K, Thijs LG. Challenges in end-of-life care in the ICU: Statement of the 5th International Consensus Conference in Critical Care: Brussels, Belgium, April 2003: Executive summary. *Crit Care Med* 2004; **321**: 781–4.

(6) Rietjens JAC, van der Heide A, Onwuteaka-Philipsen B, van der Maas PJ, van der Wal G. Preferences of the Dutch general public for a good death and associations with attitudes towards end-of-life decision making? *Palliat Med* 2006; **20**: 685–92.

(7) Singer PA, Martin DK, Kelner M. Quality end-of-life care: Patients' perspectives. *JAMA* 1999; **281**: 163–8.

(8) Teno JM, Casey VA, Welch LC, Edgman-Levitan S. Patient-focused, family-centered end-of-life medical care: Views of the guidelines and bereaved family members. *J Pain Symptom Manage* 2001; **22**: 738–51.

(9) Patrick DL, Curtis JR, Engelberg RA, Nielsen E, McCown E. Measuring and improving the quality of dying and death. *Ann Intern Med* 2003; **139**: 410–15.

(10) Patrick DL, Engelberg RA, Curtis JR. Evaluating the quality of dying and death. *J Pain Symptom Manage* 2001; **22**: 717–26.

(11) Van der Maas PJ, Pijnenborg L, van Delden JJM. Changes in Dutch opinions on active euthanasia, 1966 through 1991. *JAMA* 1995; **273**: 1411–14.

(12) Rietjens JA, van der Maas PJ, Onwuteaka-Philipsen B, van Delden JJM, van der Heide A. Two decades of research on euthanasia from the Netherlands. What have we learnt and which questions remain? *Bioethical Inquiry* 2009; **6**: 271–83.

(13) van der Maas PJ, van Delden JJM, Pijnenborg L. *Euthanasia and Other Medical Decisions Concerning the End of Life*. Health Policy Monographs. Elsevier: London, 1992.

(14) van der Maas PJ, van Delden JJM, Pijnenborg L, Looman CWN. Euthanasia and other medical decisions concerning the end of life. *Lancet* 1991; **338**: 669–74.

(15) van der Maas PJ, van der Wal G, Haverkate I, de Graaff CL, Kester JG, Onwuteaka-Philipsen BD, van der Heide A, Bosma JM, Willems DL. Euthanasia, physician-assisted suicide, and other medical practices involving the end of life in the Netherlands, 1990–1995. *N Engl J Med* 1996; **335**: 1699–705.

(16) Onwuteaka-Philipsen B, van der Heide A, Koper D, Keij-Deerenberg I, Rietjens JA, Rurup ML, Vrakking AM, Georges JJ, Muller MT, van der Wal G, van der Maas PJ. Euthanasia and other end-of-life decisions in the Netherlands in 1990, 1995, and 2001. *Lancet* 2003; **362**: 395–9.

(17) van der Heide A, Onwuteaka-Philipsen BD, Rurup M, Buiting H, van Delden JM, Hanssen-de Wolff H, Janssen A., Pasman HR, Rietjens JA, Prins C, Deerenberg I, Gevers JC, van der Wal G. End-of-life practices in the Netherlands under the euthanasia act. *N Engl J Med* 2007; **356**: 1957–65.

(18) Deliens L, Mortier F, Bilsen J, Cosyns M, Vander Stichele R, Vanoverloop J, Ingels K. End-of-life decisions in medical practice in Flanders, Belgium: A nationwide survey. *Lancet* 2000; **356**: 1806–11.

(19) Kuhse H, Singer P, Baume P, Clark M, Rickard M. End-of-life decisions in Australian medical practice. *Med J Aust* 1997; **166**: 191–6.

(20) Seale C. National survey of end-of-life decisions made by UK medical practitioners. *Palliat Med* 2006; **20**: 3–10.

(21) van der Heide A, Deliens L, Faisst K, et al. End-of-life decision-making in six European countries: Descriptive study. *Lancet* 2003; **362**: 345–50.

(22) http://www.oregon.gov/DHS/ph/pas/. Annual report 2007.

(23) Sprung CL, Cohen SL, Sjokvist P, Baras M, Bulow HH, Hovilehto S, Ledoux D, Lippert A, Maia P, Phelan D, Schobersberger W, Wennberg E, Woodcock T. Ethicus Study Group. End-of-life practices in European intensive care units: the Ethicus Study. *JAMA* 2003; **290**: 790–7.

(24) Bilsen J, Cohen J, Chambaere K, Pousset G, Onwuteaka-Philipsen BD, Mortier F, Deliens L. Medical end-of-life practices under the euthanasia law in Belgium. *N Engl J Med* 2009 10; **361**: 1119–21.

(25) Bilsen J, Norup M, Deliens L, Miccinesi G, van der Wal G, Löfmark R, Faisst K, van der Heide A. Drugs used to alleviate symptoms with life shortening as a possible side effect: end-of-life care in six European countries. *J Pain Symptom Manage* 2006; **31**: 111–21.

(26) Miccinesi G, Rietjens JA, Deliens L, Paci E, Bosshard G, Nilstun T, Norup M, van der Wal G, on behalf of the EURELD Consortium. Continuous deep sedation: Physicians' experiences in six European countries. *J Pain Symptom Manage* 2006; **31**: 122–9.

(27) Fainsinger RL, Waller A, Bercovici M et al. A multicentre international study of sedation for uncontrolled symptoms in terminally ill patients. *Palliat Med* 2000; **14**: 257–65.

(28) Sykes N, Thorns A. Sedative use in the last week of life and the implications for end-of-life decision making. *Arch Intern Med* 2003 Feb 10; **163** (3): 341–4.

(29) Chiu TY, Hu WY, Lue BH, Cheng SY, Chen CY. Sedation for refractory symptoms of terminal cancer patients in Taiwan. *J Pain Symptom Manage* 2001; **21**: 467–72.

(30) Muller-Busch HC, Andres I, Jehser T. Sedation in palliative care—A critical analysis of 7 years experience. *BMC Palliat Care* 2003; **2**: 2.

(31) Bosshard G, Nilstun T, Bilsen J, Norup M, Miccinesi G, Delden JJM, Faisst K, van der Heide A. Forgoing treatment at the end of life in 6 European countries. *Arch Intern Med* 2005; **165**: 401–7.

(32) Buiting HM, van Delden JJ, Rietjens JA, Onwuteaka-Philipsen BD, Bilsen J, Fischer S, Löfmark R, Miccinesi G, Norup M, van der Heide A; EURELD-Consortium. Forgoing artificial nutrition or hydration in patients nearing death in six European countries. *J Pain Symptom Manage* 2007; **34**: 305–14.

(33) Delden JJM van, Lofmark R, Deliens L, Bosshard G, Norup M, Cecioni R, van der Heide A. Do-not-resuscitate decisions in six European countries. *Crit Care Med* 2006; **34**: 1886–90.

(34) Hofmann JC, Wenger NS, Davis RB, et al. Patient preferences for communication with physicians about end-of-life decisions. *Ann Intern Med* 1997; **127**: 1–12.

(35) Teno J, Lynn J, Wenger N, et al. Advance directives for seriously ill hospitalized patients: effectiveness with the patient self-determination act and the SUPPORT intervention. *J Am Geriatr Soc* 1997; **45**: 500–7.

(36) Rietjens JAC, Bilsen J, van der Heide A, van der Maas PJ, Miccinesi G, Norup M, Onwuteaka-Philipsen B, Vrakking AM, van der Wal G. Using drugs to end life without an explicit request of the patient. *Death Studies* 2007; **31**: 205–21.

(37) Rietjens J, van Delden J, Onwuteaka-Philipsen B, Buiting H, van der Maas P, van der Heide A. The use of continuous deep sedation for patients nearing death in the Netherlands: A descriptive study. *Br Med J* 2008; **336**: 810–13.

(38) Cherny NI, Radbruch L; Board of the European Association for Palliative Care. European Association for Palliative Care (EAPC) recommended framework for the use of sedation in palliative care. *Palliat Med* 2009; **23**: 581–93.

(39) Claessens P, Menten J, Schotsmans P, Broeckaert B. Palliative sedation: A review of the research literature. *J Pain Symptom Manage* 2008; **36**: 310–33.

(40) Battin MP, van der Heide A, Ganzini L, van der Wal G, Onwuteaka-Philipsen BD. Legal physician-assisted dying in Oregon and the Netherlands: Evidence concerning the impact on patients in 'vulnerable' groups. *J Med Ethics* 2007; **33**: 591–7.

Chapter 5

Economic and health-related consequences of individuals caring for terminally ill cancer patients in Canada

Konrad Fassbender and Lindsey Sutherland

Introduction

We have yet to prepare adequately for the 'silver tsunami' (1). Increasing numbers of people are expected to die each year. Caregivers currently expend great effort to care for the elderly and dying. Rapidly changing demographics and social trends however suggest that caregivers may not be prepared to care for the increasing numbers of dying. Caregiving may have health consequences for those who do it and therefore economic consequences for society.

Dying is costly. Researchers in Manitoba, Canada, found that decedents (i.e. 1.1% of the population) consumed 21.3% of health care costs in the last 6 months of life (2). This number is comparable to the 27% of the Medicare budget spent on care at end of life in the United States (3). In response, policy- and decision-makers continue to shift health care resources from institutional to community settings for terminally ill patients as a cost-effective health reform strategy. As in many countries, end-of-life care policies in Canada are targeted to individuals that are expected to die within a 6-month time period. The rationale for this fact is based largely on an average 6-month decline in functional status and potential cost savings from reducing utilization of unnecessary treatments in inappropriate settings for the cancer population (4;5). A study in Canada (6) has managed to generate and synthesize costing data from a societal viewpoint. Numerous other costing studies exist but omit one or more categories of costs, thereby rendering comparisons meaningless. This point is evident when one synthesizes costing information from a recent review of end-of-life care in Canada (7). In that review, indirect costs varied from 7.4% to 71.1% of total costs.

To evaluate the costs of end-of-life care for society, we cannot focus strictly on the costs (i.e. economic consequences) of publicly-provided end-of-life care (e.g. palliative care services). This chapter therefore purposely chooses to extend that focus on contributions and consequences associated with caregivers. This review includes both the health and economic consequences of providing unpaid care to the dying, assess whether governmental support helps alleviate these consequences, and identify appropriate levels of financing and delivery of services directed to caregivers.

Dying and demographics

In Canada about 76,200 people die each year. Both the sheer numbers of those dying and the experience of dying are rapidly changing. Demographic trends for example tell us that the population is aging and the numbers dying each year will increase. Social trends as well will alter the way in which people are cared for prior to dying. Smaller families mean that fewer children will be available to care for their parents. An increase in two-income families exacerbates this reality. Globalization results in highly mobile families and decreases the likelihood that children are in a geographic position to look after their parents. Increased mobility also means that those requiring care are less likely to have formed long term relationships or social networks with friends and neighbours.

Caregiving effort

For most Canadians dying is an experience which involves many other people (8). The lives of family, friends, colleagues, and neighbours are irrevocably changed throughout the illness trajectory. These individuals provide varying levels of care for the dying. Expressions of this care include various activities including 'housekeeping, meal preparation, home and yard maintenance and repairs, transportation, financial management, care management (making appointments, arranging for formal services, etc.), personal care (feeding, dressing, toileting, medications, etc.), monitoring, and emotional support' (9).

Caring for the dying is a gradual process however that often begins earlier in life. The duration of caregiving can last from less than a year to more than 40 years. In a 2003 study, caregivers were found to spend an average of 4.3 years providing care (10). In another US national study, over 40% of caregivers had been providing assistance for five or more years, and nearly one-fifth had been doing so for 10+ years (11). As a result, a significant proportion of the population is caring for someone at any given point in time. About 1 in 4 (27.8%) employed Canadians had responsibilities for the care of an elderly dependant in 2009. The proportion of working-age adults providing care to older adults is growing at a significant rate estimated at 2% each decade (as of 2006). A significant portion (25%) of caregiving to seniors is provided by fellow seniors (12). In total, older people, the chronically ill and the dying are cared for by approximately three million Canadians (12).

Estimates of caregiving effort vary. 'According to the Canadian Health Consumer Survey (2009), the average caregiver spent 20 hours a week caring for four years, with 25 per cent of caregivers spending 40 hours a week. One in four caregivers has no help; one in four has paid help; and 61 per cent need more help' (12). One in five caregivers provides more than 40 hours of care per week (10). Caregiving intensity is not a constant and increases as death approaches. In the last few months of life, an Alberta study found that per person being cared for, on average 1.82 people provided 91.6 hours of care per week (approximately 50 hours per caregiver) (13). A study of California Caregiver Resource Center caregiving clients yielded an even higher estimate of an average 81 weekly hours each (14).

Caregivers have less time for leisure activities and report missing more days of work, taking more personal days and retiring earlier to provide care (12). As with working adults, retired people 65 and over who spend their time caregiving, experience poorer quality of life and less life satisfaction. In Canada, about half of caregivers take time off work and report significant reductions in domestic work (69.3%), personal care (46.3%), and leisure (73.2%) (13). Prolonged decline in personal care and leisure may result in poorer health. Productivity losses translate to a decline in personal finances which is also correlated with poorer health.

Mental and physical health outcomes

Caregiving effort results in significant time losses and in conflict resulting in adverse consequences for their mental and physical health. In Canada, a high proportion of females (22.7%) and males (16.6%) are conflicted. These individuals experience lowered satisfaction, higher levels of stress, lower self-reported physical and lower emotional wellbeing. Additional consequences have been identified and include: higher levels of anxiety and depression, sleep disturbances, infectious disease and suppressed immune functioning, poor dietary habits, a lack of physical exercise and obesity, increased dependence on cigarettes, alcohol, medications and drugs, hypertension, high cholesterol, coronary, musculo-skeletal and digestive problems, allergies and migraine headaches, burnout, and increased costs for medical consultations and prescription drugs (12).

Even when caregivers rate their own health as excellent (38%) or good (43%), almost half (43%) believe that caregiving influenced their health negatively (15). These beliefs have been characterized as personality characteristics or a disposition toward optimism (16). Others have categorized subjective stressors as primary and secondary (17); primary subjective stressors include role overload, role captivity, and loss of intimate exchange, whereas secondary stressors include impact on schedule, financial impact, and family support. In this model, primary stressors predict caregiver depression and poor health through the exacerbation of secondary stressors; 'overload', 'exhaustion', and 'overwhelming' are words used to describe the transition to poor health.

Positive benefits arising from caregiving have nonetheless been postulated for some caregivers (18). In a recent study, a distinction was made between caregiving and volunteering for non-caregiving activities (12); unpaid caregivers were more likely to report poor health, depressive symptoms, and high risk health behaviours. On the other hand, volunteering for non-caregiving activities resulted in improved physical health, longer life, and better mental health. In another study, caregivers were found to experience lower levels of depression and higher life satisfaction if they appraised their tasks as less stressful, found meaning and subjective benefits in their activities, and possessed more social resources (19). The findings from these studies however are not representative of the majority of caregivers or studies.

Economic impact

Economic impact refers to the dollar value of resources consumed by persons diagnosed with cancer. Economic impact data may be used for pricing, budgeting or to help inform resource allocation decisions and can be obtained from burden of illness studies, cost analyses and cost-effectiveness analyses. Variability of estimates arise from methodological differences which often trade-off precision and bias. Societal costs include direct medical, direct non-medical (travel and other out-of-pocket), indirect (caregiving and other time-related), and intangible costs. Sources of costing data can be obtained from national statistical databases; provincial, regional or institutional administrative databases; surveys and expert opinion. Costs may be directly observed or modelled. Cost estimates may be obtained using gross costing or micro-costing methods and subject to a multitude of statistical manipulations. In summary, economic data are not readily amenable to syntheses and comparison.

Due to convenience, most studies focus on direct medical costs which include hospitalizations, ambulatory care, physician and other professional services, home care, nursing home care, and outpatient medications. As a general rule of thumb, direct medical costs for end-of-life cancer patients represent a ten-fold increase over population-wide per-capita health expenditures. Of these costs, conventional wisdom further equates 2/3 to 3/4 of all direct medical costs arising from hospitalization, despite efforts to limit these costs.

Although roughly equal in magnitude to direct medical costs, indirect costs are understudied. This lack of attention represents a public health care liability. Although indirect costs include patients' waiting and treatment time, we choose to focus on caregivers. Economic estimates of caregiving differentiate the cost from the consequences of caregiving. The costs of caregiving are, in turn, based on estimates of caregiving effort as described earlier. Economic consequences are an important outcome in their own right and include financial impact, also described as a secondary stressor in the causal pathway for poor caregiver health. Valuing economic costs and consequences depends on the nature of time displaced by the caregiving effort.

Costs of caregiving

Caregiving costs are reached by multiplying caregiving effort by an appropriate wage. Seemingly straightforward estimates in the literature may, astonishingly, differ a hundredfold. At the low end, a Canadian study estimated $2 billion to $22 billion annually based on an average caregiving effort of 7.9 hrs per week for 49–64 year olds and 10.4 hrs per week for those over 65 (20). Unpaid costs for an estimated two million caregivers of older people, also in Canada, were valued as the equivalent of 276,509 full-time employees, at a cost of between $5 billion and $6 billion (9). On the high end, services provided by unpaid caregivers were estimated at $257 billion (at the rear 2000 values) which exceeds the costs associated with home health care ($32 billion) and nursing home care ($92 billion) combined (21). While explaining these differences is not important in the current context, the point is that societal costs are significant.

Caregiver effort valuation should also include the amount of time for each category of activity displaced. While labour–leisure trade-off theory in economics values all time equally, societal norms may dictate otherwise; taking time off work may be easier to value than taking time away from unpaid work. Many studies in fact are limited to measuring 'productivity losses' (time lost from paid work), which exemplifies this issue. A more careful examination of the issues involved may help to explain these differences.

Consequences of caregiving

The economic consequences of caregiving should take into account loss of income and governmental benefits in addition to increased health care costs. Increased health care costs include direct medical, direct non-medical, indirect and intangible losses. Direct medical costs include hospital stays, ambulatory care visits, visits to a doctor, laboratory tests, nursing homes, home care, hospice, and prescription medications. Direct non-medical costs include travel costs. Out of pocket costs can be medical (e.g. medical supplies and over the counter medications) or non-medical (e.g. parking). Indirect costs are those for which payment is not typically observed and includes productivity and other time-related losses. Intangible losses represent the decreased intrinsic value of both quality and length of life.

Income, governmental benefits and education may be expressed as a composite measure called socio-economic status (SES). A positive association indicates that those with fewer resources are not as able to cope with their situation. Both fewer problems and an inability to cope are associated with lower SES (22,23). A primary limitation of these studies stems from the fact that it is not known if a low SES preceded the life-limiting diagnosis or vice versa. These associations are variously reported as increased odds (OR = odds ratio) of achieving a low SES; losing family savings for example has been associated with poverty (OR = 2.11), poor health status (OR = 1.87), being married (OR = 1.75), providing care for a long time (OR = 2.29), poor performance status (OR = 1.35), and high medical expenses (OR = 1.70) (24).

Loss of income and governmental benefits may be assessed directly. Income loss has been reported by 39% of caregivers and 42% of patients (25–27). Reported income loss was expressed as using up savings (33%), changes in lifestyle (29%), and sacrificing discretionary expenditures such as vacations (54%). Income supplementation from non-governmental sources was reported as borrowing money (18%) and depending on others for money (12%). An additional US study by the National Alliance for Caregiving and the National Center on Women and Aging examined governmental benefits and estimated an average loss of $25,494 in Social Security benefits, $67,202 in pension benefits and an average of $566,433 in wage wealth (total = $659,139 per person) (28). Long-distance caregivers spend an average of $392/month on travel and out-of-pocket expenses as part of their caregiving duties (10).

During the final three months of life, family caregivers experience reductions in motivation to work (29%), productivity at work (16%), quality of work (12%), and time at work (42%) (25–27). Studies suggest that the cost of unpaid caregiving in terms of lost productivity to US businesses is $11 to $29 billion annually (29).

The need for and provision of public policy intervention

Caregivers are often unable to manage the additional responsibilities associated with caregiving (30–32). The burden associated with providing this additional care to the dying is not only significant for the caregivers (33) but also for dying patients in their knowledge of the burden they place on caregivers (34). Through the displacement of work time, there is an indirect impact on family finances resulting in the need for economic support (35–37). Williams et al. (31,37) argue that the financial benefits foregone by the family comprise a significant proportion of the total care and require systematized public intervention.

Assessing the net economic impact of caregiving requires that directed government resources be factored into the equation. Governmental resources naturally include all medical care provided to caregivers. Some of the medical services however target caregivers with the aim of alleviating adverse mental and physical consequences. These services can be provided by regional health authorities, provincial ministries of health or federal ministries. Community-based palliative care consultations and outpatient clinic services are services provided by regional health authorities. Resources may also be directed towards the provision of palliative home care. The aim of these programmes is to provide respite care in addition to care that would not otherwise be available. Federal jurisdiction includes the maintenance of income. In Canada, the Federal caregiver legislation is an example of this type of governmental support.

In 1981, the National Hospice Study was conducted in the US to analyse whether hospice care (hospital-based or home care, with and without reimbursement) conferred benefits to the patient, family and health care system as compared to conventional care (outpatient or inpatient oncology care or mix of both) (38). The study found a reduction in the use of aggressive therapies (39), modest costs savings (40) despite similar levels of reported pain (41), increased use of analgesics (42), and a reduction in secondary morbidity of caregivers (43).

Palliative medicine is unique in that it provides services directed towards the caregiver, not just the patient as in most other disciplines. The term 'melancholia' has a long and well-documented history. First described by Hippocrates in the fifth century bce (44), it has been further studied and defined by others, such as Freud who wrote that it is a prolonged period of mourning associated with unresolved relationships between the bereaved and deceased (45). Psychotherapeutic interventions were found to be effective as early as 1978 (46). Mental health interventions such as crisis intervention, suicide hot lines, and information and referral services can be provided to the caregiver with an efficacy comparable to those provided to the patient (47).

There is strong public support for postponing residential care and bringing health care services to the home, even when costs are taken into account (48). A couple of Canadian studies in fact show that this care may be cost effective (49,50). Hollander (49, pp. 149–61) demonstrated that home care can be a lower-cost alternative to residential care for clients with standardized for equivalent care needs. Rapidly transitioning care levels and dying were however associated with higher costs in the home. Another Canadian study compared the direct medical and indirect costs associated with care of the elderly at home versus in residential care facilities (50). They found that even after accounting for indirect caregiver time valued at replacement wages, home care was still provided at a significantly lower cost than residential care.

Canada's Compassionate Care Benefit (CCB) was launched in 2004 with the goal of assisting family members to take temporary leave from work in order to care for an individual at the end of their life. The programme provides up to 55% of the applicant's average insured earnings at a maximum of CDN$435 per week. The CCB provides cover for a 6-week period of care for a family member at risk of death within a 6-month period, requiring a medical certificate as proof (51). In 2008, Crooks and Williams outlined their plan to interview family caregivers of palliative or end-of-life patients, front-line palliative care practitioners (FLPCPs), and human resources personnel and employers (52). Only the results of the FLPCP interviews have been published at this time; however they present a very compelling and informative insight into the expectations and experiences of the CCB. The most common expectation discussed ($n = 35/50$) by the FLPCPs was time expectation. The FLPCPs felt that the CCB should provide adequate time for the caregivers during the end-of-life and bereavement periods and that 6 weeks was not enough. Also, FLPCPs felt that they were expected to advise the caregivers on when to start the leave and the current length of time allowed made it difficult to do this effectively. Another major concern was that the CCB stopped immediately upon the death of the patient and that caregivers could benefit greatly if it were to continue for the first week or so of the bereavement period to assist with grieving and attending to estate dealings. Other expectations expressed by 29–33 of the FLPCPs was that the financial compensation was inadequate for the caregivers, that the information provided to the FLPCPs was insufficient to ensure proper dissemination to caregivers by the FLPCPs, and that the administration application processes and procedures for the CCB should be simplified to reduce the risk of caregiver burden (53).

A 2010 analysis of the Canadian CCB program once again highlighted the problems associated with having the CCB under the Employment Insurance programme (54). It was identified in a 2005 report by the Health Council of Canada that women, especially if unemployed or of low income, are commonly ineligible for the CCB and that this population is the one that would often benefit greatly (55). In 2010, authors of a critical analysis of the Canadian CCB continued to find this issue was a major deterrent for many caregivers and felt that unless the CCB is removed from the Employment Insurance Program many caregivers in need will continue to go without assistance (54).

Conclusion

The evidence reviewed in this chapter demonstrates that the health and economic consequences for unpaid caregivers are significant. In light of rapidly changing demographics, a silver tsunami requires urgent action. Caregivers will require more health care due to increased morbidity or may themselves face increased risk of dying. Understanding these phenomena is a prerequisite to optimal resource allocation. In particular, we need to be able to help caregivers maintain their health and reduce the burden on our health care system. In part, we propose to explore whether referral to palliative care programmes, use of palliative home care and use of federal caregiver benefits is beneficial. Without adequate knowledge and support, we argue that caregivers will suffer and cause an inefficient use of health care resources. More studies are required to increase our knowledge and understanding of the costs and consequences of providing unpaid care to the dying, to assess whether governmental supports help alleviate these consequences, and to identify appropriate levels of financing and delivery of caregiver-directed services.

References

(1) Fox, S., Rainie, L., Larsen, E., Horrigan, J., Lenhart, A., Spooner, T., Carter, C. (2001). Wired seniors: A fervent few, inspired by family ties. Washington, DC: Pew Internet and American Life Project.

(2) Menec, V, Lix, L, Steinbach, C, Ekuma, O, Sirski, M, Dahl, M, Soodeen, R. (2004). *Patterns of Health Care Use and Cost at the End of Life*. Winnipeg, MB: Manitoba Centre for Health Policy.

(3) Lubitz, JD. Riley, GF. (1993). Trends in Medicare payments in the last year of life. *New England Journal of Medicine*, **328** (15): 1092–6.

(4) Teno, JM. Weitzen, S. Fennell, ML. Mor, V. (2001). Dying trajectory in the last year of life: Does cancer trajectory fit other diseases? *Journal of Palliative Medicine*, **4** (4): 457–64.

(5) Lunney, JR Lynn, J. Foley, DJ. Lipson, S. Guralnik, JM. (2003). Patterns of functional decline at the end of life. *JAMA*, **289** (18): 2387–92.

(6) Health Canada. (2011). Economic Burden of Illness in Canada, 1998. Ottawa: Health Canada; 2002. Available at: http://www.phac-aspc.gc.ca/publicat/ebic-femc98/pdf/ebic1998.pdf, accessed 14 April 2011.

(7) Barbera, L., Burge, F., De, P., Dumont, S., Fassbender, K., Grunfeld, E., Johnston, G., F Lau. (2010). Special Topic: Care at the End of Life for cancer patients in Canada. Canadian Cancer Society's Steering Committee: Canadian Cancer Statistics 2010. Toronto: Canadian Cancer Society.

(8) Carstairs, S. (2010). Raising the Bar: A Roadmap for the Future of Palliative Care in Canada. The Senate of Canada. Retrieved 12 July 2010, from http://sen.parl.gc.ca/scarstairs/PalliativeCare/Raising%20the%20Bar%20June%202010%20(2).pdf.

(9) Fast, J. (2005). Caregiving: A fact of life. *Transition Magazine*, **35**(2): 6.

(10) National Alliance for Caregiving and AARP. (2004). *Caregiving in the U.S.* Bethesda: National Alliance for Caregiving, and Washington, DC: AARP.

(11) Donelan, K., Hill, C.A., Hoffman, C., Scoles, K., Feldman, P.H., Levine, C., Gould, D. (2002). Challenged to care: Informal caregivers in a changing health system. *Health Affairs*, **21**, 222–31.

(12) Fam, M., Purdy, L. (2010). Treating patients as consumers: 2009 Canadian health care consumer survey report. Deloitte Canada 2010. Retrieved 12 July 2010, from www.deloitte.com.

(13) Fassbender, K., Aguilar, C., Brenneis, C., Fainsinger, R. (2008). Paying to die: The economic burden of care faced by patients and their caregivers. A plenary presentation at the 5th Research Forum of the European Association for Palliative Care (EAPC). Trondheim, Norway, 28–31 May 2008. *Palliative Medicine*, **22** (4), 400.

(14) Family Caregiver Alliance. (2005). A 20-year partnership in caring. San Francisco: Family Caregiver Alliance. Retrieved July 12, 2010, from http://www.caregiver.org/caregiver/jsp/content/pdfs/anniv_rpt_20th.pdf.

(15) Aranda, S.K., Hayman-White, K. (2001). Home caregivers of the person with advanced cancer–An Australian perspective. *Cancer Nursing*, **24** (4), 300–7.

(16) Kurtz, M.E., Kurtz, J.C., Given, C.W., Given, B. (1995). Relationship of caregiver reactions and depression to cancer patients' symptoms, functional states and depression—A longitudinal view. *Social Science and Medicine*, **40** (6), 837–46.

(17) Gaugler, J.E., Linder, J., Given, C.W., Kataria, R., Tucker, G., Regine, W.F. (2009). Family cancer caregiving and negative outcomes: The direct and mediational effects of psychosocial resources. *Journal of Family Nursing*, **15** (4), 417–44.

(18) Nijboer, C. (1998). Tempelaar R. Sanderman R. Triemstra M. Spruijt RJ. van den Bos GA. Cancer and caregiving: The impact on the caregiver's health. *Psycho-Oncology*, **7** (1), 3–13.

(19) Haley, W.E., LaMonde, L.A., Han, B., Burton, A.M., Schonwetter, R. (2003). Predictors of depression and life satisfaction among spousal caregivers in hospice: Application of a stress process model. *Journal of Palliative Medicine*, **6** (2), 215–24.

(20) Hollander MJ (2009). Costs of end-of-life care: Findings from the province of Saskatchewan. *Healthc Q*, **12** (3): 50–8.

(21) Arno, P.S. (2002) Well being of caregivers: The economic issues of caregivers. In T. McRae (Chair), *New Caregiver Research. Symposium conducted at the annual meeting of the American Association of Geriatric Psychiatry*. Orlando, FL. Data from 1987/8 National Survey of Families and Households (NSFH).

(22) Mor, V., Guadagnoli, E., Wool, M.S. (1987). An examination of the concrete service needs of advanced cancer patients. *J Psychosoc Oncol*, **5** (1), 1–17.

(23) Oberst, M.T., Thomas, S.E., Gass, K.A., Ward, S.E. (1989). Caregiving demands and appraisal of stress among family caregivers. *Cancer Nurs*, **12**, 209–15.

(24) Yun, Y.H., Rhee, Y.S., Kang, I.O., Lee, J.S., Bang, S.M., Lee, W.S., Kim, J.S., Kim, S.Y., Shin, S.W., Hong, Y.S. (2005). Economic burdens and quality of life of family caregivers of cancer patients. *Oncology*, **68**, 107–14.

(25) Ferrell, B.R., Grant, M., Borneman, T., Juarez, G., ter Veer, A. (1999). Family caregiving in cancer pain management. *J Palliat Med*, **2** (2), 185–95.

(26) Grunfeld, E., Coyle, D., Whelan, T., Clinch, J., Reyno, L., Earle, C.C., Willan, A., Viola, R., Coristine, M., Janz, T., Glossop, R. (2004). Family caregiver burden: results of a longitudinal study of breast cancer patients and their principal caregivers. *CMAJ*, **170** (12), 1795–1801.

(27) Juarez, G., Ferrell, B., Uman, G., Podnos, Y., Wagman, L.D. (2008). Distress and quality of life concerns of family caregivers of patients undergoing palliative surgery. *Cancer Nursing*, **31** (1), 2–10.

(28) Metlife Mature Market Institute. (1999). The Metlife Juggling Act Study: Balancing Caregiving with Work and the Costs Involved. New York: Metropolitan Life Insurance Company. Retrieved 13 July 2010, from www.caregiving.org/data/jugglingstudy.pdf.

(29) Metlife Mature Market Group. (1997). The Metlife Study of Employer Costs for Working Caregivers. Westport: Metlife Mature Market Group. Retrieved 13 July 2010, from www.caregiving.org/data/employercosts.pdf.

(30) Stajduhar, K.I., Davies, B. (1998). Death at home: Challenges for families and directions for the future. *J Palliat Care*, **14** (3), 8–14.

(31) Williams, A.M. (2004). Shaping the practice of home care: Critical case studies of the significance of the meaning of home. *Int J Palliat Nurs*, **10** (7), 333–42.

(32) MacBride-King, J. (1999). Caring about caregiving: The eldercare responsibilities of Canadian workers and the impact on employers. Ottawa, ON: Conference Board of Canada. Retrieved 13 July 2010, from www.conferenceboard.ca/documents.asp?rnext=154.

(33) Kissane, D.W., Bloch, S., Burns, W.I., McKenzie, D., Posterino, M. (1994). Psychosocial morbidity in the families of patients with cancer. *Psycho-Oncology*, **3**, 47–56.

(34) Cohen, S.R., Leis, A. (2002). What determines the quality of life of terminally ill cancer patients from their own perspective? *J Palliat Care*, **18** (1), 48–58.

(35) Greaves, L., Hankivsky, O., Livadiotakis, G., Cormier, R., Saunders, L., Galvin, L., Vissandjee, B., Carlier, P., Zanchetta, M., Amaratunga, C., Gahagan, J., Reynolds, A. (2002). Final payments: Socioeconomic costs of palliative home caregiving in the last months of life. Vancouver, BC: Centres of Excellence for Women's Health. Retrieved 12 July 2010, from www.cewh-cesf.ca/pdf/cross_cex/final-payments.pdf.

(36) Scott, G., Whyler, N., Grant, G. (2001). A study of family carers of people with life-threatening illness. 1: The carers' need analysis. *Int J Palliat Nurs*, **7** (6), 290–7.

(37) Williams, A.M. (2010). Evaluating Canada's Compassionate Care Benefit using a utilization-focused evaluation framework: Successful strategies and prerequisite conditions. *Eval Program Plann*, **33**, 91–7.

(38) Greer, D.S., Mor, V., Sherwood, S., Morris, J.N., Birnbaum, H. (1983). National Hospice Study Analysis Plan. *J Chron Dis*, **36** (2), 737–80.

(39) Greer, D.S., Mor, V., Sherwood, S., Morris, J.N., Kidder, D., Birnbaum, H. (1986). An alternative in terminal care: Results of the National Hospice Study. *J Chron Dis*, **39** (1), 9–26.

(40) Mor, V., Kidder, D. (1985). Cost savings in hospice: Final results of the National Hospice Study. *HSR*, **20** (4), 407–22.

(41) Morris, J.N., Mor, V., Goldberg, R.J., Sherwood, S., Greer, D.S., Hiris, J. (1986). The effect of treatment setting and patient characteristics on pain in terminal cancer patients: A report from the National Hospice Study. *J Chronic Dis*, **39** (1), 27–35.

(42) Goldberg, R.J., Mor, V., Wiemann, M., Greer, D.S., Hiris, J. (1986). Analgesic use in terminal cancer patients: report from the National Hospice Study. *J Chronic Dis*, **39** (1), 37–45.

(43) Greer, D.S., Mor, V. (1986). An overview of National Hospice Study Findings. *J Chron Dis*, **39** (1), 5–7.

(44) Hippocrates. (Originally written 400 BCE). *Of the Epidemics* [translated by Francis Adams 1994: 346–7]. Retrieved 12 July 2010, from http://classics.mit.edu//Hippocrates/epidemics.html.

(45) Freud, S. (1922). Mourning and melancholia. *J Nerv Ment Dis*, **56** (5), 543–5.

(46) Raphael, B. (1978). Mourning and the prevention of melancholia. *Br J Med Psychol*, **51**, 303–10.

(47) Skipwith, D.H. (1994). Telephone counseling interventions with caregivers of elders. *J Psychosoc Nurs*, **32** (3), 7–12.

(48) Canadian Association of Retired Persons. (2009). CARP Elder Care Poll Report 28 May 2009. Retrieved 12 July 2010, from http://www.carp.ca/advocacy/adv-article-display.cfm?documentID=4818.

(49) Hollander, M.J., Chappell, N.L. (2007). A comparative analysis of costs to government for home care and long-term residential care services, standardized for client care needs. *Can J Aging*, **26** (S1), 149–61.

(50) Chappell, N.L., Havens, B., Hollander, M.J., Miller, J.A., McWilliam, C. (2004). Comparative costs of home care and residential care. *Gerontologist*, **44** (3), 389–400.

(51) Service Canada. (2010). Employment Insurance: Compassionate Care Benefits. Retrieved 13 July 2010, from www.servicecanada.gc.ca/eng/ei/publications/compassionate.pdf.

(52) Crooks, V.A., Williams, A. (2008). An evaluation of Canada's Compassionate Care Benefit from a family caregiver's perspective at end of life. *BMC Palliat Care*, **7** (1).

(53) Giesbrecht, M., Crooks, V.A., Williams, A. (2010). Perspectives from the frontlines: Palliative care providers' expectations of Canada's compassionate care benefit programme. *Health Soc Care Comm* [Epub ahead of print], doi.10.1111/j.1365–2524.2010.00937.x.

(54) Flagler, J., Dong, W. (2010). The uncompassionate elements of the Compassionate Care Benefits Program: a critical analysis. *Global Health Promotion*, **17** (1), 50–9.

(55) Osborne, K., Margo, N. (2005). Analysis and Evaluation Compassionate Care Benefit. Report from the Health Council of Canada. Retrieved 13 July 2010, from http://healthcouncilcanada.ca/docs/papers/2005/Compassionate_Care_BenefitsEN.pdf.

Part III

End-of-life care: Provision, access, and characteristics

Chapter 6

Aggressive treatment and palliative care at the end of life

Kirsten Wentlandt and Camilla Zimmermann

Introduction

The use of palliative care services has been increasing for the last few decades. Despite this, many cancer centres and general hospitals still do not have palliative care services, and there is continuation of aggressive treatment at the end of life (defined broadly as treatments and settings designed for prolonging life, rather than improving quality of life) (1,2). An aggressive approach is often sustained even in patients who are close to death, and in countries such as the United States, Belgium, and Canada, more than 40% of all deaths still occur in hospital acute care units (3–5). The purpose of this chapter is to review the literature pertaining to aggressiveness of care and use of palliative care and hospice services near the end of life. We review characteristics associated with aggressiveness of care or hospice/palliative care use on the level of the physician, patient, and health care system, and discuss implications for quality of care and quality of life for patient and family.

End-of-life quality indicators and aggressiveness of care

Governments across the developed world are increasingly faced with the challenge of how best to provide health care for people with life-limiting illnesses and how to measure the quality and outcomes of that care. Administrative data provide a convenient means of assessing quality of care, because they are computerized, readily available for large populations, and inexpensive. In the United States (US), three measures of poor quality of end-of-life cancer care are readily accessible using administrative data: institution of new anticancer therapies or continuation of ongoing treatments very near death, a high number of emergency department (ED) visits, inpatient hospital admissions, or intensive care unit (ICU) days near the end of life, and a high proportion of patients never enrolled in hospice, only admitted in the last few days of life, or dying in an acute-care setting (rather than at home or in a hospice) (6). In Canada, these quality indicators were expanded on and endorsed by relevant stakeholder groups, including cancer care professionals, patients, and surviving family members and caregivers (7).

Although there remains controversy among stakeholders regarding some of these indicators, particularly in Japan (8,9) but also in countries such as Canada (7), there is a growing consensus that they reflect not only aggressive care but also poor quality of care and poor quality of death (10). While subjective evaluations by patients, families and professional caregivers are particularly important for assessing the quality of life, quality of care, and quality of death (10), the focus of this chapter is primarily on administrative quality indicators, specifically those related to aggressiveness of care.

Aggressiveness of end-of-life care

Measuring rates of aggressive care at the end of life is confounded by controversy over treatment futility, the numerous available treatment options, and the wide range of life-threatening illnesses. Hospital, ICU, and ED visits are challenging to use as markers of aggressive care, because they are influenced by patient co-morbidities, which are difficult to control for. Studies of long-term survival after ICU admission have shown a five-year mortality ranging from 40% to 58% (11), and in the SUPPORT study, the majority of patients with ICU stays longer than 14 days died within 6 months (12). Death rates in older patients are particularly high, with 3-year mortality rates of 60% in patients 65 years or older compared with 40% in younger patients (13). Nevertheless, the number of patients older than 65 admitted to ICUs is increasing, and will likely continue to do so as the population ages (14).

The most informative data on aggressive treatment at the end-of-life has come from the field of oncology, where there are accepted evidence-based treatment guidelines. An extensive study by Earle et al. (2) included a cohort of 215,484 patients in the US who died as a result of a malignancy, were 65 years of age or older at death, and were enrolled in Medicare. There was an increase in intensity and aggressiveness of care over time, with the proportion of patients still receiving chemotherapy within 14 days of death rising from 9.7% in 1993 to 11.6% by 1999. In a second cohort of younger, commercially insured patients, 17.1% were still being treated within two weeks of death and 9.7% had more than one hospitalization in the last month of life (2) (Table 6.1). A prospective study examining newly-diagnosed patients with stage IIIb or IV non-small cell lung cancer (NSCLC) patients observed even higher rates (23%) of anti-cancer therapy usage, during the final weeks of life (15) (Table 6.1). Moreover, 40% received some anticancer therapy within 30 days of death and 13% received new treatment within this period.

A comprehensive study examining the frequency and appropriateness of investigations in 118 cancer patients was completed in Canada (16). There was a decrease in the number of investigations over the course of hospitalization; however, 28% of the patients had tests performed on the final day of life, despite the fact that 78% had been given a diagnosis of dying some days earlier. In addition, 38% received aggressive treatments within the last two weeks of life and 41% during the final hospitalization.

Hospice use at the end of life

The percentage of patients referred to hospice before death appears to be rising (15,17). However, recent population-based studies of male cancer patients indicate that US rates of hospice use are still only 19% to 40%, depending on the population and the State surveyed (18–20). Overall, only about one-quarter of US patients eligible for hospice receive such care (2). Similarly, a Belgian study surveying general practitioners indicated that

Table 6.1 Aggressive care and hospice care at the end of life in US cancer patients

Study	Setting	N	Population	Chemotherapy use 2 weeks before death (%)*	New chemotherapy started <1 month before death (%)	Hospitalization in last month of life (%)	Hospice Care before death (%)
Earle et al., 2004 (17)	US, 1993	7,447	≥65, cancer, enrolled in Medicare	13.8*	4.9	7.8[†]	28.3
	US, 1996	6,870		18.5*	5.7	9.1[†]	38.8
Earle et al., 2008 (2)	US, 1991–2003	18,812	Commercially insured, cancer	17.1*		9.7[†]	23.3
Temel et al., 2008 (15)	US, 2003–2005	46	Age 45–82, Stage IIIb-IV NSCLC	23	13	50	65

*among those receiving chemotherapy.

[†]more than one hospitalization.

NSCLC, non-small cell lung cancer.

specialist palliative care was provided to dying patients in 41% of cases (21). In another study, palliative care services were involved in 78% of patients dying at home in Belgium, versus 41% in the Netherlands (22); in care homes such services were involved in only 39% and 5% of cases in each respective country. As well, studies have indicated that approximately 14% of all hospice admissions were within 3 days of death in the US and 7 days in Europe (23). In fact, although the number of patients receiving palliative care has risen, the overall average length of stay in hospice is declining (15,17). This stands in contrast to the recommendations of international and national agencies for early specialized palliative care involvement (24,25).

Physician characteristics associated with aggressive care

Judgements of futility and decisions about aggressiveness of care are influenced by the interrelated characteristics of physicians, patients, and the health care system in which these decisions take place (Table 6.2). In a study performed in the 1980s, physicians in Australia, Brazil, Canada, Scotland, and Sweden completed a questionnaire describing vignettes of treatment choices for chronically ill older patients (26). Physicians in Brazil and the US used the most aggressive treatments, whereas Australian physicians were the most conservative. Older physicians and those in family medicine were less likely to choose aggressive treatment options. In a more recent Finnish study, younger physicians were also more likely to continue therapy for patients with terminal cancer (27). Conversely, young physicians and those who spent more time in clinical practice were more willing to withdraw life support in an American study (28). These differences may

Table 6.2 Institutional, physician, and patient characteristics associated with provision of aggressive care and palliative care

	Increased likelihood of aggressive care at end of life	Decreased likelihood of aggressive care at end of life	Increased likelihood of palliative care at end of life
Institutional Characteristics	Tertiary institution Teaching hospital Availability of specialists	Rural centre Lack of specialist care	Urban centre Availability of services Teaching hospital Managed care
Physician Characteristics	Specialist Physicians who self-identify as religious African American physicians	Older physicians Family physicians	Experience with prior services and referral Contact with critically ill patients
Patient Characteristics	Multiple co-morbidities Specific disease (e.g. haematological malignancies) Patients with children or dependants Positive religious coping	Older patients Women Non-white Unmarried Poor prognosis Do-not-resuscitate status	Higher education Higher income Higher social class Married or cohabiting Younger patients White Female

be related to physicians' training, patient base, contact with critically ill patients, and prior experience of actually withholding or withdrawing treatment (29,30).

Ethnicity and religion may also play a role in physician decision-making. In a qualitative study, key informant interviews indicated that physician religion or religiosity was a major factor influencing decisions at the end of life (31). In one study, Catholic and Jewish physicians were less willing to withdraw life support than those who did not identify themselves as religious (30), and in another study exclusively among Jewish physicians, those describing themselves as very religious were less willing to withdraw life-sustaining treatments (32). Similarly, physicians attending religious services most frequently were more likely to require a zero probability of success before terming a treatment 'futile' (33). In one study African-American physicians were six times more likely to prescribe aggressive treatments than Caucasian physicians; although it is unlikely that socio-economic status played a role, unmeasured variables such as religion or spirituality might have influenced these results (34).

Characteristics such as training, role norms, experience, and incentives may alter treatment decisions (31). The odds of ICU admission in the US are increased when there is a lack of involvement of the patient's primary outpatient physician during the admission to hospital (35). Vignette- or survey-based studies have found surgeons (33) and cardiologists (29) less willing and oncologists (36) more willing to withhold or withdraw life-sustaining treatments. Other physician characteristics that guide decision-making may not be readily measurable. In a recent study investigating 747 cancer deaths, 'individual clinician' was the only predictor of receiving chemotherapy in the last four weeks of life (37); in another study it was speculated that the extreme variability in decisions to withdraw life support among staff might be explained in part by individual values (38). Many behaviours with implications for intensity of treatment may vary by physician, including communication skills, collaboration with other care providers, beliefs around dying or quality of life, and a tendency to personalize patients' deaths (31).

The process of communication between physicians and patients can have a profound effect on the outcome of aggressive care or hospice referral. Patients' preferences for care reflect their values, their understanding of their illness, and their understanding of the risks and benefits associated with treatment choices (39,40). Studies of cancer patients' values concerning trade-offs between quality and quantity of life have shown considerable variability amongst patients (41,42) and if patients do not accurately comprehend these factors, then their decisions may not reflect their true values (43). In the SUPPORT study, less than half of physicians knew about their patients' preferences for avoidance of cardiopulmonary resuscitation (CPR), and 46% of do-not-resuscitate (DNR) orders were written within only two days of death (44). Communication training may enable physicians to better elucidate patient preferences and explain the meaning of aggressive care or palliative care options (45).

Patient characteristics associated with aggressive care

Patient characteristics associated with aggressive care are not only indicators of patient preference but also reflect variations in care at the level of the medical system and treating physician. A patient's diagnosis may influence care: in the field of oncology, for example, haematological malignancies are most strongly associated with aggressive care at the end of life (17). This may be due to the treatment culture in that medical specialty, where there is a greater initial chance of cure. Higher levels of co-morbidity are also associated with a higher probability of emergency department (ED) visits (1,17) and ICU admissions (1,46). However, independent of disease-related factors such as diagnosis and prognosis, non-disease-related factors such as age, gender, religion, and ethnicity are all related to the likelihood of receiving aggressive treatment (30,38). For example in the US, elderly, female, non-white, and unmarried patients are less likely to receive aggressive care at end-of-life, as are those with a longer duration of illness, regardless of prognosis (2).

Women near the end of life tend to be treated less aggressively, with less ED and ICU use, hospitalization, and chemotherapy (1,2,4,17). However, both men and women with advanced cancer who have dependent children are more likely to prefer aggressive treatment over palliative care and less likely to engage in advance care planning (e.g. DNR orders) (47). Similarly, patients with breast cancer who live with and support dependents are more likely to view smaller gains in length of life from adjuvant chemotherapy as worthwhile despite therapy side effects (48,49).

Ethnicity and religion may also be associated with aggressiveness of care. Studies have indicated that African American patients generally prefer more aggressive treatment at the end of life than Caucasians (50,51). As with the results for physicians, this observation may be confounded by religiosity or spirituality (52,53) or other unmeasured variables. Independent of race, positive religious coping has been associated with preference for and receipt of intensive life-prolonging medical care near death (54). Despite preferring more aggressive care, black patients and Native Americans in the US with colorectal cancer tend to receive less aggressive therapy and are more likely to die of this disease; the survival differences are eliminated when patients receive comparable treatment (55). In one study black patients were three times more likely than white patients to receive intensive end-of-life care, but white patients with a preference for such care were three times more likely to receive it than black patients with the same preference (56). Moreover, white patients who reported an end-of-life discussion or DNR order did not receive intensive end-of-life care, but this was not the case for black patients. Thus there are racial differences associated with preferences and practice of care and preferences are not necessarily congruent with practice.

Aggressiveness of end-of-life care also decreases with patient age, as shown by less frequent hospital and ICU admissions (17,57) and by markedly less use of chemotherapy (2,17,58). This may be due to overly aggressive care in younger patients, appropriate limiting of care for older patients with multiple co-morbidities, or a lack of appropriate treatment in older patients. Increased age has been independently associated with decreased guideline concordance for breast cancer surgery, adjuvant chemotherapy, and adjuvant hormonal therapy (59). Older patients are also less likely to undergo cardiac catheterization for an acute coronary syndrome, despite being high risk and most likely to benefit (60), and have less aggressive stroke care (61,62). Nevertheless, data from the US show that approximately 55% of all ICU bed stays are incurred by patients who are aged 65 or older (14). Older patients have a worse outcome when admitted to the hospital or ICU, even controlling for the less aggressive treatment that they receive (63,64); however, the effect of age on survival may be less than that of acute physiology or diagnosis (64).

Healthcare system factors associated with aggressive treatment

Some healthcare organizations and provision structures are associated with higher rates of aggressive care than others. Receiving care in a US teaching hospital, or simply living in an area with more teaching hospitals, appears to predispose to more aggressive care (2). In one study, more than two-thirds of hospital decedents transferred from general wards to the ICU were managed by house staff who did not discuss alternative care options with patients and/or surrogates (65). Similarly, tertiary care hospitals have a greater number of medical sub-specialists, who are more likely to recommend or initiate potentially ineffective therapies for hospitalized patients with chronic diseases (65).

Increasingly, hospitals are developing policies for advance care planning and completion of DNR orders. End-of-life discussions are associated with lower rates of aggressive care including ventilation, resuscitation and ICU admissions, and with earlier hospice enrollment (16,66). Some patients fear that they may not receive appropriate interventions if they agree to DNR orders, but this has not been convincingly shown. Nursing home residents with DNR orders were less likely to be hospitalized when they developed pneumonia (67), but it is difficult to know whether this association was due to undocumented concomitant morbidity, patient choice of less aggressiveness of care, or an assumption made by the treating clinician. One study showed that patients hospitalized with acute myocardial infarction were less likely to be treated with effective cardiac medications, but this was true even if the DNR order occurred late in the hospital stay (68). In another study patients with DNR orders had a higher mortality rate after adjustment for sickness at admission and other characteristics; however, patients with early DNR orders had lower adjusted mortality and shorter hospital stay rates than those with late DNR orders (69). Thus DNR orders are likely to be a marker of unmeasured illness rather than a determinant of general medical care.

Associations with hospice and palliative care referral

Similar to associations with aggressive care, factors associated with specialized palliative care referral can be loosely divided into those at the patient, health care provider, and health system level, though there is a great deal of overlap. Patients with a higher level of education, income or social class (19,70), those married or co-habiting, and those living in a wealthier area are more likely to access services (71). Conversely, patients of low socio-economic status are less likely to gain access to palliative care services, particularly palliative home care (70,71), but also inpatient hospice care (72) and specialist palliative care (73). Further variables with a negative association to access include being unmarried (70,74), living alone, or being older than 75 or 85 years (71). In a retrospective analysis of Medicare beneficiaries, hospice use was higher for patients enrolled in managed care than for patients enrolled in fee-for-service programmes (28% vs 17%) (75). Although this may indicate better care coordination, it may also reflect a financial incentive to decrease the cost of care (76).

A large US study examined hospice utilization as a function of patient characteristics, such as socio-demographic variables, geographic location, type of insurance, and year of death (19). The sample included 170,136 patients aged 67 and older who were diagnosed with breast, colorectal, lung, or prostate cancer from 1991 to 1996 and who died between 1991 and 1999. Hospice services were used by 31% of non-Hispanic whites, 27.3% of blacks, and 26.7% of other ethnicities (P <0.0001). Utilization was also higher for those enrolled in managed care and those who were younger, married, female, living in urban areas, diagnosed with lung or colorectal cancer, and living in areas with higher education and income levels. In the UK, research has similarly demonstrated that people from minority ethnic populations may be underrepresented among users of specialist palliative care services (73,77).

Care aggressiveness and provision of palliative care are both highly influenced by the accessibility of hospice and palliative care services; availability leads to greater utilization of such services and a decrease in late use of chemotherapy (2). In the US, uneven access to hospice based on geography, rural settings, and patient socio-demographic factors have been documented (76,78,79). Despite their association with more aggressive care, teaching hospitals are also associated with greater overall use of hospice in the US (2). There have also been consistent reports of rural–urban differences in hospice use (see Chapter 16). For example, it was found that in the US, hospice services were unavailable in 23% of the most rural areas, while only 1.3% of metropolitan regions were unserved by hospice (63).

Aggressive care, hospice and care quality

Hospice and specialized palliative care are associated with improvements in quality indicators of end-of-life care. In non-randomized studies, enrolment in a hospice programme has been associated with fewer cancer-related ED visits (31% of hospice patients visited the ED vs 73% of non-hospice patients) (18), and lower rates of hospitalization (80). In randomized trials, involvement of specialized palliative care has been shown to increase deaths at home (81,82), and satisfaction with care (83). However, there remains a dichotomy of care at the end of life, such that patients tend to be treated either with aggressive care and no palliative care consultation, or complete cessation of therapy and palliative care exclusively (84). Patients who receive aggressive care have delayed DNR decisions, and are less likely to receive adequate end-of-life care, palliation, or hospice services (65,85). Patients who receive palliative chemotherapy are also less likely to be referred to hospice, in part because many hospices do not accept patients who are receiving chemotherapy (15). Although the cessation of medically futile chemotherapy might be distressing for the patient (86), the provision of chemotherapy despite a lack of tumour response is obviously not the appropriate solution. Rather, patients need to be supported through the decision-making process, ideally with the help of a multidisciplinary palliative care team.

Increasingly palliative care is being instituted earlier, concomitant with disease-directed treatment. Early integration of palliative care does not have to interfere with curative or life-prolonging treatment, but rather can relieve considerable suffering that can exist throughout the disease course (84). Prospective non-randomized studies have shown that specialized palliative care clinics are feasible and can improve symptom control (87,88). Recent trials of early palliative care involvement for patients with cancer have demonstrated improvement in quality of life (89,90); in a landmark study of early palliative care clinic involvement in patients with lung cancer, there was improvement in quality of life and mood, and increased survival despite less aggressive care (90).

Conclusion

In conclusion, care at the end of life continues to be aggressive, counter to established quality indicators and practice guidelines for end-of-life care. Although hospice enrolment is rising, referrals still occur late in the disease process. There are many factors, on the patient, physician and health system levels, that are associated with this pattern. Implicit in such care is a dichotomy of aggressive versus palliative treatment, with one extreme being life at all costs and the other palliative care without disease-directed intervention. Increasingly, palliative care is being integrated into acute care services, including ICUs and oncology clinics. Such integration has already been associated with decreased aggressiveness of care and improvement of quality of life, and holds promise for the betterment of the overall quality of end-of-life care. It is clear that continued support of palliative care integration into acute and chronic care models, as well as the implementation of end-of-life practice guidelines based on culturally-sensitive quality indicators, should be public health policy priorities.

References

(1) Barbera L, Paszat L, Chartier C. Indicators of poor quality end-of-life cancer care in Ontario. *J Palliat Care.* 2006; **22**: 12–17.

(2) Earle CC, Landrum MB, Souza JM, Neville BA, Weeks JC, Ayanian JZ. Aggressiveness of cancer care near the end of life: Is it a quality-of-care issue? *J Clin Oncol.* 2008; **26**: 3860–6.

(3) Pantilat SZ, Billings JA. Prevalence and structure of palliative care services in California hospitals. *Arch Intern Med.* 2003; **163**: 1084–8.

(4) Van den Block L, Deschepper R, Drieskens K, et al. Hospitalisations at the end of life: Using a sentinel surveillance network to study hospital use and associated patient, disease and healthcare factors. *BMC Health Serv Res.* 2007; **7**: 69.

(5) Wilson DM, Truman CD, Thomas R, et al. The rapidly changing location of death in Canada, 1994–2004. *Soc Sci Med.* 2009; **68**: 1752–8.

(6) Earle CC, Park ER, Lai B, Weeks JC, Ayanian JZ, Block S. Identifying potential indicators of the quality of end-of-life cancer care from administrative data. *J Clin Oncol.* 2003; **21**: 1133–8.

(7) Grunfeld E, Urquhart R, Mykhalovskiy E, et al. Toward population-based indicators of quality end-of-life care: testing stakeholder agreement. *Cancer.* 2008; **112**: 2301–8.

(8) Miyashita M, Morita T, Ichikawa T, Sato K, Shima Y, Uchitomi Y. Quality indicators of end-of-life cancer care from the bereaved family members' perspective in Japan. *J Pain Symptom Manage.* 2009; **37**: 1019–26.

(9) Miyashita M, Sanjo M, Morita T, Hirai K, Uchitomi Y. Good death in cancer care: A nationwide quantitative study. *Ann Oncol.* 2007; **18**: 1090–7.

(10) Hales S, Zimmermann C, Rodin G. The quality of dying and death. *Arch Intern Med.* 2008; **168**: 912–18.

(11) Williams TA, Dobb GJ, Finn JC, Webb SA. Long-term survival from intensive care: A review. *Intensive Care Med.* 2005; **31**: 1306–15.

(12) Teno JM, Fisher E, Hamel MB, et al. Decision-making and outcomes of prolonged ICU stays in seriously ill patients. *J Am Geriatr Soc.* 2000; **48**: S70–4.

(13) Kaarlola A, Tallgren M, Pettila V. Long-term survival, quality of life, and quality-adjusted life-years among critically ill elderly patients. *Crit Care Med.* 2006; **34**: 2120–6.

(14) Angus DC, Barnato AE, Linde-Zwirble WT, et al. Use of intensive care at the end of life in the United States: An epidemiologic study. *Crit Care Med.* 2004; **32**: 638–43.

(15) Temel JS, McCannon J, Greer JA, et al. Aggressiveness of care in a prospective cohort of patients with advanced NSCLC. *Cancer.* 2008; **113**: 826–33.

(16) Hui D, Con A, Christie G, Hawley PH. Goals of care and end-of-life decision making for hospitalized patients at a Canadian tertiary care cancer center. *J Pain Symptom Manage.* 2009; **38**: 871–81.

(17) Earle CC, Neville BA, Landrum MB, Ayanian JZ, Block SD, Weeks JC. Trends in the aggressiveness of cancer care near the end of life. *J Clin Oncol.* 2004; **22**: 315–21.

(18) Bergman J, Kwan L, Fink A, Connor SE, Litwin MS. Hospice and emergency room use by disadvantaged men dying of prostate cancer. *J Urol.* 2009; **181**: 2084–9.

(19) Lackan NA, Ostir GV, Freeman JL, Mahnken JD, Goodwin JS. Decreasing variation in the use of hospice among older adults with breast, colorectal, lung, and prostate cancer. *Med Care.* 2004; **42**: 116–22.

(20) Locher JL, Kilgore ML, Morrisey MA, Ritchie CS. Patterns and predictors of home health and hospice use by older adults with cancer. *J Am Geriatr Soc.* 2006; **54**: 1206–11.

(21) Van den Block L, Deschepper R, Bossuyt N, et al. Care for patients in the last months of life: The Belgian Sentinel Network Monitoring End-of-Life Care study. *Arch Intern Med.* 2008; **168**: 1747–54.

(22) Abarshi E, Echteld MA, Van den Block L, et al. Use of Palliative Care Services and General Practitioner Visits at the End of Life in The Netherlands and Belgium. *J Pain Symptom Manage.* 2010.

(23) Costantini M, Toscani F, Gallucci M, et al. Terminal cancer patients and timing of referral to palliative care: a multicenter prospective cohort study. Italian Cooperative Research Group on Palliative Medicine. *J Pain Symptom Manage.* 1999; **18**: 243–52.

(24) World Health Organization. WHO definition of palliative care. Cited 2003. Available from: www.who.int/cancer/palliative/definition/en.

(25) American Society of Clinical Oncology. Palliative Care.

(26) Alemayehu E, Molloy DW, Guyatt GH, et al. Variability in physicians' decisions on caring for chronically ill elderly patients: An international study. *CMAJ.* 1991; **144**: 1133–8.

(27) Hinkka H, Kosunen E, Metsanoja R, Lammi UK, Kellokumpu-Lehtinen P. Factors affecting physicians' decisions to forgo life-sustaining treatments in terminal care. *J Med Ethics.* 2002; **28**: 109–14.

(28) Christakis NA, Asch DA. Biases in how physicians choose to withdraw life support. *Lancet.* 1993; **342**: 642–6.

(29) Kelly WF, Eliasson AH, Stocker DJ, Hnatiuk OW. Do specialists differ on do-not-resuscitate decisions? *Chest.* 2002; **121**: 957–63.

(30) Christakis NA, Asch DA. Physician characteristics associated with decisions to withdraw life support. *Am J Public Health.* 1995; **85**: 367–72.

(31) Larochelle MR, Rodriguez KL, Arnold RM, Barnato AE. Hospital staff attributions of the causes of physician variation in end-of-life treatment intensity. *Palliat Med.* 2009; **23**: 460–70.

(32) Wenger NS, Carmel S. Physicians' religiosity and end-of-life care attitudes and behaviors. *Mt Sinai J Med.* 2004; **71**: 335–43.

(33) Swanson JW, McCrary SV. Doing all they can: physicians who deny medical futility. *J Law Med Ethics.* 1994; **22**: 318–26.

(34) Mebane EW, Oman RF, Kroonen LT, Goldstein MK. The influence of physician race, age, and gender on physician attitudes toward advance care directives and preferences for end-of-life decision-making. *J Am Geriatr Soc.* 1999; **47**: 579–91.

(35) Sharma G, Freeman J, Zhang D, Goodwin JS. Continuity of care and intensive care unit use at the end of life. *Arch Intern Med.* 2009; **169**: 81–6.

(36) Hanson LC, Danis M, Garrett JM, Mutran E. Who decides? Physicians' willingness to use life-sustaining treatment. *Arch Intern Med.* 1996; **156**: 785–9.

(37) Kao S, Shafiq J, Vardy J, Adams D. Use of chemotherapy at end of life in oncology patients. *Ann Oncol.* 2009; **20**: 1555–9.

(38) Cook DJ, Guyatt GH, Jaeschke R, et al. Determinants in Canadian health care workers of the decision to withdraw life support from the critically ill. Canadian Critical Care Trials Group. *JAMA.* 1995; **273**: 703–8.

(39) Forrow L, Wartman SA, Brock DW. Science, ethics, and the making of clinical decisions. Implications for risk factor intervention. *JAMA.* 1988; **259**: 3161–7.

(40) Singer PA, Choudhry S, Armstrong J, Meslin EM, Lowy FH. Public opinion regarding end-of-life decisions: Influence of prognosis, practice and process. *Soc Sci Med.* 1995; **41**: 1517–21.

(41) Singer PA, Tasch ES, Stocking C, Rubin S, Siegler M, Weichselbaum R. Sex or survival: Trade-offs between quality and quantity of life. *J Clin Oncol.* 1991; **9**: 328–34.

(42) Slevin ML, Stubbs L, Plant HJ, et al. Attitudes to chemotherapy: Comparing views of patients with cancer with those of doctors, nurses, and general public. *BMJ.* 1990; **300**: 1458–60.

(43) Weeks JC, Cook EF, O'Day SJ, et al. Relationship between cancer patients' predictions of prognosis and their treatment preferences. *JAMA.* 1998; **279**: 1709–14.

(44) Phillips RS, Wenger NS, Teno J, et al. Choices of seriously ill patients about cardiopulmonary resuscitation: Correlates and outcomes. SUPPORT Investigators. Study to Understand Prognoses and Preferences for Outcomes and Risks of Treatments. *Am J Med.* 1996; **100**: 128–37.

(45) Back AL, Arnold RM, Baile WF, et al. Efficacy of communication skills training for giving bad news and discussing transitions to palliative care. *Arch Intern Med.* 2007; **167**: 453–60.

(46) Sharma G, Freeman J, Zhang D, Goodwin JS. Trends in end-of-life ICU use among older adults with advanced lung cancer. *Chest.* 2008; **133**: 72–8.

(47) Nilsson ME, Maciejewski PK, Zhang B, et al. Mental health, treatment preferences, advance care planning, location, and quality of death in advanced cancer patients with dependent children. *Cancer.* 2009; **115**: 399–409.

(48) Duric V, Stockler M. Patients' preferences for adjuvant chemotherapy in early breast cancer: A review of what makes it worthwhile. *Lancet Oncol.* 2001; **2**: 691–7.

(49) Duric VM, Stockler MR, Heritier S, et al. Patients' preferences for adjuvant chemotherapy in early breast cancer: What makes AC and CMF worthwhile now? *Ann Oncol.* 2005; **16**: 1786–94.

(50) Garrett JM, Harris RP, Norburn JK, Patrick DL, Danis M. Life-sustaining treatments during terminal illness: Who wants what? *J Gen Intern Med.* 1993; **8**: 361–8.

(51) Hopp FP, Duffy SA. Racial variations in end-of-life care. *J Am Geriatr Soc.* 2000; **48**: 658–63.

(52) Johnson KS, Elbert-Avila KI, Tulsky JA. The influence of spiritual beliefs and practices on the treatment preferences of African Americans: A review of the literature. *J Am Geriatr Soc.* 2005; **53**: 711–19.

(53) Song MK, Hanson LC. Relationships between psychosocial-spiritual well-being and end-of-life preferences and values in African American dialysis patients. *J Pain Symptom Manage.* 2009; **38**: 372–80.

(54) Phelps AC, Maciejewski PK, Nilsson M, et al. Religious coping and use of intensive life-prolonging care near death in patients with advanced cancer. *JAMA.* 2009; **301**: 1140–7.

(55) Hodgson DC, Fuchs CS, Ayanian JZ. Impact of patient and provider characteristics on the treatment and outcomes of colorectal cancer. *J Natl Cancer Inst.* 2001; **93**: 501–15.

(56) Loggers ET, Maciejewski PK, Paulk E, et al. Racial differences in predictors of intensive end-of-life care in patients with advanced cancer. *J Clin Oncol.* 2009; **27**: 5559–64.

(57) Teno JM, Mor V, Ward N, et al. Bereaved family member perceptions of quality of end-of-life care in U.S. regions with high and low usage of intensive care unit care. *J Am Geriatr Soc.* 2005; **53**: 1905–11.

(58) Braga S, Miranda A, Fonseca R, et al. The aggressiveness of cancer care in the last three months of life: a retrospective single centre analysis. *Psychooncology.* 2007; **16**: 863–8.

(59) Giordano SH, Hortobagyi GN, Kau SW, Theriault RL, Bondy ML. Breast cancer treatment guidelines in older women. *J Clin Oncol.* 2005; **23**: 783–91.

(60) Bagnall AJ, Goodman SG, Fox KA, et al. Influence of age on use of cardiac catheterization and associated outcomes in patients with non-ST-elevation acute coronary syndromes. *Am J Cardiol.* 2009; **103**: 1530–6.

(61) Basu J, Mobley LR. Trends in racial disparities among the elderly for selected procedures. *Med Care Res Rev.* 2008; **65**: 617–37.

(62) Rudd AG, Hoffman A, Down C, Pearson M, Lowe D. Access to stroke care in England, Wales and Northern Ireland: the effect of age, gender and weekend admission. *Age Ageing.* 2007; **36**: 247–55.

(63) Covinsky KE, Fuller JD, Yaffe K, et al. Communication and decision-making in seriously ill patients: Findings of the SUPPORT project. The Study to Understand Prognoses and Preferences for Outcomes and Risks of Treatments. *J Am Geriatr Soc.* 2000; **48**: S187–93.

(64) Hamel MB, Davis RB, Teno JM, et al. Older age, aggressiveness of care, and survival for seriously ill, hospitalized adults. SUPPORT Investigators. Study to Understand Prognoses and Preferences for Outcomes and Risks of Treatments. *Ann Intern Med.* 1999; **131**: 721–8.

(65) Rady MY, Johnson DJ. Admission to intensive care unit at the end-of-life: Is it an informed decision? *Palliat Med.* 2004; **18**: 705–11.

(66) Wright AA, Zhang B, Ray A, et al. Associations between end-of-life discussions, patient mental health, medical care near death, and caregiver bereavement adjustment. *JAMA.* 2008; **300**: 1665–73.

(67) Zweig SC, Kruse RL, Binder EF, Szafara KL, Mehr DR Effect of do-not-resuscitate orders on hospitalization of nursing home residents evaluated for lower respiratory infections. *J Am Geriatr Soc.* 2004; **52**: 51–8.

(68) Jackson EA, Yarzebski JL, Goldberg RJ, et al. Do-not-resuscitate orders in patients hospitalized with acute myocardial infarction: the Worcester Heart Attack Study. *Arch Intern Med.* 2004; **164**: 776–83.

(69) Wenger NS, Pearson ML, Desmond KA, Brook RH, Kahn KL. Outcomes of patients with do-not-resuscitate orders. Toward an understanding of what do-not-resuscitate orders mean and how they affect patients. *Arch Intern Med.* 1995; **155**: 2063–8.

(70) Walshe C, Todd C, Caress A, Chew-Graham C. Patterns of access to community palliative care services: a literature review. *J Pain Symptom Manage.* 2009; **37**: 884–912.

(71) Grande GE, Addington-Hall JM, Todd CJ. Place of death and access to home care services: Are certain patient groups at a disadvantage? *Soc Sci Med.* 1998; **47**: 565–79.

(72) Wood DJ, Clark D, Gatrell AC. Equity of access to adult hospice inpatient care within north-west England. *Palliat Med.* 2004; **18**: 543–9.

(73) Rees WD. Immigrants and the hospice. *Health Trends.* 1986; **18**: 89–91.

(74) Lackan NA, Ostir GV, Kuo YF, Freeman JL. The association of marital status and hospice use in the USA. *Palliat Med.* 2005; **19**: 160–2.

(75) Virnig BA, Morgan RO, Persily NA, DeVito CA. Racial and income differences in use of the hospice benefit between the medicare managed care and medicare fee-for-service. *J Palliat Med.* 1999; **2**: 23–31.

(76) McCarthy EP, Burns RB, Ngo-Metzger Q, Davis RB, Phillips RS. Hospice use among Medicare managed care and fee-for-service patients dying with cancer. *JAMA*. 2003; **289**: 2238–45.

(77) O'Neill J, Marconi K. Underserved populations, resource-poor settings, and HIV: Innovative palliative care projects. *J Palliat Med*. 2003; **6**: 457–9.

(78) Keating NL, Herrinton LJ, Zaslavsky AM, Liu L, Ayanian JZ. Variations in hospice use among cancer patients. *J Natl Cancer Inst*. 2006; **98**: 1053–9.

(79) Virnig BA, Ma H, Hartman LK, Moscovice I, Carlin B. Access to home-based hospice care for rural populations: Identification of areas lacking service. *J Palliat Med*. 2006; **9**: 1292–9.

(80) Gozalo PL, Miller SC. Hospice enrollment and evaluation of its causal effect on hospitalization of dying nursing home patients. *Health Serv Res*. 2007; **42**: 587–610.

(81) Brumley R, Enguidanos S, Jamison P, et al. Increased satisfaction with care and lower costs: results of a randomized trial of in-home palliative care. *J Am Geriatr Soc*. 2007; **55**: 993–1000.

(82) Jordhoy MS, Fayers P, Saltnes T, Ahlner-Elmqvist M, Jannert M, Kaasa S. A palliative-care intervention and death at home: a cluster randomised trial. *Lancet*. 2000; **356**: 888–93.

(83) Zimmermann C, Riechelmann R, Krzyzanowska M, Rodin G, Tannock I. Effectiveness of specialized palliative care: A systematic review. *JAMA*. 2008; **299**: 1698–1709.

(84) Zimmermann C, Wennberg R. Integrating palliative care: A postmodern perspective. *Am J Hosp Palliat Care*. 2006; **23**: 255–8.

(85) Lynn J, Teno JM, Phillips RS, et al. Perceptions by family members of the dying experience of older and seriously ill patients. SUPPORT Investigators. Study to Understand Prognoses and Preferences for Outcomes and Risks of Treatments. *Ann Intern Med*. 1997; **126**: 97–106.

(86) Zimmermann C, Burman D, Swami N, et al. Determinants of quality of life in patients with advanced cancer. *Support Care Cancer*. 2010.

(87) Follwell M, Burman D, Le LW, et al. Phase II study of an outpatient palliative care intervention in patients with metastatic cancer. *J Clin Oncol*. 2009; **27**: 206–13.

(88) Temel JS, Jackson VA, Billings JA, et al. Phase II study: Integrated palliative care in newly diagnosed advanced non-small-cell lung cancer patients. *J Clin Oncol*. 2007; **25**: 2377–82.

(89) Bakitas M, Lyons KD, Hegel MT, et al. Effects of a palliative care intervention on clinical outcomes in patients with advanced cancer: the Project ENABLE II randomized controlled trial. *JAMA*. 2009; **302**: 741–9.

(90) Temel S, Greer J, Gallagher E, et al. Effect of early palliative care (PC) on quality of life (QOL), aggressive care at the end-of-life (EOL), and survival in stage IV NSCLC patients: Results of a phase III randomized trial. *J Clin Oncol*. 2010; **28**.

Chapter 7

Access to palliative care

Gunn Grande

Introduction

Equity in access is central to palliative care policy (1). This means that people of equal need should have the same access to care, and that the level of care available should depend only on a patient's level of need and not on factors irrelevant to that need (2).

In practice, level of access is often difficult to establish, and realistically what will be discussed in this chapter will mainly be referral and utilization of palliative care services, which will relate to, but not be identical with, access. Differences in referral and utilization may not reflect inequity in access, as they may reflect underlying differences in need (2). Alternatively, individuals with similar needs and similar opportunity to obtain palliative care (i.e. similar access) may exercise different choices in their use of such care.

By palliative care in this chapter is meant specialist palliative care or palliative care services that may not consist of specialists, but whose sole remit is palliative care. This is in contrast to generalist services in which palliative care may be a component of the care provided. This chapter will describe who uses palliative care, and particularly review the factors affecting access to palliative care.

Use of palliative care

Few studies have looked, at a population level, at what proportion of patients potentially benefitting from palliative care actually use palliative care services. A study in the USA reported an overall hospice utilization rate for persons 65 years and older of 28.6% in 2002, with the highest hospice utilization found for individuals with cancer (65%), kidney disease and nephritis (55%), and Alzheimer's disease (41%) (3). Reliable recent data from the UK are lacking, but in 1990 a nationwide survey found that 28% of deaths received care from a specialist palliative care nurse (4). In Italy, 14% of those dying from cancer were found to have used home palliative care services and 20% of hospitalized cancer patients used hospital palliative care (5). A nationwide study in Belgium found that in 2005, 25% of all patients who died non-suddenly from non-cancer conditions and 61% of those who died from cancer used specialist palliative care services, a figure higher than that found in other European countries (6,7). Studies looking at trends have suggested that the proportion of cancer patients using palliative care is increasing over time (8). However, it seems that still a fairly large proportion of patients are not using palliative care, while they may benefit from it.

Factors affecting access

2.1 Availability of palliative care services

A prerequisite for access to palliative care is the availability of palliative care services to meet the palliative care needs of a population. It is difficult to arrive at an estimate of what the level of palliative care provision should be and therefore at what point availability can be said to affect access. Higginson et al. (9) outline three approaches to assessment of population need: the epidemiological, the corporate and the comparative approach.

The epidemiological approach combines information on number of deaths by cause with estimates of symptom prevalence for each disease to estimate the number of people in a population likely to require palliative care. Using this approach Franks et al. (10) report estimates that among 2,800 cancer deaths per million people per year, 2,400 suffer pain, 1,300 breathing difficulties, 1,400 vomiting and nausea, and 700 acute anxiety, with 930 families also suffering severe anxiety. Among 6,900 per million deaths from progressive non-malignant disease, 3,400 suffer pain, 3,400 breathing problems, 1,900 nausea and vomiting, and 1,600 acute anxiety, with 2,200 families suffering severe anxiety. In their work on the minimal size of a potential palliative care population, Rosenwax et al. (11), estimate that at least half of all dying patients would benefit from palliative care services. However, the figures attained through either approach may not equate to perceived need by recipients.

A corporate approach may achieve closer approximation of actual need by asking the receiving population about their needs and priorities (9). Currow et al. (12) conducted a population survey in South Australia of people who had experienced a recent death of someone close to them due to a terminal illness. Their findings suggest that 38–53% of people with terminal illness did not access palliative care, but that this was rarely due to unavailability or lack of knowledge of such services. The most important reasons cited for not accessing palliative care included that family or friends already provided the care and that the service was not wanted. Problems with this approach include the possibility that respondents may not be aware of the patient's needs, and study conclusions were affected by missing information.

A comparative approach compares service provision between areas and concludes that areas of lower provision have greater need for service development (9). If countries with the highest palliative care availability serve as a benchmark, countries and locations that fall below this level arguably have worse access on the basis of service provision. Wright et al. (13) reviewed palliative care worldwide and outlined four levels of national provision: 1) no identified palliative care activity (33% of countries); 2) capacity building, but no services (18%); 3) localized provision (34%); 4) palliative care approaching integration with mainstream service providers (15%). Of Level 4 countries those with the best ratios of service (regardless of type and size) to population numbers were the UK (1:43,000), Iceland (1:49,000), Australia (1:63,000), and Canada (1:65,000), and the findings of Currow et al. for Australia (12), above, need to be seen in this context. People in countries with levels substantially below this will clearly have worse access to palliative care, including many Level 4 countries (e.g. Kenya at 1:4.28 million). We should note that the remaining discussion of this chapter refers to countries at Level 3 and 4 for whom palliative care is a realistic option.

Even within Level 4 countries there are large local variations in availability (14) that are unlikely to be randomly distributed. Palliative care provision has typically evolved in an unplanned manner (12) and there is concern that it is most likely to develop within resourceful communities, in accord with the Inverse Care Law (15), whereby the most deprived communities have lowest provision. Pragmatics also means that rural communities, in terms of distance to services, will have less access to palliative care than urban communities (2). This factor will have a particularly high impact in countries with larger geographical distances and more rural communities.

2.2 Diagnostic and demographic variables

Under conditions of similar service availability, it also appears that different groups of patients do not access palliative care to a similar extent.

Originally palliative care focused on the needs of patients with cancer and has only relatively recently broadened its remit to patients with non-malignant diseases. Although the proportion of referrals for patients with non-malignant diseases may to some extent increase with active encouragement, patients with cancer still make up the vast majority of referrals to palliative care (2;10).

The majority of studies suggest that older patients, particularly the oldest old, are less likely to be referred to palliative care than are younger patients (2;16;17).

There is also strong evidence that socio-economic status affects access to palliative care, in that those on higher incomes, who live in their own homes, live in less deprived areas have better access as possibly do those with higher education (2;16). This could in part be due to people with lower socio-economic status living in areas with worse service provision (15). However, research by Campbell et al. (18) suggests that socio-economic differences in access to palliative home care persist even in areas with identical provision.

While we should avoid considering people from black and ethnic minority (BEM) populations to be a uniform group, there appears to be consistent evidence that BEM patients are less likely to access palliative care (2).

Those who are married or have a live-in lay carer are more likely to be referred to palliative home care. Indeed some home services stipulate the presence of such a carer as a precondition before a referral can be made (2;16). Demographic changes in the developing world are likely to lead to increases in people living alone, particularly within some groups, e.g. older people (19), in turn affecting the options of palliative care provision available.

While these above patterns have been repeatedly shown, there has been little research to establish the factors behind the observed patterns. Some of the above patient groups will be considered in detail in subsequent chapters. In the present chapter we will move on to consider general factors that may affect timely access to palliative care, and only refer back to particular groups in so far as a factor may affect one group more than another.

2.3 **Challenges of defining patients as suitable for palliative care**

Palliative care is by definition holistic and encompasses management of pain and other symptoms and psychological, social, and spiritual support both for patients and their families (20), and should be gradually phased in alongside curative treatment (21). However, this also means that that a firm trigger point or criterion for referral to palliative care is lacking. While palliative care should ideally begin early in the patient's disease trajectory, in practice its initiation is often based on the patient's proximity to death. This is lent further emphasis by referral criteria for many palliative care services and by access to funding (Medicare in the US, Disability Living Allowance in the UK) being linked to survival.

Moreover, options of palliative or compassionate leave for families are in many countries also linked to a relatively short predicted survival time.

Prediction and communication of prognosis

Key prerequisites for timely referral to palliative care are the ability of health professionals to recognize and acknowledge that the patient is 'for palliative care' and the communication of this to the patient.

Murray et al. (21) outline three trajectories of functional decline towards the end of life to help professionals and patients plan for palliative care: 1) death following a rapid decline or distinct terminal phase of illness, most characteristic of cancer patients; 2) long-term limitations with a gradual decline interspersed with serious, potentially fatal acute episodes, e.g. COPD and heart failure, and 3) 'prolonged dwindling' where there is 'progressive disability from an already low baseline of cognitive or physical functioning'. Palliative care delivery has, in the UK as in many other countries, traditionally been based on the cancer trajectory where intervention has been confined mainly to the terminal phase (22). It can be argued that it is more difficult to define patients as 'for palliative care' for non-malignant conditions with a less predictable progression and a less distinct and time limited terminal phase.

Empirical research into dying trajectories using aggregate data has generally confirmed the above trajectories (23). However, aggregate data mask considerable individual variation in the trajectories of both function and symptoms, both for patients with non-malignant and with malignant disease (22;24). While service planning may be based on aggregate trajectories, health professionals still face the challenge of anticipating what will happen to an individual patient to inform individual discussion and referral recommendations.

Dying trajectories suggest that estimation of prognosis, particularly towards the end, should be easier for cancer than for other conditions. Nevertheless, the literature shows that physicians are usually inaccurate in predicting survival in cancer patients and that they are more likely to give over-optimistic than over-pessimistic prognoses (25), which are likely to delay referral.

Prediction of survival in non-malignant progressive disease may pose still greater challenges for health professionals (26) in the prediction of both short- and long-term prognoses (e.g. (24), on COPD), and professionals may have particular difficulty in deciding when to move to palliative care and initiate discussions about patient concerns and preferences e.g. in patients with COPD and heart failure (27;28). Research by Gott et al. (29) seems to confirm that non-cancer-hospital patients may less easily be labelled as palliative compared to cancer patients. Research by Christakis and Lamont (30) suggests that physicians may be least accurate in predicting survival in AIDS patients, and that they are more likely to make over-optimistic predictions for cancer patients than for AIDS patients and those with other conditions. However, this study was based on patients already referred to palliative care and had a relatively small proportion of patients with non-malignant disease.

Different groups of health professionals differ considerably in the accuracy of their prognosis or willingness to see the patient as suitable for palliative care (29). More experienced doctors make more accurate prognoses than less experienced colleagues, but perhaps surprisingly, prognoses become less accurate the more familiar the doctor is with the patient (30). General practitioners have been found to be more reluctant to label patient as palliative compared to oncologists (31), while hospital nurses may favour earlier referral to palliative care than hospital doctors and general practitioners (32).

Even if an accurate prediction of prognosis could be made in theory, physicians may find it psychologically difficult to 'give up' on the patient and may regard a switch to palliative care as a failure, and dealing with a patient's potential distress over a poor prognosis may pose additional challenges (33). This may again lead to bias towards over-optimistic prognoses.

Although health professionals may believe that a patient is 'for palliative care', transition depends largely on this information being communicated to the patient. Lamont and Christakis (34) report that only 37% of physicians would give cancer patients an estimate of survival, 40% would give an estimate different from and usually more optimistic than the one they have formulated, and 23% would give no estimate.

Research by Gott et al. (27) in COPD suggests that even if professionals may agree that end of life discussion should be initiated, they disagree as to which professional group should take responsibility for this, though with a general tendency to agree that the responsibility is somebody else's.

Acknowledgement of the prognosis by patients

Patients themselves may clearly have considerable barriers to acknowledging their prognosis. Schofield at al (32) review evidence that patients with advanced disease often underestimate its extent and are over-optimistic about their prognosis. Furthermore, the evidence suggests there is limited agreement between doctors and patients whether the terminal nature of the disease had been communicated by the doctor: in nearly half of cases where doctors reported that they had told the patient, the patient reported no communication (32).

Although the majority of patients (85%) have been reported as wanting to know both good and bad information (32), a graded approach to discussion of palliative care may be necessary. Research reported by Schofield et al.'s review found that only one third of patients wanted to discuss dying and palliative care when first told that their cancer had spread, 19% in the next few consultations, 33% said later, upon their request, 11% never, and 10% were unsure (32).

Desire to know may furthermore differ between groups. Older people may prefer not to have overt awareness of dying (32;35), while in some BEM cultures there may be a lack of open discussion of dying with the family controlling the information (36). While there is public awareness that cancer may be fatal, there may be less awareness of the terminal nature of some non-malignant diseases such as COPD (27), although these may have less likelihood of cure, which makes initiation of discussion of palliative care more difficult for such conditions.

Defining need

While open acknowledgement of the incurable nature of the patient's disease is important for the planning of appropriate care and referral, this does not necessarily mean that a palliative care referral is required. Not all deaths from terminal disease are associated with symptoms requiring palliative care (10) and lack of referral to palliative care does not necessarily equate with unmet need (12).

On the basis of symptom prevalence (10) patients with non-malignant conditions should be referred to palliative care on a more similar level to cancer patients than is currently the case. A review by Solano et al. (37) of symptoms in cancer, AIDS, heart disease, COPD, and renal disease found high symptom prevalence across cancer and non-cancer diagnoses, with pain, breathlessness and fatigue being particularly universal and frequent, and with insomnia and anorexia also as common symptoms in all conditions. However, the wide range of study designs, sampling criteria and measures used makes direct comparison difficult.

On a similar basis, research on symptom prevalence indicates that older patients should be referred to palliative care at a similar level to younger patients (2). However, a recent study by Burt et al. (38) concludes that differential referral between older and younger patients is based on need. Nevertheless, the relationship between need and referral for older patients is not clear, as suggested by Gott et al.'s (29) study which found that the majority of hospital patients identified as having palliative care needs were older patients, but that, for whatever reason, this did not translate into greater likelihood of referral to a palliative care bed.

There is relatively little research on the actual triggers for palliative care referral, but evidence gives prominence to symptom control (32): pain is reportedly the most common reason for referral and is perceived to be the symptom that palliative care is most suited to addressing, followed by nausea, fatigue, and dyspnoea. However, what may drive referral is the complexity of needs, i.e. when there is more than one symptom or problem, and when the scale of problems goes beyond the ability to cope of the generalist professionals and families. These may include psychosocial and practical problems that surround the physical demise of the patient (39). This highlights the complex nature of defining a need for palliative care support, in that it is not just a matter of establishing the prevalence and severity of patients' problems per se, but also the existing professional and family resources to cope with the problem.

Higginson et al. (9) further highlight some of the complexities of identifying need. Need can be based on what individuals feel they need, where 'felt need' by patients and carers in response to similar challenges may differ considerably depending on existing resources and ability to cope. Need may also be 'expressed need', where individuals may differ in the needs they are able and willing to express, something we will return to in a subsequent section.

Need may also be what professionals think an individual wants and requires. Gott et al. (29) found hospital doctors and nurses identified similar numbers of patients as having palliative care needs, but there was only 'fair' agreement between them as to which patients these were, although correspondence increased with closer proximity to death.

However, Gott et al. (29) found that defining patients as having such needs does not necessarily translate into referral to palliative care, and suggest this may in part reflect a lack understanding of the remit of palliative care services. This links to a final definition noted by Higginson et al. (9) where palliative care needs would be defined in relation to the availability of effective palliative care solutions. That is, for health professionals to define the patients as having a palliative care need requiring referral they must perceive there to be a palliative care service to meet that need.

2.4 Interface between palliative care services and other health professionals

Health professionals may have varying levels of knowledge of the availability and remit of palliative care services (39). Burt et al. (40), for instance, found that general practitioners differed in their awareness of local out of hours palliative care services, with 33–47% not being aware of availability of such services in evenings, at nights or at weekends. They may furthermore hold misperceptions about the role and remit of palliative care services which will further affect their likelihood of referral (29;41).

Generalist providers may also differ considerably in the extent to which they see palliative care as part of their own remit and in their willingness to share provision of palliative care with more specialist providers. Burt et al. (40) found that 72% of general practitioners saw palliative care as a central part of their role, while 27% wanted to hand over such care fully to specialists. Many general practitioners may also have a general reluctance to accept expertise or direction from others outside their own profession (42), a reluctance which is probably not limited to general practitioners. Furthermore, district nurses reportedly often see palliative care as an essential and satisfying part of their role (14). These factors are all likely to affect referral patterns.

Walshe et al. (43) also highlight how referral to palliative care is only partly determined by patient need (however defined) and depends on generalists' sense of 'ownership' and perceived skill and time to provide palliative care themselves. Actual referral is furthermore not only dependent on the formal remit of the palliative care services, but on the perceived skills and personal characteristics of palliative care team members. From the perspective of specialist palliative care providers, the acceptance of referrals may in turn depend on the perceived skills and resources of generalists, i.e. how well they are likely to manage on their own, while preservation of good interprofessional relationships regarding referral may take precedence over immediate needs of individual patients. The latter strategy may improve referrals longer term as generalists are more likely to refer to specialist palliative care providers that take a collaborative approach than to those perceived to be 'elitist' (43).

2.5 **Patient characteristics**

Other important influences on referral and access may be found in the communication between health professionals and patients or families and in the characteristics and contexts of patients and families themselves.

Patients and their families may differ in the extent to which they share a culture and language with health professionals. A basic level of ability is required to formulate and articulate the need or problem for which help is being sought, and e.g. middle class people may be more articulate and confident in requesting support compared with patients of lower class backgrounds (44). Similarly, patients who share a common, 'proto-professionalized' language with general practitioners may be more likely to be referred on to specialists than those who do not (45). Patients may also differ in their ability to take on board information regarding prognosis and options available, and such understanding cannot be assumed but needs to be ascertained (46).

Patients with whom professionals are better able to identify may also trigger different responses, e.g. patients of a similar generation may produce a greater sense of urgency to help as opposed to those of an older generation (47). General practitioners are also more likely to refer if the recipient is economically active and has dependants (44). Such factors may form part of the explanation for why older patients or those with older carers may be less likely to be referred to palliative care (48).

While there may be different degrees of 'language barriers' between professionals and different groups in society, these problems are most acute where the patient is a foreign language speaker and may be dependent on a family or official interpreter for communication (36;49). As noted, communication with patients from black and ethnic minority groups may be further hampered by cultural preferences for less open discussion of dying and for withholding the prognosis from the patient (36;49).

A patient's own knowledge of palliative care may differ considerably between demographic groups. People who live in more deprived circumstances may be more likely to lack awareness of palliative care services or resources to utilize them (44;50). Knowledge about palliative care is also associated with age, ethnicity and possibly gender (50). Lack of awareness of different types of palliative care services and how they work makes it difficult to make informed choices (43). In recent years access to information about support available may be further influenced by age differences in the use of internet resources.

Patients' attitudes to palliative care may also differ considerably and affect acceptance of it. Older patients have been found to have different attitudes from younger people (51). People from black and ethnic minority groups may be more likely to consider hospice as somewhere you go to die (36), and their families may furthermore be more likely to see support from outsiders as a sign of failure (36). Patients and family carers may also be reluctant to accept palliative care in an effort to preserve normal aspects of life and independence and prevent intrusion (52). Patients may differ in the level of psychological distress from a terminal prognosis, and it has been suggested that, e.g., older patients may be less troubled by a cancer diagnosis than younger patients (41).

3 **Conclusions and ways forward**

It is difficult to estimate what the appropriate level of palliative care provision in a population should be. However, such provision varies considerably between countries and it is clear that many patients across the world have little or no access to palliative care due to lack of service provision. Even within nations with good palliative care provision there is considerable local variation. Patients differ in their access to palliative care on the basis of diagnosis, age, socio-economic status, ethnic background and the presence of a family carer. Some of the factors underlying these differences are poorly understood and require further research.

Timely referral to palliative care is in part due to difficulties of establishing prognosis. Although improved understanding of disease trajectories and better prediction of survival would help, this is unlikely ever to become an exact science. Murray et al. (53) propose that health professionals should ask themselves the question 'Would I be surprised if my patient were to die in the next 12 months?' and initiate discussion of palliative care with patients if the answer is 'no'. Improved communication with patients and increased use of Advance Care Planning (ACP) are likely to facilitate appropriate referral. Wright et al. (54) found that ACP did not lead to increased patient anxiety and depression, which may be the fear of many health professionals, but reduced aggressive treatment and lead to earlier referral to palliative care and better patient and carer quality of life. Schofield et al. (32) outline key components of this process including provision of a supportive environment, understanding of the patient's perspective, ascertaining of preferences, introduction of palliative care options and rebuilding of morale. Ascertaining patient preferences includes establishing how much they want to know and at what point, as patients will differ in this respect.

There may also be difficulty in establishing when need should trigger a palliative care referral, which is partly dependent on expression and identification of need, the ability of generalist professionals' and families' ability to cope, and an awareness and understanding of existing palliative care provision. Solutions here include clearer referral criteria and guidelines (39) and the use of palliative care frameworks and pathways to aid appropriate palliative care timing and management. Examples include the Gold Standards Framework (described in Chapter 9) and the Liverpool Care Pathway, both of which have been widely adopted in England as part of a national strategy for palliative care (55). Research also suggests that the building of good relationships between generalist and specialist care, not just guidelines and criteria, may be important for timely referral.

Finally some language and cultural differences in the broadest sense may leave some patient and carer groups at a disadvantage in being heard and obtaining palliative care to suit their needs. Some of these difficulties have been overcome through advocacy on the patient's behalf in the case of black and ethnic minority groups (36), but may also be relevant in the case of other disadvantaged groups.

Timely referral to palliative care can significantly improve patients' quality of life and psychological wellbeing, and may in certain situations improve survival (56). It is therefore of substantial importance to ensure there are adequate levels of palliative care provision within countries and to develop effective means for improving early and appropriate referral to palliative care.

References

(1) Department of Health (2008) *End of Life Care Strategy: Promoting High Quality Care for All Adults at the End of Life*. Crown copyright.

(2) Walshe C, Todd C, Caress A, Chew-Graham C (2009) Patterns of access to community palliative care services: A literature review. *J Pain Symptom Manage* 37 (5): 884–912.

(3) Connor SR, Elwert F, Spence C, Christakis NA (2007) Geographic variation in hospice use in the United States in 2002. *J Pain Symptom Manage* Sep; 34 (3): 277–85.

(4) Addington-Hall J. & Altmann D (2000) Which terminally ill patients in the United Kingdom receive care from community specialist palliative care nurses? *Journal of Advanced Nursing* 32 (4): 799–806.

(5) Beccaro M, Costantini M, Merlo DF; ISDOC Study Group (2007) Inequity in the provision of and access to palliative care for cancer patients. Results from the Italian survey of the dying of cancer (ISDOC). *BMC Public Health* Apr 27; 7: 66.

(6) Van den Block L, Deschepper R, Bossuyt N, Drieskens K, Bauwens S, Van Casteren V, Deliens L (2008) Care for patients in the last months of life: The Belgian Sentinel Network Monitoring End-of-Life Care study. *Arch Intern Med* Sep 8; 168 (16): 1747–54.

(7) Abarshi E, Echteld MA, Van den Block L, Donker G, Bossuyt N, Meeussen K, Bilsen J, Onwuteaka-Philipsen B, Deliens L (2011) Use of palliative care services and general practitioner visits at the end of life in The Netherlands and Belgium. *J Pain Symptom Manage* Feb; 41 (2): 436–48.

(8) Earle CC, Neville BA, Landrum MB, Ayanian JZ, Block SD, Weeks JC (2004) Trends in the aggressiveness of cancer care near the end of life. *J Clin Oncol* Jan 15; 22 (2): 315–21.

(9) Higginson IJ, Hart S, Koffman J, Selman L, Harding R (2007) Needs assessments in palliative care: an appraisal of definitions and approaches used. *J Pain Symptom Manage* 33 (5): 500–5.

(10) Franks PJ, Salisbury C, Bosanquet N, Wilkinson EK, Lorentzon M, Kite S, Naysmith A, Higginson IJ (2000) The level of need for palliative care: A systematic review of the literature. *Palliat Med* 14 (2): 93–104.

(11) Rosenwax LK, McNamara B, Blackmore AM, Holman CD (2005) Estimating the size of a potential palliative care population. *Palliat Med* Oct; 19 (7): 556–62.

(12) Currow DC, Abernethy AP, Fazekas BS (2004) Specialist palliative care needs of whole populations: A feasibility study using a novel approach. *Palliat Med* 18 (3): 239–47.

(13) Wright M, Wood J, Lynch T, Clark D (2008) Mapping levels of palliative care development: A global view. J Pain Symptom Manage 35 (5): 469–85.

(14) Shipman C, Addington-Hall J, Richardson A, Burt J, Ream E, Beynon T (2005) Palliative care services in England: A survey of district nurses' views. *British Journal of Community Nursing* 10 (8): 381–6.

(15) Tudor-Hart J (1971) The inverse care law. *The Lancet*, Feb 27; 1 (696): 405–12.

(16) Grande GE, Addington-Hall JM, Todd CJ (1998) Place of death and access to home care services: Are certain patient groups at a disadvantage? *Social Science and Medicine*, 47 (5): 565–79.

(17) Burt J, Raine R (2006) The effect of age on referral to and use of specialist palliative care services in adult cancer patients: A systematic review. *Age and Ageing* 35 (5): 469–76.

(18) Campbell M, Grande G, Wilson C, Caress A-L, Roberts D (2010) Exploring differences in referrals to a Hospice at Home Service in two socio-economically distinct areas of Manchester. *Palliat Med* 24 (4): 403–9.

(19) Seale C (2000). Changing patterns of death and dying. *Social Science & Medicine* **51**: 917–30.

(20) NICE (2004) *Guidance on Cancer Services Improving Supportive and Palliative Care for Adults with cancer*. Oxford: NICE. http://guidance.nice.org.uk/CSGSP/Guidance/pdf/English.

(21) Murray SA, Kendall M, Boyd K, Sheikh A (2005). Illness trajectories in palliative care, *BMJ* **330**: 1007–11.

(22) Gott M, Barnes S, Parker C, Payne S, Seamark D, Gariballa S, Small N (2007) Dying trajectories in heart failure. *Palliat Med* **21**: 95–9.

(23) Teno JM, Weitzen S, Fennell ML, Mor V (2001) Dying trajectory in the last year of life: Does cancer trajectory fit other diseases? *Palliat Med* **4** (4): 457–64.

(24) Bausewein C, Booth S, Gysels M, Kühnbach R, Haberland B, Higginson IJ (2010) Individual breathless trajectories of not match summary trajectories in advanced cancer and chronic obstructive pulmonary disease: Results from a longitudinal study. *Palliat Med* **24**(8): 777–86 10.1177/0269216310378785. http://pmj.sagepub.com/cgi/content/abstract/0269216310378785v1.

(25) Glare P, Virik K, Jones M, Hudson M, Eychmuller S, Simes J, Christakis N (2003) A systematic review of physicians' survival predictions in terminally ill cancer patients. *BMJ* **327**: 195–8.

(26) Coventry PA, Grande GE, Richards DA, Todd CJ (2005) Prediction of appropriate timing of palliative care for older adults with non-malignant life-threatening disease: A systematic review. *Age & Ageing* **34** (3): 218–27.

(27) Gott M, Gardiner C, Small N, Payne S, Seamark D, Barnes S, Halpin D, Ruse C (2009) Barriers to advance care planning in chronic obstructive pulmonary disease. *Palliat Med* **23**: 642–8.

(28) Boyd KJ, Worth A, Kendall M, Pratt R, Hockley J, Denvir M, Murray SA (2009) Making sure services deliver for people with advanced heart failure: A longitudinal qualitative study of patients, family carers, and health professionals. *Palliat Med* **23** (8): 767–76.

(29) Gott MC, Ahmedzai SH, Wood C (2001) How many inpatients at an acute hospital have palliative care needs? Comparing the perspectives of medical and nursing staff. *Palliat Med* **15** (6): 451–60.

(30) Christakis NA, Lamont EB (2000) Extent and determinants of error in doctors' prognoses in terminally ill patients: Prospective cohort study. *BMJ* **320**: 469–72.

(31) Farquhar M, Grande G, Todd C, Martin A, Barclay S (2002) Defining patients as palliative: Hospital doctors' versus General Practitioners' perceptions. *Palliat Med* **16** (3): 247–50.

(32) Schofield P, Carey M, Love A, Nehill C, Wein S (2006) 'Would you like to talk about your future treatment options?' Discussing the transition from curative cancer treatment to palliative care. *Palliat Med* **20**: 397–406.

(33) Meier DE, Back AL, Morrison S (2001) The inner life of physicians and care of the seriously ill. *JAMA* **286** (23): 3007–14.

(34) Lamont EB, Christakis NA (2001) Prognostic disclosure to patients with cancer near the end of life. *Annals of Internal Medicine* **34**: 1096–105.

(35) Gott M, Small N, Barnes S, Payne S, Seamark D (2008) Older people's views of a good death in heart failure: Implications for palliative care provision. *Social Science & Medicine* **67**: 1113–21.

(36) Worth A, Irshad T, Bhopal R, Brown D, Lawton L, Grant E, Murray S, Kendall M, Adam J, Gardee R, Sheikh A (2009) Vulnerability and access to care for South Asian Sikh and Muslim patients with life limiting illness in Scotland: Prospective longitudinal qualitative study. *BMJ* **338**: b183: doi:10.1136/bmj.

(37) Solano JP, Gomes B, Higginson IJ (2006) A comparison of symptom prevalence in far advanced cancer, AIDS, heart disease, chronic obstructive pulmonary disease and renal disease. *J Pain Symptom Manage* **31** (1): 58–69.

(38) Burt J, Plant H, Omar R, Raine R (2010) Equity of use of specialist palliative care by age: Cross-sectional study of lung cancer patients. *Palliat Med* **24**(6): 641–50 DOI: 10.1177/0269216310364199; pmj. sagepub.com.

(39) Bestall JC, Ahmed N, Ahmedzai SH, Payne S, Noble B, Clark D (2004) Access and referral to specialist palliative care: Patients' and professionals' experiences. *International Journal of Palliative Nursing* **10** (8): 381–9.

(40) Burt J, Shipman C, White P, Addington-Hall J (2006) Roles, service knowledge and priorities in the provision of palliative care: A postal survey of London GPs. *Palliat Med* **20**: 487–92.

(41) Ahmed N, Bestall JC, Ahmedzai SH, Payne SA, Clark D, Noble B (2004) Systematic review of the problems and issues of accessing specialist palliative care by patients, carers and health and social care professionals. *Palliat Med* **18** (6): 525–42.

(42) Walshe C, Todd C, Caress AL, Chew-Graham C (2008a) Judgements about fellow professionals and the management of patients receiving palliative care in primary care: A qualitative study. *British Journal of General Practice* **58** (549): 264–72.

(43) Walshe C, Chew-Graham C, Todd C, Caress A (2008) What influences referrals within community palliative care services? A qualitative case study. *Social Science & Medicine* **67** (1): 137–46.

(44) Dixon-Woods M, Cavers D, Agarwal S, Annandale E, Arthur A, Harvey J, Hsu R, Katbamna S, Olsen R, Smith L, Riley R, SuttonAJ (2006) Conducting a critical interpretive synthesis of the literature on access to healthcare by vulnerable groups. *BMC Medical Research Methodology* **6**: 35.

(45) Alberts JF, Sanderman R, Gerstenbluth I, van den Heuvel WJ (1998) Sociocultural variations in help-seeking behaviour for everyday symptoms and chronic disorders. *Health Policy* **44** (1): 57–72.

(46) Silverman J, Kurtz S, Draper J (1998) *Skills For Communicating With Patients*. Abingdon, UK: Radcliffe Medical Press.

(47) Lawton J (2000) *The Dying Process: Patients' Experiences of Palliative Care*. London: Routledge.

(48) Grande GE, Farquhar MC, Barclay SIG, Todd CJ (2006) The influence of patient and carer age in access to palliative care. *Age and Ageing* **35**: 267–73.

(49) Karim K, Bailey M, Tunna K (2000) Nonwhite ethnicity and the provision of specialist palliative care services: Factors affecting doctors' referral patterns. *Palliat Med* **14**: 471–8.

(50) Koffman J, Burke G, Dias A, Raval B, Byrne J, Gonzales J, Daniels C (2007) Demographic factors and awareness of palliative care and related services. *Palliat Med* **21**: 145–53.

(51) Catt S, Blanchard M, Addington-Hall J, Zis M, Blizard R, King M (2005) Older adults' attitudes to death, palliative treatment and hospice care. *Palliat Med* Jul; **19** (5): 402–10.

(52) Grande GE, Todd, CJ, Barclay SIG (1997) Support needs in the last year of life: Patient and carer dilemmas. *Pallia Med* **11**: 202–8.

(53) Murray SA, Boyd K, Sheikh A (2005) Palliative care in chronic illness. *BMJ* **330** (7492): 611–12.

(54) Wright AA, Zhang B, Ray A, Mack JW, Trice E, Balboni T, Mitchell SL, Jackson VA, Block SD, Maciejewski PK, Prigerson HG (2008b) Associations between end-of-life discussions, patient mental health, medical care near death, and caregiver bereavement adjustment. *JAMA* **8**; **300** (14): 1665–73.

(55) Hughes PM, Bath PA, Ahmed N, Noble B (2010) What progress has been made towards implementing national guidance on end of life care? A national survey of UK general practices. *Palliat Med* **24** (1): 68–78.

(56) Temel JS, Greer JA, Muzikansky A, Gallagher ER, Admane S, Jackson VA, Dahlin CM et al. (2010) Early palliative care for patients with metastatic non-small-cell lung cancer. *N Engl J Med* **363**: 733–42.

Chapter 8

Communication between patient and caregiver

Linda Emanuel

Introduction

The last communications of a dying person may be valued as the most important in a lifetime. Similarly, the decisions a person makes, including medical care decisions, as he or she negotiates the last chapter of life may be so meaningful that they are remembered for the rest of the lives of the bereaved. On a concrete level, care near the end of life can be so costly that the surviving family may shoulder the consequences for years or even generations. (1) With decisions of such significance, communication of the information and other factors that go into them and communication of the decisions themselves, should be clear and reliable. And yet, communication at a time of serious illness and high emotions is both notoriously difficult and often further complicated by social taboos and interpersonal dynamics.

This chapter identifies communications of importance and reviews some of the mechanisms involved in processing and managing them; the goal is to provide clinicians, patients and their families and communities with a framework for understanding the issues, and with approaches that can optimize communications near the end of life.

What is communication and what characterizes it in end-of-life settings?

Communication is the exchange of meaning between people. The exchange can involve information, concepts, thoughts—conscious or unconscious—and feelings.

Interaction between people often involves the exchange of several or all of these types of meaning, and they are not always aligned.

A clinician or any involved person who listens to one aspect of any exchange of meaning, say about factual information, to the exclusion of the others, say mood, will miss important meaning. Similarly, failure to ask oneself what is the significance of any misalignment between the aspects of meaning risks incomplete communication. Inattention to the way people process information and feeling risks distorting communication.

Communication near the end of life characteristically involves exchanges about at least the following: information about the illness, including its manifestations, prognosis, and care; preferences and decisions about care; implementation of care for the ill person; conditions of the family care providers and others; and relationships between the patient and care providers.

Because the information involved in terminal illness is often of grave significance, communication near the end of life needs to be conducted with sensitivity to and a deep understanding of the psychological processes entailed in taking in, adapting to, and making use of difficult, usually highly undesirable, information.

Communicating across cultural or personal barriers

Most people seek the information they need to accurately understand their circumstances. At the same time, if information is so difficult for a person to handle that their psychological defence mechanisms come into play, it may be preferable for that person to not be over-exposed to the news until coping seems possible. These balances are highly culture-, individual-, and situation-specific. It is almost impossible to assess how people like to handle communication without getting to know them; in the limited time available to clinicians it is usually best to ask (e.g. how do you like to handle information and decisions? Should I talk directly with you? Are there topics that you prefer to avoid?).

Some cultures, and probably many people at some level, believe that simply speaking the word 'cancer' or 'AIDS' or another diagnostic word that implies a terrible outcome can bring about the fate that they wish to eschew. However, even in such settings, people have found ways of talking about unwanted things. Some talk about the matter indirectly, saying for instance 'if someone were to have cancer, I think that . . . '. So when a clinician is caring for a person for whom frankness is counter-cultural or counter-intuitive, the clinician can start with such indirect communication and, gently erring on the side of candour without triggering withdrawal or superstitious fear, attain the best communication possible for that patient.

Additional considerations regarding culture and diversity are provided in section 5 of this textbook.

Taking in and adapting to new, terminal, illness circumstances

Sharing information in optimal ways

Clinicians, like many people, are reluctant to share bad news with patients. An abundance of data documents how limited are the necessary conversations about illness information, as illustrated in Table 8.1. Barriers exist in all parties on many levels. The distress of the patients and their family members is readily transmitted to the clinician and all concerned. It is common to say to oneself that shielding the person (or oneself) from the truth protects from distress. But studies also suggest that even across cultures, people need to have the information at some level and in some fashion, so clinicians need to overcome their distress and share appropriate information with the appropriate parties, using whatever communication methods work. The goal of this communication is to first optimize the ability to take it in and then optimize the transition to realistic hope. Most people with any cognizant time left to live will seek to take command of their situation by doing the

Table 8.1 Selected studies on communication about end-of-life matters

Citation	Study	Key finding
Azoulay 2000 (10)	ICU patients and families	54% of designated representatives of ICU patients failed to comprehend diagnosis, prognosis, or treatment after discussion with a physician. Numerous statistically significant factors were associated with lack of comprehension.
Covinsky 2000 (11)	Terminal patients	Physician, nurse, and surrogate understanding of preferences was found to be only moderately better than chance. Only half of patients who do not want CPR receive do-not-resuscitate orders. Care provided to patients was often inconsistent with their preferences.
Bradley 2001 (12)	Terminal cancer patients	Only 38% of patients had a documented discussion about prognosis; physicians and patients were both present during these discussions only 52% of the time.
Ditto 2001 (13)	Patients and proxies	Four interventions testing scenario- or value-based advance directives failed to produce significant improvement in the accuracy of surrogate predictions of patient preferences, compared to no intervention.
Wenger 2001 (14)	AIDS patients	In a cross-sectional, probability sample of the US population half of all persons with HIV did not discuss any aspect of end-of-life care with their physicians.
Phipps 2003 (15)	Caregivers and patients	A racial disparity in end-of-life care preferences was found. Roughly 50% of patient–caregiver pairs disagreed in each scenario regarding patient preferences about end-of-life care.
Knauft 2005 (16)	COPD patients	Only 32% of patients reported communication with their physician about end-of-life care. Patient-identified barriers included: Patient not wanting to discuss death, being concerned about continuity of care if transitioned into a palliative program, and not knowing what kind of care they would want.
Zapka 2006 (17)	Advanced heart failure and cancer patients	Only 30% of patients discussed advance directives, and only 22% reported inquiry by their physician about spiritual support. African-American patients under the care of African-American physicians were the least likely of any racial pairing to report management of pain and/or symptoms.
Ozanne 2009 (18)	Breast cancer patients	75% of patients had learned about, and 55% had written, advance directives, but only 14% of physicians were aware of the presence of an advance directive.
Thornton 2009 (19)	Families of ICU patients with non-English speakers	Family conferences requiring interpretation were shorter by an average of ~20%. Physicians spoke only 42.7% of the time during interpreted conferences, compared to 60.5% during non-interpreted conferences. Statistically significantly fewer statements were made by the physician supporting the family during interpreted conferences.
Gattellari 2002 (20)	Australian cancer patients	Alternatives to cancer treatment were presented only in 44.1% of consultations, and patients were informed about the impact of anticancer therapy on quality of life only 36.4% of the time. 29.7% of patients were offered a choice in the management of their disease, and oncologists checked patient understanding only 10.2% of the time. Greater information disclosure was not found to increase levels of anxiety in patients, but greater patient participation in decisions was associated with increased anxiety levels over a two-week period.

Table 8.1 (*continued*) Selected studies on communication about end-of-life matters

Citation	Study	Key finding
Lamont 2001 (21)	Hospice patients	22.7% of physicians surveyed would not communicate a survival estimate they made, and 40.3% would communicate a different survival estimate than the one they made, in most cases (70.2%) optimistically. Physicians reported providing a frank survival estimate only 37% of the time.
Ptacek 2001 (22)	Cancer patient perspectives	Patients reported high levels of satisfaction with communications with their physicians, with the following factors differentiating the most satisfied: physicians giving special attention to environmental comfort, taking their time with the patient, and empathizing.

best they can with the time they have. Physicians have a proclivity to overestimating the patient's prognosis (2),(3), which is not helpful for people trying to make good use of a short amount of remaining time, so clinicians should take this into account and attempt to counterbalance their inclinations with self-awareness and objective data.

Buckman has developed a step-wise approach for clinicians sharing difficult information, which is a useful guide (4). This or a similarly systematic approach should be used.

In 9 out of 10 life-ending illnesses, people have a moderately predictable trajectory with successive losses along the way. The inaccuracies of prediction have received much attention recently, particularly the proclivity of clinicians to overestimate the time a patient has left to live(3). Appreciating that people need to be able to plan and to accomplish whatever they want to in the time they have left should encourage clinicians to give a suitable range of estimated time left and a description of the functions they may loose during the illness trajectory. Time can be addressed using units such as 'hours to days'; 'days to weeks'; 'weeks to months'; or 'months to years'. Regarding loss of function, it is helpful, if hard, to say something like 'most people progressively lose the ability to think and recognize people' or 'the tumor is encasing the spinal cord; she is likely to lose more of her ability to move'.

Providing people with diagnoses and prognoses in such a way that they can use them and in a fashion that gives them purpose rather than loss of hope depends not only on optimizing their ability to take it in, which may be accomplished by Buckman's or similar approaches, but also depends on how people take in, understand, and respond to life-altering situations. Figure 8.1 provides a depiction by Knight et al. of one model describing this process. It recognizes three phases in a dynamic, reiterative process of initial intake of information, creative adaptation, and reintegration.

Receiving serious information

Initially, people tend to be stunned when they are confronted by bad news e.g. a new diagnosis or an event that makes clear their loss, and the immediate loss is of their expectations for the future. Consider the experience immediately after a stroke of being unable to speak; there is immediate loss of a physical capacity that has many implications for one's life. Family members have a similar sense of shock as they take in their loss of expectations,

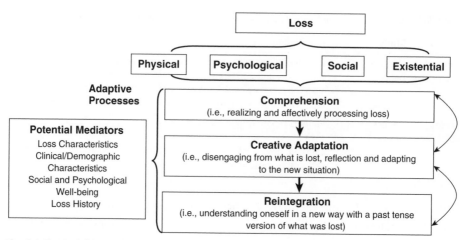

Fig. 8.1 The Knight reintegration model. Reprinted with permission from *Journal of Palliative Medicine*, Volume 10, Issue 5, published by Mary Ann Liebert, Inc., New Rochelle, NY.

trying to understand what their future will be with their loved one changed by illness or no longer there. This stunned or shocked state is refractory to new input for many people and suspends their normal thought processes and can be observed by clinicians and others as the person appears to be unfocused, unhearing or responds to comments in a distracted or incomplete or unconnected fashion. Sometimes a person has dissociated the information and seems 'too normal'. It is useful to ask what it is they just heard, saying something like 'this is hard information to take in; what are you thinking right now?'

The refractory period can last moments or days. Clinicians and all involved should allow time to pass while realization develops and wait before introducing significant new issues if at all possible. For instance, informed consent for a procedure (e.g. reducing intracerebral pressure due to a tumour) for which there is little time to loose may feel pressing but not be valid in the sense that the patient will not have taken in the significance of the procedure if he or she is still in the refractory period.

Creative adaptation

As the new situation dawns on the individual, he or she enters a new phase, that of creative adaptation. Thoughts about how to live without speech (can I still write?) or with little time left to live (can I still see my sister in the time I have?) start to take centre stage.

During this phase a person is likely to try out various ideas, some of which may be unrealistic. Clinicians and others can be helpful in brainstorming ideas (if the individual welcomes that) about what may work. Hitting on a plan that is realistic can infuse a person with a new type of hope and a goal that organizes their time and effort. This should be welcomed and supported.

Creative adaptation can entail a wide range of emotions, including anger and frustration. Grief and mourning for functions and relationships and capacities and dreams lost is important for returning to an acceptable state of mind. However, the losses can be overwhelming. Supportive acknowledgment of the reasons why such feelings are normal can be helpful.

Integration

For those with a chronic, stable condition, integration entails living in a manageable way, having made peace with the loss. Arrival at and maintenance of this state, especially for those who have adjusted to significant losses, usually requires people to have done a great deal of personal, interpersonal, and practical work.

For those with the expectation that death is soon, integration entails bringing one's personal story to closure. Often this entails making peace with others and making a baton-pass to those who will survive. Essentially, integration involves vesting parts of the dying person in the surviving people. Those parts may be wisdoms ('When it gets hard, think of something you forgot to appreciate, appreciate it and keep smiling'), the means for doing familiar things ('Take my tool box'; 'You have the cooking recipes'), values ('Be a good person, the way we taught you'), material gifts ('The grandfather clock is yours'), memorabilia ('I want you to have the photographs') role transfers ('You'll look after the children, won't you?'), or messages of love.

Clinicians need to be aware of the importance of these communications and to make time and space for them amidst the medical hubbub. A person's dying is the last stage of life that they have and they should be able to make of it what they need or want to, not what medicine dictates.

Often a clinician is in a position to notice that the tasks of understanding, creative adaptation, or integration are not happening. If this is the case, the help of a counsellor—especially one experienced in counselling for the terminally ill and their families—can be helpful.

Models of shared decision-making

As set out in Table 8.2, various models of decision making are available. One framework provides four types. In the paternalistic type, now largely discredited, the physician knows best and makes decisions that are in the best interest of the patient. In the informative type, the physician provides information to the patient and allows the patient to make all decisions.

Table 8.2 Models of the patient–clinician interaction around information transmittal and decision-making

Emanuel & Emanuel 1998 (23)	*JAMA*	4 models	Paternalistic, Informative, Instructional, Deliberative
Botelho 1992 (24)	*Fam Pract*	1 model	Negotiation
Hantho 2002 (25)	*Scand J Prim Health*	1 model	Mutual understanding
Rowan 2003 (26)	*Health Commun*	1 model	CAUSE
Kiesler 2003 (27)	*Soc Sci Med*	1 model	Interpersonal circumplex
Slingsby 2004 (28)	*Soc Sci Med*	2 models	Omakase/entrusting
			Participatory
Fredericks (29)	*J Natl Med Assoc*	1 model	Society, Culture and Personality model
Finset 2009 (30)	*Patient Educ Couns*	1 model	Value Chain model

In the instructional type, the physician provides information to the patient but also tells them what the best decision is. In the deliberative type, the physician provides information and then enters into deliberation with the patient to discern the best decision, both learning from the patient and offering advice.

For some decisions, such as which anti depressant to use, it may be that the paternalistic or instructional type of decision making is suitable. For others, such as which setting of care the patient prefers, the informative type may be appropriate. The deliberative type is the most suitable in many situations in present day society, and even more so for the overarching decisions, such as goals of care. If the patient is unable to participate in decision making, the family and/or proxy decision maker can participate. The deliberative model is most suitable because of the great complexity of the decisions and their personal significance, not only to the patient but to the family and community. An algorithm based on science or on some privileged knowledge on the part of the physician that would allow him or her to make a good decision under the paternalistic, informative, or instructional type, is highly unlikely for larger decisions such as goals of care.

Topics that matter to patients nearing the end of life

People with serious illness are often in unknown territory. Not only have they not experienced these current illness circumstances before nor faced their imminent mortality but, in present day western culture, many people have not witnessed another person's death. They may feel disoriented and unsure of what is important and what is less important.

A clinician can help by knowing what tends to be important to people in similar situations. Data from surveys documents what these areas are, as shown in Table 8.3. Use of a screening instrument can help validate for patients and families their common concerns and can guide clinicians and family members to suitable responses.

Screening questions

Several instruments exist for screening patient needs in the palliative care setting. One is the Needs near the End of life Screening Tool or NEST. Derived from surveys of terminally ill people and their family caregivers, NEST screens for needs in each of the main domains of a person's experience of illness—physical and mental symptoms, social, spiritual, and therapeutic relationships—and if needs are detected, it provides more specific screening questions (5). It can be adapted to different settings and programmed to lead to possible recommended interventions to address the needs detected (6). Some of the initial screening questions are included in the relevant domains below.

Physical function and symptoms

Making clear by explicit statement and action that freedom from physical suffering is a priority helps most patients. A screening question such as that from NEST, namely: 'How much do you suffer from physical symptoms such as pain, shortness of breath, fatigue, bowel or urination problems?' can open the inquiry.

Table 8.3 Studies on areas that matter to patients

Citation	Study	Areas patient find important
Emanuel 1998 (31)	Representative sample of terminally ill patients in the USA	Management of: physical and psychological symptoms, economic and caregiving needs, social relationships and support, spiritual beliefs and hopes, and advance care planning.
Singer 1999 (32)	Dialysis, HIV, and Long-Term Care patients	(1) Receiving adequate pain and symptom management; (2) avoiding inappropriately prolonging dying; (3) a sense of control; (4) relieving burden; (5) strengthening relationships with loved ones.
Steinhauser 2000 (33)	Seriously ill patients, recently bereaved family, physicians, and other care providers	26 items rated as important by >70% of each of the four groups, including management of pain and symptoms, preparation for death, a sense of completion, being able to decisions about treatment preferences, and being treated as a whole person. The patient group also rated being mentally aware, having funeral arrangements, not being a burden, helping others, and peace with God highly.
Gardner 2009 (34)	Terminally ill elders and their family caregivers	Experiencing decline, managing pain/discomfort, living with uncertainty, receiving quality care, being treated with dignity and respect, avoiding unnecessary life-sustaining treatment, desire to be prepared for death, desire to avoid being a burden.

Psychological states associated with illness

Terminal illness almost always entails mental as well as physical symptoms. The NEST instruments screens for this with the question: 'How often do you feel confused or anxious or depressed?'

Social stresses due to illness, including economic ones

Suffering due to illness in the social context of life usually arises from multiple sources. Often the illness causes significant financial concern and too often it causes real hardship as well. Even without financial limitations, for many it is hard to access good palliative or other types of care. The clinician can ask the NEST questions: 'How much of a financial hardship is your illness for you or your family?' and: 'How much trouble do you have getting the medical care you need?'

Spiritual needs related to serious illness

Birth and death are the ultimate existential events. Spirituality is our relationship with existence. It is expressed in various ways, only one of which is in denominationally identified religious expression. All people face questions about existence, and this aspect comes to the fore when death is anticipated.

For many, their existential concern is to be able to complete the tasks of dying. One of these is, for many people, tending to their personal narrative and providing a narrative legacy for those they leave behind. This was discovered by Chochinov as a young psychiatrist as he was being asked to consult on terminally ill patients whose attending physicians believed to be depressed (7). He could diagnose depression rarely, but he could make them feel much better by asking them questions about their life. Dignity therapy has been developed into a manual so that any trained individual can provide it for patients. It entails inviting the patient to respond to the prompts identified in Box 8.1. The taped responses are transcribed, edited, and returned to the patient within two to three days so that they can offer it as a legacy gift to their loved ones. Because dignity therapy requires training in psychology or related fields, the clinician should seek someone trained in the process to provide it.

Therapeutic relationships—communicating about care relationships

Clinicians enter a dying person's life at a most intimate time in his or her life cycle. Other care relationships also take on heightened significance. It is important that they go as well as possible, so it is helpful to ask. NEST provides a question: 'How much do you feel your doctors and nurses respect you as an individual?' It also asks about how well information is being communicated: 'How clear is the information from us about what to expect regarding your illness?' Patients, like most people, are remarkably good at guiding us in the type of relationship and communication they want if we just ask.

Box 8.1 Dignity therapy prompts

- Tell me a little about your life history; particularly the parts that you either remember most, or think are the most important. When did you feel most alive?
- Are there specific things that you would want your family to know and remember about you?
- What are the most important roles you have played in life (family, vocational, community service roles, etc.)? Why were they so important to you, and what do you think you accomplished in those roles?
- What are your most important accomplishments, and what do you feel most proud of?
- What are your hopes and dreams for your loved ones?
- What have you learned about life that you would want to pass along to others?
- What advice or words of guidance would you wish to pass along to your [family member(s), other(s)]?
- Are there things you want to say to your loved ones, or that you want to take the time to say once again?
- Are their words or instructions you want to offer your family, to provide help to prepare them for the future?
- In creating this permanent record, are their other things that you would like included?

Decisions that matter to patients nearing the end of life

Goals of care

If people do not communicate about critical issues, assumptions are made. A case in point for modern medicine has been the failure to communicate about goals of care for illness with limited prognosis. In the middle to second half of the twentieth century it was assumed that, in the scientific enthusiasm of the era, the ends of medicine were to save lives and stamp out disease. Patients were admitted for all diagnoses with interventions and they were provided with the assumption that the goals were cure at all costs. Starting little by little in the 1960s and then gathering steam, by the dawn of the twenty-first century citizens made it apparent that this assumption was not fully valid. Perhaps at all times of illness, but especially near the expected end of life, people have a range of goals.

A fair proportion of people do want curative intervention if it is available; others want palliative care and an emphasis on quality of life; others want something in between or something unique. One review study identified six goals (8).

(1) To be cured

(2) To live longer

(3) To improve or maintain functionality/quality of life/independence

(4) To be comfortable

(5) To achieve life goals

(6) To provide support for the family/caregiver.

Clinicians should periodically ask their patients something like the following: 'Your illness has changed since we last talked so it is important to review your goals for our care so that we can be sure you are receiving from us the type of care that you want. In your circumstances people may have goals ranging from wanting all possible disease modifying treatments regardless of cost or invasiveness to wanting treatments that prioritize comfort and quality of life in what time remains. Here are some of the goals that people choose. How are you thinking about this now?'

Goals are known to predict relatively accurately the specific interventions that a person would want, so if the clinician and the patient's family know what the patient's goals are, they can be strongly guided by them in the treatment decisions they bring up for discussion.

Thresholds

Indeed, patients mostly have an identifiable threshold, prior to which they want disease-modifying intervention and after which they want palliative care. By setting out a series of scenarios and asking about goals for care (9) the clinician team and family can see where that threshold is in most cases.

Proxy designation

Terminal illness usually entails a period of time when the patient has become too ill to speak for him or herself and medical decisions must be made. One way to accomplish this with as much respect for patient autonomy as the situation allows is to designate ahead of time a proxy decision maker. This designation is honoured by state and federal law. It is important to include this proxy in as many communications as possible so that decision making with the proxy can be accomplished with the proxy speaking in lieu of the patient with as accurate as possible a representation of what the patient would have said. The clinician should establish by asking directly of the patient and the proxy whether the patient wants the proxy to be guided as much as possible by the patient's prior wishes or for the proxy to use his or her judgment more liberally.

Can communication improve palliative care from a public health perspective?

In view of the reality that the vast majority of health care expenditures occur near the end of life and that serious illnesses cause severe economic blows to households which can have a major impact on family member's lives, it is appropriate to ask whether expenditures are being optimally used. Some studies have demonstrated reduced use of resources by patients using palliative care (see Chapter 6 of this book). Absence of randomized controlled trials makes it difficult to establish whether palliative care as an intervention might rationalize or reduce costs of care near the end of life for those who still seek disease-modifying intervention. However, it seems that patients with goals that prioritize palliative care do consume fewer direct cost health care resources. If it is the case that communication about the topics that are covered in this chapter promotes existential maturity, completion of the tasks of the dying role, and comfort with palliative goals of care, then it may well be that communication can drive optimization of medical resource use among the dying. Public health efforts to aid optimal communication across society can include augmented dissemination and implementation projects to ensure skill and adequate comfort among clinicians in leading the communications and, perhaps using separate but coordinated programming, to ensure familiarity and openness to discussing mortality among patients, patients' families, and members of the public generally. Suitable costing and reimbursement policies that provide balanced encouragement for clinicians to take the time to enter such discussions are essential if the skills of communication are to be used appropriately.

In the meantime, for its independent merit, its ability to foster optimal team work around common goals, its ability to yield quality of life, and its possible ability to drive optimized use of resources (something we can call 'warranted care'), communication is a cornerstone of palliative care for individuals, families, communities, and populations.

Acknowledgement

I am indebted to Brian Joyce for his excellent literature search and assistance with manuscript preparation.

References

(1) *Growing Older in America: The Health and Retirement Study.* Income and wealth. Unexpected health events. Available at: http://hrsonline.isr.umich.edu/docs/sho_refs.php?hfyle5index&xtyp57. Accessed 20 Jan. 2011.

(2) Glare, P, Virik, K, Jones, M, et al. (2003) A systematic review of physicians' survival predictions in terminally ill cancer patients. *BMJ*, **327** (7408): 195–8. PMID: 12881260.

(3) Stiel, S, Bertram, L, Neuhaus, S, et al. (2009) Evaluation and comparison of two prognostic scores and the physicians' estimate of survival in terminally ill patients. *Support Care Cancer*, **18** (1): 43–9. PMID: 19381693.

(4) Buckman, R (1992) *How to Break Bad News: A Guide for Health Care Professionals*. Baltimore: Johns Hopkins University Press, 65–97.

(5) Emanuel, LL, Alpert, HR, and Emanuel, EE (2001) Concise screening questions for clinical assessments of terminal care: The needs near the end-of-life care screening Tool. *J Palliat Med*, **4** (4): 465–74. PMID: 11798478.

(6) Richards CT, Gisondi MA, Chang CH, et al. Palliative care symptom assessment for patients with cancer in the emergency department: validation of the Screen for Palliative and End-of-life care needs in the Emergency Department instrument. *J Palliat Med*. 2011; **14**(6): 757–764. Epub 2011 May 6. PMCID: PMC3107583.

(7) Chochinov, HM, Hack, T, Hassard, T, Kristjanson, LJ, McClement, S, and Harlos, M (2005) Dignity therapy: A novel psychotherapeutic intervention for patients near the end of life. *J Clin Oncol*, **23** (24): 5520–5. PMID: 16110012.

(8) Kaldjian, LC, Curtis, AE, Shinkunas, LA, and Canon, KT (2008) Goals of care toward the end of life: A structured literature review. *Am J Hosp Palliat Care*, **25** (6): 501–11. PMID: 19106284.

(9) Emanuel, L (1991) The health care directive: Learning how to draft advance care documents. *J Am Geriatr Soc*, **39** (12): 1221–8. PMID: 1960367.

(10) Azoulay, E, Chevret, S, Leleu, G, et al. (2000) Half the families of intensive care patients experience inadequate communication with physicians. *Crit Care Med*, **28** (8): 3044–9. PMID: 10966293.

(11) Covinsky, KE, Fuller, JD, Yaffe, K, et al. (2000) Communication and decision-making in seriously ill patients: Findings of the SUPPORT project. *J Am Geriatr Soc*, **48** (5 Suppl): S187–93. PMID: 10809474.

(12) Bradley, EH, Hallemeier, AG, Fried, TR, et al. (2001) Documentation of discussions about prognosis with terminally ill patients. *Am J Med*, **111** (3): 218–23. PMID: 11530033.

(13) Ditto, PH, Danks, JH, Smucker, WD, et al. (2001) Advance directives as acts of communication: A randomized controlled trial. *Arch Intern Med*, **161** (3): 421–30. PMID: 11176768.

(14) Wenger, NS, Kanouse, DE, Collins, RL, et al. (2001) End-of-life discussions and preferences among persons with HIV. *JAMA*, **285** (22): 2880–7. PMID: 11401609.

(15) Phipps, E, True, G, Harris, D, et al. (2003) Approaching the end of life: Attitudes, preferences, and behaviors of African-American and white patients and their family caregivers. *J Clin Oncol*, **21** (3): 549–54. PMID: 12560448.

(16) Knauft, E, Nielsen, EL, Engelberg, RA, Patrick, DL, and Curtis, JR (2005) Barriers and facilitators to end-of-life care communication for patients with COPD. *Chest*, **127** (6): 2188–96. PMID: 15947336.

(17) Zapka, JG, Carter, R, Carter, CL, Hennessy, W, Kurent, JE, and DesHarnais, S. (2006) Care and the end of life: Focus on communication and race. *J Aging Health*, **18** (6): 791–813. PMID: 17099134.

(18) Ozanne, EM, Partridge, A, Moy, B, Ellis, KJ, and Sepucha, KR. (2009) Doctor–patient communication about advance directives in metastatic breast cancer. *J Palliat Med*, **12** (6): 547–53. PMID: 19508141.

(19) Thornton, JD, Pham, K, Engelberg, RA, Jackson, JC, and Curtis, JR (2009) Families with limited English proficiency receive less information and support in interpreted intensive care unit family conferences. *Crit Care Med*, **37** (1): 89–95. PMID: 19050633.

(20) Gattellari, M, Voigt, KJ, Butow, PN, and Tattersall, MH (2002) When the treatment goal is not cure: Are cancer patients equipped to make informed decisions? *J Clin Oncol*, **20** (2): 503–13. PMID: 11786580.

(21) Lamont, EB, and Christakis, NA (2001) Prognostic disclosure to patients with cancer near the end of life. *Ann Intern Med*, **134** (12): 1096–105. PMID: 11412049.

(22) Ptacek, JT, and Ptacek, JJ. Patients' perceptions of receiving bad news about cancer. *J Clin Oncol*, **19** (21): 4160–4. PMID: 11689584.

(23) Emanuel, EJ, and Emanuel, LL (1998) Four models of the patient–physician relationship. *JAMA*, **267** (16): 2221–6. PMID: 1556799.

(24) Botelho, RJ (1992) A negotiation model for the doctor–patient relationship. *Fam Pract*, **9** (2): 210–18. PMID: 1505712.

(25) Hantho, A, Jensen, L, and Malterud, K (2002) Mutual understanding: A communication model for general practice. *Scand J Prim Health Care*, **20** (4): 244–51. PMID: 12564578.

(26) Rowan, KE, Sparks, L, Pecchioni, L, Villagran MM (2003) The CAUSE model: A research-supported aid for physicians communicating with patients about cancer risk. *Health commun*, **15** (2): 235–48. PMID: 12742774.

(27) Kiesler, DJ, and Auerbach, SM (2003) Integrating measurement of control and affiliation in studies of physician–patient interaction: the interpersonal circumplex. *Soc Sci Med*, **57** (9): 1707–22. PMID: 12948579.

(28) Slingsby, BT (2004) Decision-making models in Japanese psychiatry: Transitions from passive to active patterns. *Soc Sci Med*, **59** (1): 83–91. PMID: 15087145.

(29) Fredericks, M, Odiet, JA, Miller, SI, and Fredericks, J (2006) Toward a conceptual reexamination of the patient–physician relationship in the healthcare institution for the new millennium. *J Natl Med Assoc*, **98** (3): 378–85. PMID: 16573302.

(30) Finset, A, and Mjaaland, TA (2009) The medical consultation viewed as a value chain: A neurobehavioral approach to emotion regulation in doctor–patient interaction. *Patient Educ Couns*, **74** (3): 323–30. PMID: 19153023.

(31) Emanuel, EJ, and Emanuel, LL (1998) The promise of a good death. *Lancet*, **351** (Suppl 2): SII21–29. PMID: 9606363.

(32) Singer, PA, Martin, DK, and Kelner, M. Quality end-of-life care: Patients' perspectives. *JAMA*, **281** (2): 163–8. PMID: 9917120.

(33) Steinhauser, KE, Christakis, NA, Clipp, EC, McNeilly, M, McIntyre, L, and Tulsky, JA (2000) Factors considered important at the end of life by patients, family, physicians, and other care providers. *JAMA*, **284** (19): 2476–82. PMID: 11074777.

(34) Gardner, DS, and Kramer, BJ (2009) End-of-life concerns and care preferences: Congruence among terminally ill elders and their family caregivers. *Omega*, **60** (3): 273–97. PMID: 20361726.

Part IV

End-of-life care settings

Chapter 9

Palliative care in primary care

Lieve Van den Block

Introduction

Many people prefer to be cared for and die at home in their familiar surroundings (1–3). However, previous research has shown that many patients are not able to die at their place of choice and experience inappropriate hospital admissions at the very end of life, leading to a high number of hospital deaths in many countries (4;5). Developing palliative care services in primary care in such a way that people's aspirations about where they would like to die can be met is an important challenge in contemporary health care for many countries in the world. Primary care physicians, nurses, and other health care workers in general practice often have long-standing relationships with patients, initiated early in the disease course of the patient—and often before a patient has become seriously ill—which make them key figures in starting up an early palliative care approach (6).

In this chapter we will focus on palliative care delivered in the home. We explore the mutual values of palliative and primary care, outline different models of primary palliative care organization, focus in particular on the Gold Standard Framework in the UK, and outline the major challenges and barriers to effective palliative care in primary care today.

Mutual values in palliative care and primary care

Many of the principles formulated by the European Academy of Teachers in General Practice (7), a network within the European regional branch of the World Organization of National Colleges, Academies and Academic Associations of General Practitioners/ Family Physicians (WONCA Europe) coincide with the principles set forth in the WHO definition of palliative care (8). Communication, integrated care of the patient and family, focus on physical as well as psychological and social concerns and symptom control, providing holistic care, emphasis on quality of life and respecting patient values, person-centredness, anticipation of problems and advance care planning, and working closely with other professionals and teamwork are some of the core values shared across both disciplines (6;9). Thus, palliative care and primary care share many mutual values and the attitudes and competencies required to provide high-quality palliative care overlap to a large extent with those required to provide good primary care. As mentioned in the *Oxford Handbook of Palliative Care* (10): 'good palliative care is appreciated by GPs' patients and their families and is at the core of good primary care'.

Caring for dying patients in the community is also seen by many general practitioners as an important and intrinsic part of their work which is often rewarding and satisfying (11;12), even if many might feel discomfort about their competence to perform palliative care adequately (13). Furthermore, patients themselves and their families often view their GPs as important professional caregivers and hope to maintain their relationships at the end of life. Patients mostly appreciate that the GP is accessible, takes time to listen, and allows patient and carers to ventilate their feelings (13;14). In the UK, national directives have emphasized the vital role of community palliative care (10;12). This is described in detail in a later part of this chapter.

Different models of organization of palliative care in primary care

Primary care models differ widely across the world and the role of the GP varies considerably. It is not possible to summarize all these differences here, but most models have in common their focus on primary care being provided by a team of which the practitioner is often just one member, albeit with an important coordinating role. In some countries GPs are gatekeepers to secondary care while in others patients can access any part of health care without GP referral. The position of general practitioners—also called family physicians in North America—differs widely across the world, but in reasonably well-developed health care systems these GPs are physicians who see their patients in or near their home rather than in hospitals (13;15). Primary care nurses' titles also differ greatly across the world but in general these nurses are professional carers who assist in the care of the person at home and work closely with the GP (15).

GPs and district nurses know their patients well and are in a key position to provide the best support for them and their families, especially in the final stages of life. Research has shown that 90% of the final year of life for most patients is spent at home in many countries. Hence, GPs—within a primary health care team or as individuals—deliver the majority of palliative care to patients in the last year of life (10;13;16;17). GPs have always been and will remain the main providers of palliative care for most patients.

Palliative care provided by the usual professional carers of the patient and family with low to moderate complexity of palliative care need, is sometimes called general palliative care. *General palliative care* is a vital and integral part of routine clinical practice following the following principles (10):

◆ Focus on quality of life including good symptom control

◆ Whole person approach, taking into account someone's past and current experiences

◆ Care for the person with life-threatening illness as well as for the family or significant others

◆ Respect for patient autonomy and choice with attention to advance care planning and exploration of wishes and preferences

◆ Open and sensitive communication, involving patients, informal and professional carers.

However, since most GPs have only a few terminally ill patients they care for each year—albeit variable across countries and individual GPs—it cannot be expected that all GPs and nurses in regular home care are equipped to provide *specialist palliative care*. Support from specialist, organized palliative care teams with a high expertise level when it comes to palliative care provision can back up primary caregivers, provide advice and resources, and share knowledge when needed (10;13;17). The relationship between general and specialist palliative care is also outlined in Figure 9.1. Research has shown that formal arrangements engaging GPs to work with specialist teams can improve functional outcomes, patient satisfaction, effective use of resources and effective physician behaviour in other areas of medicine (13). The use of specialist palliative care collaborating with community health care professionals has also been shown to increase home deaths in a cluster randomized trial (18).

Within and outside Europe, there are many names and models of palliative home care provision (19;20). The way primary care professionals use specialist palliative care support also varies a great deal, from some referring patients systematically to specialist services to some completely ignoring them. An overall trend in most countries with good palliative care provision is to achieve adequate geographical coverage across the country, and to organize specialist palliative care services as advisory and complementary services aimed at supporting the GP and not acting as the primary responsible caregiver. Palliative day care centres are also part of the facilities of patients residing at home in some countries, but these have been mainly developed in the UK, providing daytime psycho-social support and nursing treatments. Studies have also shown differences between countries in evolution of palliative care (19;20). While in some countries palliative care development is only in its infancy, with several pioneering professionals or institutions promoting palliative care on a voluntary basis, there are other countries where governments have acknowledged its importance and finance its provision. However, few countries worldwide have been able to integrate palliative care within the health system, broadly disseminating palliative care

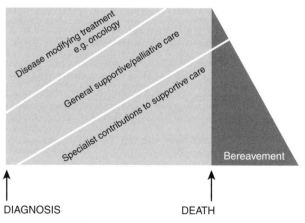

Fig. 9.1 General and specialist palliative care.
Republished from Watson, Lucas, Hoy, and Wells, *Oxford Handbook of Palliative Care*, Second Edition, 2009, with permission from Oxford University Press.

principles in all health care services, have added it to undergraduate and graduate university programmes and have developed research programmes on it (19;20).

One important model of community palliative care delivery that deserves further attention concerns the *Gold Standards Framework (GSF) in the UK* (12). Developed in 2000, the GSF is a systematic evidence-based approach to improve and optimize the organization and quality of supportive or palliative care for patients in their last 6 to 12 months of life. A key goal is to enable more to die where they choose, reducing hospitalizations and the numbers who inappropriately die on acute hospital wards. Programmes have been developed for primary care, care homes and acute hospitals. Table 9.1 outlines the GSF

Table 9.1 The Gold Standard Framework for primary care (10;12)

Central processes are to	1) **identify** the patients who may be in the last year of life and identify their stage (use of the question 'would you be surprised if the patient was to die within the year?', and needs-based coding)
	2) **assess** main needs, physical and psycho-social, and needs of carers
	3) **plan** ahead of problems using a proactive instead of reactive approach to care, including out-of-hours.
The 5 goals that enable patients to die well are to die	G1) symptom-free
	G2) in the preferred place of care
	G3) feeling safe and supported with fewer crises
	G4) with carers feeling supported, involved and empowered, satisfied with care
	G5) with staff feeling more confident, satisfied, with better communication and team working with specialists.
The 'gold standards' of community palliative care identified in this framework are	C1) communication: via a supportive care register patient care is monitored and planned; the home care team meets monthly and focuses on advance care planning, measurement and regular evaluation
	C2) coordination: each team nominates a GSF coordinator (e.g. district nurse) ensuring good organization and coordination of care
	C3) control of symptoms: holistic needs assessment tools are used and identified symptoms, problems, concerns are discussed and acted upon
	C4) continuity, including out-of-hours: transfer of information to out-of-hours services using a handover form and use of an out-of-hours protocol, in order to reduce crises and inappropriate hospitalizations. Information is also passed on to the other relevant services involved, keeping the number of different professionals minimal
	C5) continued learning: based on a 'learn as you go' idea, advocating reflection and continuous practice improvement
	C6) carer support: provision of practical and emotional support to informal carers, including bereavement counselling, and to professional carers
	C7) care in the dying phase by using the Liverpool Integrated Care Pathway for patients who are in the terminal phase or last days of life (minimum protocol).

primary care programme currently being used and tested extensively across the UK to improve the delivery of primary palliative care (10;12).

These seven Cs perfectly summarize the core tasks of primary palliative care. Even though developed within one country only, the GSF provides important opportunities for other countries to improve the organization of palliative care in the community. More information can be found at www.gsf.org.uk. Within the UK, large-scale implementation and evaluation projects are being performed and further results are expected in the near future.

Challenges and barriers to optimal primary palliative care

Care at home can become suboptimal for many different reasons. Several challenges and barriers to optimal palliative care in the home care are described.

Competency and knowledge of GPs

Most GPs are exposed to only a small number of palliative care patients each year. Combined with the rapid advances in the evidence-base for palliative care, it might be hard for GPs to keep their competence and knowledge concerning palliative care up to date. While GPs seem to have a fundamentally sound knowledge of basic symptom relief and have developed important basic communication skills, in most countries the training of GPs in palliative care is not part of the standard curriculum and dependent on local initiatives. Defining a minimum set of palliative care skills to be taught to all physicians at undergraduate and intern level and embedding them into the standard curriculum in medical schools is a major challenge for many countries (9;13;21;22).

Time constraints and work load

In some countries there seems to be a shortage of GPs in the community, or at least in certain areas, putting serious time constraints on GPs' consultation behaviour. Also, an increasing proportion of female GPs is increasingly opting for part-time work, and GPs are less willing to perform home visits and work after-hours. However, time is a fundamental component of palliative care (21;22). Important of course—without minimizing the important role of GPs devoting time to communicate with palliative care patients—is that GPs can also receive support from specialist community nurses who may have more time available, underlining the importance of multidisciplinary team work in palliative care.

The economic costs of providing palliative care might also be a barrier for some GPs. In countries such as Belgium GPs are paid per performance regardless of the time devoted to it, which does not support a time-consuming palliative care consultation model.

Out-of-hours services and cooperation between other health care and social care services

The fact that in many countries home care is not available out-of-hours can cause significant breakdown in home care and inappropriate admissions to hospitals. The availability and coordination of night sitters, Marie Curie nurses or other social services might therefore play a vital role in maintaining home care (10;23). Research in the UK has shown that more terminally ill patients are kept at home where 24-hour district nursing is available. Maintaining clear communication lines between GPs and hospitals has also been identified as important, but is, unfortunately, not always done well (13).

Early identification of palliative care needs and continuous care planning

As the WHO advocates, palliative care is no longer regarded as being applicable exclusively at the point when death is imminent but at a much earlier stage in the course of progressive disease, when disease modifying and life-prolonging treatments are still possible (8). Although the GP can be seen as a key figure in identifying palliative care needs or recognizing the palliative phase among patients, this seems difficult for many (17). Palliative care is often still seen as terminal care, which might prevent early and timely identification of palliative needs.

A main barrier to effective community palliative care is also the lack of an organized system or plan of care (10). It is important to prevent discontinuous care and reduce hospital deaths to plan ahead, to agree with all health care professionals involved on the plan of care, and to find effective ways of sharing and transferring information. Important here is to take into account patient preferences in determining the plan and goals of care. Advance care planning is also preferably started up early in the disease course in order to explore patient preferences in case they lose competence (24).

Collaboration and referral criteria for specialist palliative care

Whereas specialist teams have been set up in most countries to assist GPs, these professionals need to have confidence in each other and good working relationships to ensure that GPs will call upon them when needed (15;22). While there are many examples of this working well in Europe, there are also reports on GPs who are less enthusiastic about involving them (13). The relationship between local community nurses and GPs is also of great importance since all have different complementary clinical and diagnostic skills and different perspectives on a patient's needs (13;25). Delineation of the role of GPs, community nurses, and specialist palliative care teams is different in different countries but also an issue of discussion in many.

One particularly relevant aspect of referral concerns the referral criteria to specialist palliative care. GPs need to acknowledge the boundaries of their own competence, but also need to be able to refer to or consult specialist services on the basis of more or less objective criteria. However, in many countries specialist palliative care services are still very much orientated towards cancer patients (17;26) and referral criteria vary across countries or are not always made explicit. One important attempt concerns the recently implemented Gold Standards Framework in the UK (12) where referral criteria are clearly defined and which might be useful for all countries. Closely related to this issue however concerns the specific challenge of identifying the palliative care needs of non-cancer diseases.

The challenge of non-cancer patients

While people live longer in Western societies, they also experience longer periods of chronic illness. Infectious diseases are no longer the main cause of death but are replaced by deaths caused by chronic life-limiting diseases such as cancer, cardiovascular, respiratory, or neuro-degenerative diseases. Within the current population of people with serious, progressive, and eventually fatal chronic illnesses, three trajectories have been identified (27;28): patients with a short period of evident decline, often from cancer; patients with long-term limitations with intermittent serious episodes, mostly heart and lung failure; and patients with prolonged dwindling, such as frailty and dementia which is expected to increase considerably with population aging. Palliative care needs and challenges within these populations might be very different. Cancer patients, for instance, benefit from intense but relatively brief specialist palliative care, while patients who have organ system failure require long-term standby support to live with their uncertain prognosis. Those who succumb to frailty and dementia will need intense personal care through a long period of dependency (21;27–29). These patients will be cared for mainly in the community and therefore pose specific challenges to future community palliative care, in terms of length of care provision, referral criteria to specialist palliative care, hospital transitions, etc. While it is generally agreed that palliative care should be extended to patients with non-malignant diseases, issues remain concerning what is the most effective model of care and concerns about pressure on specialist services. GPs and community nurses can lead the way by identifying patients who might benefit from an early palliative or supportive care approach (6).

Ethical issues

A major challenge for physicians and other professional carers working in palliative care—but also for patients and informal carers—concerns the different ethical dilemmas they might be confronted with. While educational curricula often lack a thorough approach to the ethics of end-of-life care giving, decisions about forgoing life-prolonging treatments e.g. withdrawal of feeding tubes, intensifying symptom medication in such a way that life might be shortened, palliative or terminal sedation, but also request for euthanasia—i.e. the ending of life upon explicit patient request—are prevalent in primary care in many European countries (30;31) Euthanasia requests have also been found to be expressed most often to GPs (32). The legal status and frequency of use of advance directives and living wills and how to deal with them when patients are no longer able to speak for themselves also differ greatly between countries and will increasingly have an impact in primary palliative care.

Conclusion

Developing palliative care services in primary care in such a way that people can stay and die at home—as is preferred by many—is an important challenge in contemporary health care for many countries in the world. While many different models of primary care delivery and palliative community care exist all over the world, there are a number of mutual

Box 9.1 Key public health challenges for palliative care in primary care

◆ High number of patients not dying at the place of wish and experiencing inappropriate hospital admissions at the very end of life

◆ Increasing number of people with chronic and serious illnesses need to be taken care of in the community setting

◆ Lack of sufficient experience and equipment of GPs to provide specialist palliative care, and the need for support from specialist, organized palliative care teams as a back-up for primary caregivers.

◆ Competency and knowledge level of GPs regarding palliative care

◆ Referral criteria and collaboration between general and specialist palliative care

◆ Timely recognition of palliative care needs and timely initiation of a palliative care approach.

challenges concerning the training of GPs in palliative care, the lack of time and high workload of GPs in many health care systems, the organization and coordination of care including out-of-hours, the early identification of palliative care needs and the referral from general to specialist palliative care services when needed, in relation to cancer patients but also to those suffering from non-cancer illnesses, and there are also ethical dilemmas confronting primary care teams at the end of life. (See Box 9.1.)

References

(1) Higginson IJ, Sen-Gupta GJ. Place of care in advanced cancer: a qualitative systematic literature review of patient preferences. *J Palliat Med* 2000; **3** (3): 287–300.

(2) Meeussen K, Van den Block L., Bossuyt N, et al. GPs' awareness of patients' preference for place of death. *Br J Gen Pract* 2009; **59** (566): 665–70.

(3) Townsend J, Frank AO, Fermont D, et al. Terminal cancer care and patients' preference for place of death: A prospective study. *BMJ* 1990; **301** (6749): 415–17.

(4) Van den Block L., Deschepper R, Bilsen J, Van Casteren V, Deliens L. Transitions between care settings at the end of life in belgium. *JAMA* 2007; **298** (14): 1638–9.

(5) Cohen J, Bilsen J, Addington-Hall J, et al. Population-based study of dying in hospital in six European countries. *Palliat Med* 2008; **22** (6): 702–10.

(6) Murray SA, Boyd K, Sheikh A, Thomas K, Higginson IJ. Developing primary palliative care. *BMJ* 2004; **329** (7474): 1056–7.

(7) Allen J, Gay B, Crebolder H, Heyrman J, Svab I, Ram P. The European Definition of General Practice/Family Medicine. Evans P, editor. 2005. WONCA Europe.

(8) World Health Organization. *Palliative Care: The Solid Facts*. Copenhagen, Denmark: 2004.

(9) Block SD, Bernier GM, Crawley LM, et al. Incorporating palliative care into primary care education. National Consensus Conference on Medical Education for Care Near the End of Life. *J Gen Intern Med* 1998; **13** (11): 768–73.

(10) Watson M, Lucas C, Hoy A, Wells J. *Oxford Handbook of Palliative Care*, 2nd edn. New York: Oxford University Press, 2009.

(11) Field D. Special not different: General practitioners' accounts of their care of dying people. *Soc Sci Med* 1998; **46** (9): 1111–20.

(12) The National GSF Centre. Gold Standards Framework. NHS Walsall Community Health. 2009.

(13) Mitchell GK. How well do general practitioners deliver palliative care? A systematic review. *Palliat Med* 2002; **16** (6): 457–64.

(14) Grande GE, Farquhar MC, Barclay SI, Todd CJ. Valued aspects of primary palliative care: Content analysis of bereaved carers' descriptions. *Br J Gen Pract* 2004; **54** (507): 772–8.

(15) Doyle D, Jeffrey D. *Palliative Care in the Home*. Oxford: Oxford University Press, 2000.

(16) Addington-Hall J, Higginson I. *Palliative Care for Non-cancer Patients*. New York: Oxford University Press, 2001.

(17) Van den Block L, Deschepper R, Bossuyt N, et al. Care for patients in the last months of life: The Belgian Sentinel Network Monitoring End-of-Life Care study. *Arch Intern Med* 2008; **168** (16): 1747–54.

(18) Jordhoy MS, Fayers P, Saltnes T, hlner-Elmqvist M, Jannert M, Kaasa S. A palliative-care intervention and death at home: a cluster randomised trial. *Lancet* 2000; **356** (9233): 888–93.

(19) Rocafort J, Centeno C. *EAPC Review of Palliative Care in Europe*. Rocafort J, editor. Milano: EAPC Press, 2008.

(20) Wright M, Wood J, Lynch T, Clark D. Mapping levels of palliative care development: A global view. *J Pain Symptom Manage* 2008; **35** (5): 469–85.

(21) Yuen KJ, Behrndt MM, Jacklyn C, Mitchell GK. Palliative care at home: General practitioners working with palliative care teams. *Med J Aust* 2003; **179** (6 Suppl): S38–40.

(22) Mitchell GK, Reymond EJ, McGrath BP. Palliative care: Promoting general practice participation. *Med J Aust* 2004; **180** (5): 207–8.

(23) Murray SA, Boyd K, Sheikh A. Developing primary palliative care: Primary palliative care services must be better funded by both day and night. *BMJ* 2005; **330** (7492): 671.

(24) Royal College of Physicians, National Council for Palliative Care, British Society of Rehabilitation Medicine, et al. *Advance Care Planning*. Concise Guidance to Good Practice series, No. 12. 1-2-2009. London: RCP.

(25) Grande GE, Barclay SI, Todd CJ. Difficulty of symptom control and general practitioners' knowledge of patients' symptoms. *Palliat Med* 1997; **11** (5): 399–406.

(26) Eve A. National Survey of Patient Activity Data for Specialist Palliative Care Services: MDS Full Report for the year 2005–2006. The National Council for Palliative Care, ed. London, 2006.

(27) Lunney JR, Lynn J, Foley DJ, Lipson S, Guralnik JM. Patterns of functional decline at the end of life. *JAMA* 2003; **289** (18): 2387–92.

(28) Lynn J, Adamson D. *Living Well at the End of Life: Adapting Health Care to Serious Chronic Illness in Old Age*. Santa Monica, CA: Rand, 2003.

(29) Murray SA, Kendall M, Boyd K, Sheikh A. Illness trajectories and palliative care. *BMJ* 2005; **330** (7498): 1007–11.

(30) Miccinesi G, Rietjens JA, Deliens L, et al. Continuous deep sedation: Physicians' experiences in six European countries. *J Pain Symptom Manage* 2006; **31** (2): 122–9.

(31) van der Heide A, Deliens L, Faisst K, et al. End-of-life decision-making in six European countries: Descriptive study. *Lancet* 2003; **362** (9381): 345–50.

(32) Marquet RL, Bartelds A, Visser GJ, Spreeuwenberg P, Peters L. Twenty five years of requests for euthanasia and physician assisted suicide in Dutch general practice: Trend analysis. *BMJ* 2003; **327** (7408): 201–2.

Chapter 10

Palliative care in institutional long-term care settings

Jenny van der Steen, Margaret R. Helton,
Philip D. Sloane, and Miel W. Ribbe

In Western countries, institutional long-term care settings increasingly provide end-of-life care for their residents, mostly older people with chronic illness. Providing affordable and high-quality end-of-life care poses universal challenges and drives development of new care models, which we illustrate using examples from the US and the Netherlands.

Demographic developments

The world population aged 80 and over will more than double between 2010 and 2050 (1) (Table 10.1). In Western societies, in a few decades nearly a quarter of citizens will be 65 and older. These demographic developments will tremendously increase the number of people needing long-term care (2–6) (Table 10.2). In Western countries in particular, many people spend their last days, or years, in long-term care settings, including nursing homes and residential homes that provide nursing services. Currently, up to a quarter of deaths occur in long-term care settings including most of the deaths of people with dementia (Table 10.2). Long-term care settings, therefore, are a common site for the provision of end-of-life care and will become even more so in the future. As such, the way this care is delivered, organized, and financed is a major public health issue.

Long-term care challenges that may affect end-of-life care

Difficulties in providing long-term care are not limited to end-of-life care. Nursing home care has a poor public image (7) and several studies have shown that many, if not most, people prefer to die at home. Still, even care-dependent older people recognize that long-term care may be necessary for people with dementia (7). Policies restricting access have resulted in *fewer* people entering long-term care over recent decades (Table 10.3) (4,13,28–30) which may be consistent with people wanting to stay at home as long as possible. Consequently, care needs for patients in long-term care have become increasingly complex (4,16) making staff skills and qualifications even more important.

It is challenging to attract, train, and maintain an adequate and skilled work force to care for people with complex needs (16,27,28). Most care is provided by nursing assistants with modest training, relatively low pay and a physically demanding workload (31).

Table 10.1 Aging across the globe

Mid-year population in millions	World	US	Western Europe	Netherlands
Total population				
- in 2010	6853,0	310,2	409,4	16,8
- in 2050 (estimate)	9284,1	439,0	412,2	17,3
Population aged 65 and older (% of total population)				
- in 2010	532,8 (7.8%)	40,3 (13.0%)	73,6 (18.0%)	2,5 (15.2%)
- in 2050 (estimate)	1555,6 (16.8%)	89,1 (20.3%)	117,2 (28.4%)	4,6 (26.3%)
Population aged 80 and older (% of total population)				
- in 2010	106,6 (1.6%)	11,6 (3.7%)	20,8 (5.1%)	0,6 (3.9%)
- estimate in 2050	445,9 (4.8%)	33,1 (7.5%)	46,9 (11.4%)	1,9 (10.7%)

Source: US Census Bureau, 2010 (1)

Nurses' time per resident has already decreased (32), which is concerning since staff shortage and turnover are related to decreased quality of care (33,34). Moreover, care for dying patients, although often rewarding to staff, may be more labour intensive and emotionally burdensome than 'regular' care (35).

Nursing home residents generally have high care needs because admission to a long-term care facility is usually the result of cognitive and functional decline with progressive dependency on care that cannot be provided at home (36–38). In nursing homes, almost all residents are dependent in activities of daily living (98% US 2004) (13) and even in residential homes, most have severe disabilities (4). This dependency is strongly related to mortality (e.g. 39), and dementia is an independent predictor of mortality in nursing home residents (40).

In the last phase of life, nursing home residents with dementia, who account for about half of the nursing home population in the US and the Netherlands (4,41), will typically experience episodes of acute illness and medical complications that require decision-making that considers a range of options from palliation to aggressive and invasive measures (42–44). Such episodes of acute illness make it difficult to predict death accurately

Table 10.2 Long-term care challenges in the USA and the Netherlands

USA	Netherlands
Long-term care needs are projected to double between 2000 and 2050 (2)	Nursing care needs are expected to rise 49% between 2010 and 2020, with a 42% increase in admissions to nursing homes and a 53% increase in the need for home care (4)
28% of deaths of people 65 and over occur in nursing homes (data of 2001 (3))	One in five deaths occurs in a nursing home. For people over 80 years old, half die in a nursing or residential home (data of 2003 (5))
67% of people with dementia die in a nursing home (data of 2001 (3))	92%* of people with dementia die in a nursing home or residential home (6)

*Some over-reporting is likely because in the Netherlands, dementia is more likely to be under diagnosed in the community than in nursing homes (or residential homes).

Table 10.3 Long-term care models in the US and the Netherlands

	US	Netherlands
A. Current and dominant care models		
% of population 65 and older that resides in nursing homes (1990s) (8)	5.0	2.5
(2006) (9)	4.3	2.8
% of population 65 and older that resides in residential homes (1990s) (8)	1.5*	6.5
Funding sources (nursing homes)	Mixture of private (out-of-pocket, private insurance, and other private funds), and public funding (federal, state, and local) (10). Most of the coverage is Medicaid which is a mixture of state and federal funds. Medicare (exclusively federal funds) only pays for short-term stays and does not cover long-term care.	All citizens are covered by the Exceptional Medical Expenses Act (AWBZ), which pays for chronic and mental health care services such as home care and care in nursing homes (11).
% of total health care spending on long-term nursing care,		
- 1996 (9)	7.8	17.0
- 2006 (9)	6.2	13.3
Specialized wards	Approximately 1/3 of nursing homes and assisted living facilities have specialized dementia units, mostly for people in earlier stages of dementia. In addition, some state and private psychiatric facilities serve persons with dementia.	Nursing homes beds are designated for rehabilitation and 'somatic' patients with physical handicaps (45%), and 'psychogeriatric patients' (55%, almost all dementia). Day care is also provided (4). Some residential homes have special units for psychogeriatric patients (12).
Medical services	Nursing homes use different and multiple arrangements to provide medical services, including using private physicians from the community (85.9%), contracting with physician group practices (30.1%), and employing physicians on staff (19.6%). Medical care is provided by geriatricians, internists, and family physicians (13). In assisted living the predominant model has been taking patients to the physician's office. However, both models are changing rapidly, with specialized long-term care practices taking over an increasing proportion of long-term care.	Medical care is provided by elderly care physicians who are on-staff, employed by the nursing home on an average ration of 1 fte per 100 nursing home beds (12,14,15).

Table 10.3 (*continued*) Long-term care models in the US and the Netherlands

	US	Netherlands
Nursing staff	A total of 936,000 persons (registered nurses, licensed practical nurses, certified nursing assistants, nurse aides, and orderlies) provided nursing care in nursing homes. Certified nursing assistants (CNA, 600,800), who have only a few months of training, represent the majority of all nursing staff employed in nursing homes. (data of 2004 (13)).	Nurses: almost all with limited education (2 years with most time spent in practice; comparable to CNAs), and nurse aids; related to difficulty attracting registered nurses (16).
Palliative services	Hospice team supports local staff (17).	Palliative care units are not for those needing long-term care, but for brief admissions for people living in the community (18).

Quality improvement and new care models

	US	Netherlands
Quality indicators	Several quality reviews are in place, including the general Minimum Data Set, and after-death family evaluations of nursing home care and Hospice care, some of which are processed online (19).	The Minimum Data Set is not generally used. Consumer choice is promoted by online quality data on nursing homes. Quality indicators specific to palliative care are being developed.
New general care models	New models include the culture change movement and the home-like Green House model with emphasis on autonomy, individuality, fewer procedures, and quality of life (20). The Evercare Programme assigns residents to a managing nurse practitioner. The Programme for All-Inclusive Care for the Elderly (PACE), recently became generally available as a Medicare option for nursing home-eligible seniors. PACE provides comprehensive, capitated services for persons who would qualify for nursing home care but prefer to continue living at home. Care is centered around a comprehensive care team, a medical day facility, and often applies palliative care principles throughout the course of care, with PACE serving the role of Hospice in persons who are in the terminal stages of illness (21,22).	Elderly care physicians are reaching out to the community ('Gerimedica' project). Nursing homes increasingly employ nurse practitioners. Small-scale group homes for residents with dementia have been implemented (23).

(Continued)

Table 10.3 (*continued*) Long-term care models in the US and the Netherlands

	US	Netherlands

New palliative care models in long-term care	Examples include:
	
	- a method to communicate treatment preferences (Physician Orders for Life-Sustaining Treatment (POLST) which was implemented in Oregon. Results include better documentation of preferences but no change in symptom relief (24)
	
	- the Palliative Excellence in Alzheimer Care Efforts (PEACE) is a disease management model that incorporates advance planning, patient-centered care, family support, and a palliative care focus (25,26)
	
	- a report on palliative care practices in a group of progressive US nursing homes revealed the emergence of four models:
	
	  - Outside palliative care consultants
	
	  - Hospice staff providing non-hospice palliative care services
	
	  - Improved training of nursing home staff so they are comfortable with palliative care
	
	  - Increased use of the Medicare Hospice benefit (27).
		New postgraduate training programmes in palliative care and other such developments have probably resulted in an increasing awareness that palliative care applies to dementia.

*Residential care homes not group facilities such as board and care homes.

more than a week in advance (45,46). This unpredictable disease trajectory is common in chronic illnesses and has important implications for providing end-of-life care, because residents often have high care needs for long periods, yet it is unclear when to prepare for death.

Palliative care in long-term settings

Palliative care is appropriate for many long-term care residents who have chronic, incurable, and progressive diseases such as dementia and heart failure. This is reflected in a recent definition of geriatric palliative medicine as 'the medical care and management of older patients with health-related problems and progressive, advanced disease for which the prognosis is limited and the focus of care is quality of life' (47). It differs from the WHO definition (48) of palliative care in that it goes beyond 'life-threatening disease'.

Palliative care extends to care for families (WHO) as they deal with grief and caregiver burden. Since many patients in long-term settings have cognitive impairment and therefore lack decision-making capacity, physician–family interactions are important in end-of-life care. Proactive assessment and advance care planning are also relevant to palliative care in nursing home populations (49).

However, some long-term care settings may be insufficiently prepared to care for dying patients (e.g. 50). Staff may focus on cure or rehabilitation which can lead to burdensome treatments while potentially under-treating symptoms (51–53). Newer work has shown encouraging trends, such as an expansion of Hospice care in US nursing homes, including to dementia patients (17), an increasing awareness of appropriate symptom relief in the Netherlands (54), and no disparities between care for dementia patients and patients with other life-limiting diseases in the US (55,56).

Current models of care in the US and the Netherlands

Long-term care, including palliative care, varies across countries. Here we look at the US and the Netherlands, two systems that are well-studied and reflect a range of approaches to palliative care in long-term care settings.

Long-term care in the United States

Two types of institutional long-term care serve over a million persons in the US: nursing homes and residential care/assisted living (RC/AL) facilities. Nursing homes are federally regulated and have nurses available around the clock, with physicians typically visiting on a weekly basis, seeing individual residents at least once every 60 days, which is a federal requirement for nursing home certification (57). RC/AL facilities are largely regulated by the states, varying in both nursing and physician presence ranging from medical directors who visit frequently to physicians who provide all care in off-site offices (58).

In the US, long-term care policy has evolved from a variety of initiatives without an underlying general policy or philosophy (28). Most facilities are for-profit (Table 10.3). The US system financially rewards more aggressive care or over-treatment such as tube feeding and hospitalization (59,60). Palliative care is paid for by Medicare under the Hospice benefit and is generally available to patients with a life expectancy of six months or less, although this requirement has become more flexible and now allows Hospice enrolment of older people with dementia and other chronic diseases, as long as services are aimed at comfort rather than cure. Hospice is still relatively underused in residents with non-cancer diagnoses (17).

Long-term care in the Netherlands

The Netherlands has about 366 nursing homes, and more residential homes (4). The country is unique in that elderly care medicine (formerly nursing home medicine) is a recognized medical specialty for which physicians are trained and then employed exclusively in nursing home settings (12,14,15). The provision of palliative care in the nursing home is part of standard elderly care physician training. The branch organization that sets policy for long-term care in the Netherlands supports choice and autonomy in spite of a patient's limitations (61). About half of nursing home beds in the Netherlands are for patients with moderate to severe dementia (Table 10.3).

Nursing home costs are paid for by the government with additional medical expenses covered by mandated insurance (Table 10.3). Physicians cannot increase their income by hospitalizing patients or ordering more treatments. Relative spending on long-term care is more than that in the US (62), although in neither country has spending on nursing home care kept up with spending on other aspects of health care (Table 10.3).

System and societal influences on end-of-life care in nursing homes

Looking at the US and Dutch systems for nursing home care is a good way of illustrating how societal attitudes and the organization of health care can affect end-of-life care. While the Netherlands tends to do well on health care measures such as access, efficiency, equity, and long and healthy life expectancy, it does less well than the US in patient-centred care (63), defined as 'care delivered with the patient's needs and preferences in mind'. For example, US physicians more frequently encourage patients to ask questions and are more accessible by email. US families report a lower symptom burden in family members who are dying in nursing homes compared with Dutch families (64), reversing findings of a decade ago when symptom burden was higher in the US (65), suggesting improvement in the US, with little, or less improvement in the Netherlands. Societal issues may be at play as the Netherlands has a strong tradition of avoiding over-treatment such as feeding tubes and unnecessary hospitalization of residents with dementia and pneumonia (44,54), but may focus less on assessment and treatment of symptoms. An attitude of accepting a 'natural death' rather than actively fighting symptoms might play a role. This has not been studied well. Further, one study shows that Dutch family physicians were more willing to take risks regarding medical decision-making, including acceptance of uncertainty and not always doing everything possible, compared with Belgian and British physicians (66).

The organization of nursing home care has a significant influence on end-of-life care. Because physicians are on-site in Dutch nursing homes they serve as 'gatekeepers' and prefer not to hospitalize patients with dementia (6,67). On-staff physicians provide continuity of care, similar to care by the same family physician, which reduces the rate of hospitalization of older people with ambulatory care-sensitive conditions (68). In the US, with less physician presence overall (69) and in nursing homes, this continuity role may be served by an on-site nurse practitioner who can also lower hospitalization rates in dementia patients (43). US physicians have been described by families as 'missing in action' due to their insufficient efforts to address the needs of dying patients in nursing homes (70). Reimbursement practices also influence end-of-life care decisions in nursing homes, such as financial payment for feeding tubes in the US, so their use is not discouraged. The effect is evident in that feeding tubes are used more frequently in for-profit nursing homes than in non-profit nursing homes (59,60).

The US probably has higher rates of advance directives than the Netherlands, with ongoing efforts to make these rates even higher (27). Dutch nursing home physicians tend to focus on the patient's quality of life (71) and perceive less need for advance care planning, probably because physician presence makes written directives less important. Higher use of advance directives in the US are probably due to an emphasis on individuality as well as the desire to protect the patient from the default of curative care in the more technology-oriented US health care system.

Quality improvement and new models of care

Guidelines for improving the quality of end-of-life care affecting long-term facilities have been issued in several countries including Australia, Austria, Great Britain, and the US (PACE, Table 10.3). Best practices in palliative care in long-term care settings across the world are being identified and information about best practices is being made accessible (72). Monitoring of trends and bench-marking of treatments and outcomes cross-nationally may identify places where care needs improvement, based on proven quality indicators specific to end-of-life care in vulnerable older people or in nursing homes (73–75). In resource-poor areas, a minimum acceptable standard of end-of-life care may be implemented.

New care models that improve outcomes and provide affordable, high-quality care at the end of life for older people with long-term care needs have been developed in the US (Table 10.3). Some models are not limited to long-term care settings, but focus on 'aging in place' options, such as in retirement communities (76), and assisted living may increasingly provide end-of-life care of similar quality as in long-term care settings (77). Few new models have been extensively studied or shown to reduce costs, however (20,28). For example, the PEACE programme (Table 10.3) lacked a control group and generalizability is unclear. Some examples have been described in detail more recently (78).

Innovative models of care for those dying of cancer focus on preserving the dying patient's dignity (79). This goal is similarly appropriate for older patients in nursing homes and practices and policies that promote dignity and reduce symptom burden are likely to promote quality care in the dying process (80,81). Patient and family satisfaction with care is another important measure of quality care (65,82). These goals are consistent with the principles of palliative and patient-centred care, honouring individual wishes and promoting quality of life and dying.

New care models frequently seek to improve important aspects of care (Box 10.1). Continuity of care is particularly relevant because palliative care needs in long-term care

Box 10.1 Important aspects of high-quality end-of-life care in long-term care settings

- patient-centred care that considers personal values
- shared decision-making that includes the physician's experience with the family or patient's preferences
- continuity, communication, and coordination of care among a well-trained staff
- advance care planning and timely recognition of the dying phase is the appropriate care approach for many long-term care recipients
- financial responsibility and sustainability.

may extend over months or even years. Ideally, providers recognize evolving care needs and provide timely end-of-life care to patients and families. Informing families early is crucial to appropriate and affordable end-of-life care for residents with cognitive impairment. Patients with dementia whose families perceive dementia as a terminal disease receive less aggressive and higher comfort care at the end of life (42,51). With this in mind, models for advance care planning are being developed in a variety of countries (51) and will need testing to identify the most effective elements, taking into account the values and preferences of the now aging baby-boom generation.

While some of the principles of good end-of-life care may be universal, different cultures will emphasize different aspects of care. Financial realities will also play a role and the way health care is financed can greatly affect the way care is organized. Given the financial pressures on both health systems, it is important to recognize that directing more resources to end-of-life care in institutional settings may decrease overall spending.

Conclusion

The number of people dying in nursing homes will increase dramatically over the next decades. New models of care may combine promising elements from current models (Box 10.1) with innovations in health care policy and financing, health professional training, and societal education, and will be needed to ensure compassionate and dignified care of the dying.

Acknowledgement

The authors thank W. Elsenburg for his comments to an earlier version of the manuscript.

References

(1) U.S. Census Bureau. *International data base* (IDB) (2010). Available at: http://www.census.gov/ipc/www/idb/index.php (accessed 1 July 2010).

(2) US Department of Health and Human Services and US Department of Labor (2003). *The future supply of long-term care workers in relation to the aging baby boom generation.* Available at: http://aspe.hhs.gov/daltcp/reports/ltcwork.htm (accessed 3 August 2010).

(3) Mitchell SL, Teno JM, Miller SC, Mor V (2005). A national study of the location of death for older persons with dementia. *J Am Geriatr Soc*, **53**, 299–305.

(4) RIVM, National Institute for Public Health and the Environment (2010). *Volksgezondheid toekomst verkenning, Nationaal kompas volksgezondheid.* Version 3.22, 24 June 2010. Available at: http://www.nationaalkompas.nl/zorg/verpleging-en-verzorging/ (accessed 1 August 2010).

(5) CBS, Statistics Netherlands (2004). Een op de drie Nederlanders overlijdt in ziekenhuis. *Webmagazine*, 21 June 2004. Available at: http://www.cbs.nl/nl-NL/menu/themas/bevolking/publicaties/artikelen/archief/2004/2004-1483-wm.htm (accessed 11 December 2010).

(6) Houttekier D, Cohen J, Bilsen J, Addington-Hall J, Onwuteaka-Philipsen BD, Deliens L (2010). Place of death of older persons with dementia. A study in five European countries. *J Am Geriatr Soc*, **58** (4), 751–6.

(7) Wolff JL, Kasper JD, Shore AD (2008). Long-term care preferences among older adults: A moving target? *J Aging Soc Policy*, **20** (2), 182–200.

(8) Ribbe MW, Ljunggren G, Steel K, et al. (1997). Nursing homes in 10 nations: A comparison between countries and settings. *Age Ageing*, **26** (Suppl 2), 3–12.

(9) Anderson GF, Markovich P (2008). *Multinational comparisons of health systems data.* Commonwealth Fund publication no 1371. Available at: http://www.commonwealthfund.org/Content/Publications/Chartbooks/2010/Apr/Multinational-Comparisonsof-Health-Systems-Data-2008.aspx (accessed 3 August 2010).

(10) CMS, Centers for Medicare and Medicaid Services (2010). *National health expenditure data.* Calender years 2003–8. http://www.cms.gov/NationalHealthExpendData/downloads/tables.pdf (accessed 13 December 2010).

(11) Klazinga N (2010). The Dutch health care system. In: *International profiles of health care systems*, pp 36–8. New York: Commonwealth Fund.

(12) Conroy S, van der Cammen T, Schols J, van Balen R, Peteroff P, Luxton T (2009). Medical services for older people in nursing homes-comparing services in England and the Netherlands. *J Nutr Health Aging*, **13**, 559–63.

(13) Jones AL, Dwyer LL, Bercovitz AR, Strahan GW, National Center for Health Statistics (2009). The National Nursing Home Survey: 2004 overview. *Vital Health Stat*, **13** (167).

(14) Hoek JF, Ribbe MW, Hertogh CM, van der Vleuten CP (2001). The specialist training program for nursing home physicians: A new professional challenge. *J Am Med Dir Assoc*, **2** (6), 326–30.

(15) Koopmans RT, Lavrijsen JC, Hoek JF, Went PB, Schols JM (2010). Dutch elderly care physician: A new generation of nursing home physician specialists. *J Am Geriatr Soc*, **58** (9): 1807–9.

(16) RIVM, National Institute for Public Health and the Environment (2010). *Zorgbalans 2010: De prestaties van de Nederlandse zorg.* RIVM, Bilthoven, the Netherlands.

(17) Miller SC, Lima J, Gozalo PL, Mor V (2010). The growth of hospice care in U.S. nursing homes. *J Am Geriatr Soc*, **58** (8), 1481–8.

(18) Echteld MA, Deliens L, van der Wal G, Ooms ME, Ribbe MW (2004). Palliative care units in The Netherlands: Changes in patients' functional status and symptoms. *J Pain Symptom Manage*, **28** (3), 233–43.

(19) Nursing Home Compare. The Official US government site for Medicare. Available at: www.medicare.gov/nhcompare/ (accessed 11 December 2010).

(20) Koren MJ (2010). Person-centered care for nursing home residents: The culture-change movement. *Health Aff (Millwood)*, **29** (2), 312–17.

(21) Hirth V, Baskins J, Dever-Bumba M (2009). Program of all-inclusive care (PACE): Past, present, and future. *J Am Med Dir Assoc*, **10** (3), 155–60.

(22) Wieland D, Boland R, Baskins J, Kinosian B (2010). Five-year survival in a Program of All-inclusive Care for Elderly compared with alternative institutional and home- and community-based care. *J Gerontol A Biol Sci Med Sci*, **65** (7), 721–6.

(23) te Boekhorst S, Depla MF, de Lange J, Pot AM, Eefsting JA (2009). The effects of group living homes on older people with dementia: A comparison with traditional nursing home care. *Int J Geriatr Psychiatry*, **24** (9), 970–8.

(24) Hickman SE, Nelson CA, Perrin NA, Moss AH, Hammes BJ, Tolle SW (2010). A comparison of methods to communicate treatment preferences in nursing facilities: traditional practices versus the physician orders for life-sustaining treatment program. *J Am Geriatr Soc*, **58** (7), 1241–8.

(25) Shega JW, Levin A, Hougham GW, et al. (2003). Palliative Excellence in Alzheimer Care Efforts (PEACE): A program description. *J Palliat Med*, **6** (2), 315–20.

(26) Shega JW, Sachs GA (2010). Offering supportive care in dementia: Reflections on the PEACE programme. In Hughes J, Lloyd-Williams M, Sachs GA (eds), *Supportive care for the person with dementia*, pp 33–43. Oxford: Oxford University Press.

(27) Meier DE, Sieger CE (2007). *Improving palliative care in nursing homes.* Center to Advance Palliative Care, New York. Available at: http://www.capc.org/support-from-capc/capc_publications/nursing_home_report.pdf (accessed 11 December 2010).

(28) Lehning AJ, Austin MJ (2010). Long-term care in the United States: policy themes and promising practices. *J Gerontol Soc Work*, **53** (1), 43–63.

(29) CBS, Statistics Netherlands (2004). Aantal bewoners van instellingen en tehuizen daalt niet verder. *Webmagazine*, 19 April 2004. Available at: http://www.cbs.nl/nl-NL/menu/themas/dossiers/vrouwen-en-mannen/publicaties/artikelen/archief/2004/2004-1442-wm.htm (accessed 1 August 2010).

(30) Feder J, Komisar HL, Niefeld M (2000). Long-term care in the United States: An overview. *Health Aff (Millwood)*, **19** (3), 40–56.

(31) Sloane PD, Williams CS, Zimmerman S (2010). Immigrant status and intention to leave of nursing assistants in U.S. nursing homes. *J Am Geriatr Soc*, **58** (4), 731–7.

(32) Teno J, Gozalo P, Mitchell S, Bynum J, Dosa D, Mor V (2010). Does increasing advance care planning reduce terminal hospitalizations among nursing home residents? *Palliat Med*, **24** (Suppl), S5.

(33) Bostick JE, Rantz MJ, Flesner MK, Riggs CJ (2006). Systematic review of studies of staffing and quality in nursing homes. *J Am Med Dir Assoc*, **7** (6), 366–76.

(34) Castle NG, Engberg J, Men A (2007). Nursing home staff turnover: Impact on nursing home compare quality measures. *Gerontologist*, **47** (5), 650–61.

(35) Burack OR, Chichin ER (2001). A support group for nursing assistants: Caring for nursing home residents at the end of life. *Geriatr Nurs*, **22** (6), 299–307.

(36) Wong A, Elderkamp-de Groot R, Polder J, van Exel J (2010). Predictors of long-term care utilization by Dutch hospital patients aged 65+. *BMC Health Serv Res*, May 6, **10**, 110.

(37) Gaugler JE, Duval S, Anderson KA, Kane RL (2007). Predicting nursing home admission in the U.S: A meta-analysis. *BMC Geriatrics*, June 19, **7**, 13.

(38) de Meijer CA, Koopmanschap MA, Koolman XH, van Doorslaer EK (2009). The role of disability in explaining long-term care utilization. *Med Care*, **47** (11), 1156–63.

(39) Flacker JM, Kiely DK (2003). Mortality-related factors and 1-year survival in nursing home residents. *J Am Geriatr Soc*, **51** (2), 213–21.

(40) Naughton BJ, Mylotte JM, Tayara A (2000). Outcome of nursing home-acquired pneumonia: Derivation and application of a practical model to predict 30 day mortality. *J Am Geriatr Soc*, **48** (10), 1292–9.

(41) Magaziner J, German P, Zimmerman SI, et al. (2000). The prevalence of dementia in a statewide sample of new nursing home admissions aged 65 and older: Diagnosis by expert panel. *Gerontologist*, **40** (6), 663–72.

(42) Mitchell SL, Teno JM, Kiely DK, et al. (2009). The clinical course of advanced dementia. *New Engl J Med*, **361** (16), 1529–38.

(43) Mitchell SL, Teno JM, Intrator O, Feng Z, Mor V (2007). Decisions to forgo hospitalization in advanced dementia: A nationwide study. *J Am Geriatr Soc*, **55** (3), 432–8.

(44) van der Steen JT, Kruse RL, Ooms ME, et al. (2004). Treatment of nursing home residents with dementia and lower respiratory tract infection in the United States and The Netherlands: An ocean apart. *J Am Geriatr Soc*, **52** (5), 691–9.

(45) van der Steen JT, Mitchell SL, Frijters DH, Kruse RL, Ribbe MW (2007). Prediction of 6-month mortality in nursing home residents with advanced dementia: Validity of a risk score. *J Am Med Dir Assoc*, **8** (7), 464–8.

(46) Brandt HE, Deliens L, Ooms ME, van der Steen JT, van der Wal G, Ribbe MW (2005). Symptoms, signs, problems, and diseases of terminally ill nursing home patients: A nationwide observational study in the Netherlands. *Arch Intern Med*, **165** (3), 314–20.

(47) Pautex S, Curiale V, Pfisterer M, Rexach L, Ribbe M, Van Den Noortgate N (2010). A common definition of geriatric palliative medicine. *J Am Geriatr Soc*, **58** (4), 790–1.

(48) WHO, World Health Organization (2002). *National cancer control programmes: Policies and managerial guidelines*. Geneva: WHO.

(49) van der Steen JT, Deliens L (2009). End-of-life Care for Patients with Alzheimer's Disease, In: Bährer-Kohler S (ed.), *Self management of chronic disease: Alzheimer' disease*, pp 113–23. Heidelberg: Springer Medizin Verlag.

(50) Forbes S (2001). This is Heaven's waiting room: End of life in one nursing home. *J Gerontol Nurs*, **27** (11), 37–45.

(51) van der Steen JT (2010). Dying with dementia: What we know after more than a decade of research. *J Alzheimers Dis*, **22** (1), 37–55.

(52) Oliver DP, Porock D, Zweig S (2005). End-of-life care in U.S. nursing homes: A review of the evidence. *J Am Med Dir Assoc*, **6** (3 Suppl), S21–30.

(53) Ersek M, Wilson SA (2003). The challenges and opportunities in providing end-of-life care in nursing homes. *J Palliat Med*, **6** (1), 45–57.

(54) van der Steen JT, Meuleman-Peperkamp I, Ribbe MW (2009). Trends in treatment of pneumonia among Dutch nursing home patients with dementia. *J Palliat Med*, **12** (9), 789–95.

(55) Mitchell SL, Kiely DK, Miller SC, Connor SR, Spence C, Teno JM (2007). Hospice care for patients with dementia. *J Pain Symptom Manage*, **34** (1), 7–16.

(56) Pautex S, Herrmann FR, Le LP, et al. (2007). Symptom relief in the last week of life: is dementia always a limiting factor? *J Am Geriatr Soc*, **55** (8), 1316–17.

(57) CMS, Centers for Medicare and Medicaid Services (2009). *State operations manual. Interpretive guidelines for long-term care facilities—Appendix PP*. Available at: http://www.cms.gov/manuals/ Downloads/som107ap_pp_guidelines_ltcf.pdf (accessed 31 July 2010).

(58) Sloane PD, Zimmerman S (2010). Assisted living programmes providing supportive care for dementia. In: Hughes JC, Lloyd-Williams M, Sachs GA (eds), *Supportive care for the person with dementia*, pp. 189–97. Oxford: Oxford University Press.

(59) Mitchell SL, Teno JM, Roy J, Kabumoto G, Mor V (2003). Clinical and organizational factors associated with feeding tube use among nursing home residents with advanced cognitive impairment. *JAMA*, **290** (1), 73–80.

(60) Mitchell SL, Buchanan JL, Littlehale S, Hamel MB (2004). Tube-feeding versus hand-feeding nursing home residents with advanced dementia: A cost comparison. *J Am Med Dir Assoc*, **5** (2 Suppl), S22–9.

(61) ActiZ, branch organization for long-term care (2010). *Naar autonomie, verbondenheid en een gezond leven-een nieuwe ambitie voor de langdurige zorg*. Available at: http://www.actiz.nl/website/ actiz/publicaties (accessed 3 August 2010).

(62) Anderson GF, Squires DA (2010). Measuring the U.S. health care system: A cross-national comparison. *Issues in International Health Policy*, June. New York: The Commonwealth Fund.

(63) Davis K, Schoen C, Stremikis K (2010). *Mirror, mirror on the wall: How the performance of the U.S. health care system compares internationally*. New York: The Commonwealth Fund.

(64) Cohen LW, van der Steen JT, Reed D, Hodgkinson JC, van Soest-Poortvliet MC, Sloane PD, Zimmerman S. Family perceptions of end-of-life care for long-term care residents with dementia: Differences between the United States and Netherlands. *J Am Geriatr Soc* 2011, accepted for publication.

(65) van der Steen JT, Gijsberts M-J, Muller MT, Deliens L, Volicer L (2009). Evaluations of end of life with dementia by families in Dutch and U.S. nursing homes. *Int Psychogeriatr*, **21** (2), 321–9.

(66) Grol R, Whitfield M, De Maeseneer J, Mokkink H (1990). Attitudes to risk taking in medical decision making among British, Dutch and Belgian general practitioners. *J Gen Pract*, **40** (333), 134–6.

(67) Helton MR, van der Steen JT, Daaleman TP, Gamble GR, Ribbe MW (2006). A cross-cultural study of physician treatment decisions for demented nursing home patients who develop pneumonia. *Ann Fam Med*, **4** (3), 221–7.

(68) Menec VH, Sirski M, Attawar D, Katz A (2006). Does continuity of care with a family physician reduce hospitalizations among older adults? *J Health Serv Res Policy*, **11** (4), 196–201.

(69) OECD, Organization for Economic Co-operation and Development (2009). *Health Data 2009*. Available at: http://stats.oecd.org/Index.aspx?DataSetCode=HEALTH (accessed 3 August 2010).

(70) Shield RR, Wetle T, Teno J, Miller SC, Welch L (2005). Physicians 'missing in action': Family perspectives on physician and staffing problems in end-of-life care in the nursing home. *J Am Geriatr Soc*, **53** (1), 1651–7.

(71) The AM, Pasman R, Onwuteaka-Philipsen B, Ribbe M, van der Wal, G (2002). Withholding the artificial administration of fluids and food from elderly patients with dementia: Ethnographic study. *BMJ*, **325** (7376), 1326.

(72) Froggatt K, Heimerl K. *Palliative care and long term care settings for older people: Worldwide resources*. Available at: http://www.eolc-observatory.net/information/ltc/index.php?cat=1 (accessed 3 August 2010).

(73) Casarett DJ, Teno J, Higginson I (2006). How should nations measure the quality of end-of-life care for older adults? Recommendations for an international minimum data set. *J Am Geriatr Soc*, **54** (11), 1765–71.

(74) Lorenz KA, Rosenfeld K, Wenger N (2007). Quality indicators for palliative and end-of-life care in vulnerable elders. *J Am Geriatr Soc*, **55** (Suppl 2), S318–26.

(75) Steel K, Ljunggren G, Topinková E, et al. (2003). The RAI-PC: An assessment instrument for palliative care in all settings. *Am J Hosp Palliat Care*, **20** (3), 211–9.

(76) Wick JY, Zanni GR (2009). Aging in place: Multiple options, multiple choices. *Consult Pharm*, **24** (11), 804–6, 808, 811–12.

(77) Sloane PD, Zimmerman S, Hanson L, Mitchell CM, Riedel-Leo C, Custis-Buie V (2003). End-of-life care in assisted living and related residential care settings: comparison with nursing homes. *J Am Geriatr Soc*, **51** (11), 1587–94.

(78) Carlson MD, Lim B, Meier DE (2011). Strategies and innovative models for delivering palliative care in nursing homes. *J Am Med Dir Assoc*, **12** (2), 91–8.

(79) Chochinov HM, Hack T, McClement S, Kristjanson L, Harlos M (2002). Dignity in the terminally ill: A developing empirical model. *Soc Sci Med*, **54** (3), 433–43.

(80) Hall S, Longhurst S, Higginson I (2009). Living and dying with dignity: A qualitative study of the views of older people in nursing homes. *Age Aging*, **38** (4), 411–6.

(81) van der Steen JT, van Soest–Poortvliet MC, Achterberg WP, Ribbe MW, De Vet HCW (2011). Family perceptions of wishes of dementia patients regarding end-of-life care. *Int J Geriatr Psychiatry*, **26** (2), 217–20.

(82) Stewart AL, Teno J, Patrick DL, Lynn J (1999). The concept of quality of life of dying persons in the context of health care. *J Pain Symptom Manage*, **17** (2), 93–108.

Chapter 11

Palliative care in hospitals

Amy S. Kelley, Daniel J. Fischberg, and
R. Sean Morrison

The United Kingdom is credited with having the first palliative care programmes. Over the past four decades, the principles of palliative care have been widely adopted and now more than 90 countries around the world have palliative care services of some type (1). The palliative care needs of a population may vary widely due to different patterns of disease prevalence, local culture and religion, and the availability of resources (2). Hospital-based palliative care programmes, which remain rare in the developing world, are becoming more common across the United States, Australia, the United Kingdom, and other Western developed nations; their growth is due in large part to advances in medical therapies and the increasingly complex care needs of patients with serious and life-limiting illness. This chapter describes the organization of palliative care services in hospitals, reviews the impact of hospital-based palliative care on patient outcomes and health care costs, examines international variation in hospital-based palliative care programmes, and surveys the challenges hospital palliative care programmes may face in the future. Due to limitations in data, most of the issues examined relate to US hospitals.

Palliative care consultation teams

Beginning in the 1970s, some professionals caring for seriously ill and dying patients in hospitals began to pioneer a new type of care that was modelled on the basic precepts of the hospice movement, i.e. provision of comprehensive, compassionate, and competent care focused on the relief of suffering and promotion of quality of life for patients facing a life-threatening illness. As in a hospice, this new type of care often was delivered by interdisciplinary teams of nurses, physicians, social workers, and other allied professionals all working towards the implementation of a treatment plan concordant with the values and preferences of the patient and family. Although these teams have different names at different institutions, including terminal care support team, symptom control team, supportive care team, and comfort care team, palliative care team seems to have become the favoured term to describe these hospital-based teams (3). Hospitals with early hospital-based palliative care services included St Luke's Hospital in New York, McGill's Royal Victoria Hospital in Montreal, St Thomas's Hospital in London, and the National Cancer Institute in Milan (4,5).

While the structure, composition and focus of the palliative care team may vary across institutions due to the institution's specific needs and local culture, successful hospital-based palliative care consultation teams share many fundamental goals:

♦ to improve patient outcomes through expert pain and symptom control

♦ to facilitate communication and decision making for patients, family members, and health care providers

♦ to increase coordination among health care providers

♦ to ease patient transitions between care settings

♦ to improve staff satisfaction and retention by reducing the burden of time-intensive and complex cases

♦ to promote beneficial care, resulting in more appropriate use of hospital resources

♦ to satisfy quality, training, and accreditation requirements, including those of the US Joint Commission on Accreditation of Healthcare Organizations

Palliative care hospital units

At some institutions, the palliative care team may assume primary responsibility for seriously ill or dying patients and provide care in specialist palliative care units. Such units are typically placed in cancer centres or general hospitals. In the United States, two distinct forms of hospital unit exist – palliative care units and hospice units (6). In the United States, hospice is regulated as a Medicare benefit and most private health insurance providers offer a hospice benefit modelled after Medicare. The Medicare Hospice Benefit regulations stipulate that only patients with an expected prognosis of six months or less are eligible. Patients who receive the hospice benefit must agree to forgo curative therapies. In return, they receive comprehensive nursing, physician, and allied services, durable medical equipment, and medications related to the relief of symptoms due to their terminal illness. Inpatient hospice units provide short-term respite for patients and families. Additionally, patients with difficult to control symptom and actively dying patients whose needs exceed caregiver capacity can be admitted to inpatient hospice units. Unlike hospice, palliative care in the US has no such requirements to forgo curative therapies and is paid for in the same way as standard medical services. Palliative care may be offered at any time during the course of a chronic, serious, or potentially life-limiting illness, concurrently with curative and disease-modifying treatments. It is appropriate for patients with serious illness and complex medical and symptom problems whatever the diagnosis or prognosis. Patients with serious or life-threatening illnesses are typically admitted to hospital palliative care units for aggressive symptom control or if their needs cannot be met on regular medical wards.

Growth of hospital palliative care services

Data on the growth of hospital palliative care teams are rather limited outside the United States (7,8). A 2010 survey of hospitals in the US demonstrated that 60% of hospitals with 50 or more total facility beds reported having hospital palliative care services (9). This represents a steady rate of growth over the past decade (Figure 11.1). These data are

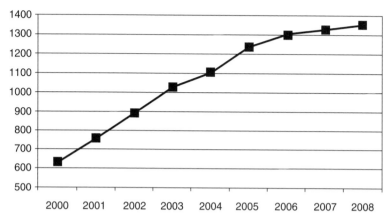

Fig. 11.1 Number of US hospitals with palliative care programmes, 2000–8 (9). Goldsmith B, Dietrich J, Du Q, Morrison RS. *Variability in access to hospital palliative care in the United States.* J Palliat Med. 2008;11(8):1094–1102.

encouraging evidence of the increasing availability of palliative care service for patients with serious illness; however some states (e.g. Mississippi, Alabama, and Oklahoma, all <20%), publicly financed hospitals (41%), and hospitals serving as the sole community hospital (30%) lag far behind. Outside the US, penetration of hospital palliative care is highly variable with relatively high penetration in Canada, Australia, New Zealand, Israel, and parts of Europe (e.g. the U.K., Belgium, Norway, Germany), more modest penetration in countries such as Taiwan, Japan, Europe (e.g. the Netherlands, Poland, Portugal), and limited penetration in Africa, south-east Asia, and eastern Europe (7).

Impact of palliative care in hospitals

Quality measurement and outcomes assessment are relatively new and rapidly developing areas of palliative care research. To date, efforts have focused on patient and family-centered outcomes and costs and healthcare utilization measures. Many hospital-based palliative care teams have collected data, as outlined in Table 11.1, for the purpose of internal evaluation and quality improvement as well as external comparison (10). These metrics can also help to demonstrate care structures, processes, and outcomes associated with improved quality (such as routine assessment of pain in the hospital), while a palliative care programme may help hospitals measure and meet Joint Commission for Accreditation of Healthcare Organizations (JCAHO) requirements in the domains of pain management, communication, family and patient education, and continuity of care, among others. The following paragraphs will discuss the effect hospital-based palliative care programmes have on patients and families and on healthcare costs and utilization.

Patient and family outcomes

Many studies have reported a range of benefits after referral to a hospital-based palliative care service or admission to a specialist palliative care unit, including reduced pain (11–13) and other symptom distress (13–16), improved health-related quality of life (17), and high

Table 11.1 Self-assessment of palliative care consultation service and inpatient unit metrics (10)

Domain	Measure	Action plan and potential barriers
Consultation service metrics		
1. Consultation Volume		
Palliative care consultations	N (%)	
Other consultations	N (%)	
2. Consultation Rate	Consults/100 admissions	
3. Patient Demographics		
Female	N (%)	
Male	N (%)	
Asian/Pacific Islander	N (%)	
African American/Black	N (%)	
Caucasian	N (%)	
Hispanic/Latino	N (%)	
Native American/Alaska Native	N (%)	
Other	N (%)	
4. Disease Distribution		
Cancer	N (%)	
Non-cancer	N (%)	
5. Location of Consult Origin		
Ward	N (%)	
Intensive Care (ICU)	N (%)	
Emergency Department (ED)	N (%)	
6. Age Distribution		
Adult programmes	N (%)	
Age 18–65	N (%)	
Age >65	N (%)	
Pediatric programmes	N (%)	
Age 0–1		
Age 2–18		
7. Consults by Referring Service and/or MD	N (%)	
8. Discharge Distribution		
Live discharges	N (%)	
Inpatient deaths	N (%)	
9. Hospice Discharges	N (%)	
10. Length of Stay (LOS)	Admission-consult, consult-d/c, los (median and mean)	
11. Length-of-Stay Outlier		
Admission-consultation >30 days	N (%)	
Consultation- death/dc >30 days	N (%)	
Inpatient unit metrics		
1. Inpatient Unit (PCU) Admissions		
Palliative care admissions	N (%)	
Other admissions	N (%)	

Table 11.1 (*continued*) Self-assessment of palliative care consultation service and inpatient unit metrics (10)

Domain	Measure	Action plan and potential barriers
2. Origin of Admission		
Outside, direct to PCU (non-hospice patient)	N (%)	
Outside, direct to PCU (hospice patient)	N (%)	
Emergency department	N (%)	
Intensive care unit	N (%)	
Ward	N (%)	
3. Type of Inpatient Unit		
a. Fixed-bed unit		
Average daily census	N	
Average % occupancy	N	
OR		
b. Swing-bed unit		
Average daily census	N	
4. Patient Demographics		
Female	N (%)	
Male	N (%)	
Asian/Pacific Islander	N (%)	
African American/Black	N (%)	
Caucasian	N (%)	
Hispanic/Latino	N (%)	
Native American/Alaska Native	N (%)	
Other	N (%)	
5. Disease Distribution		
Cancer	N (%)	
Non-cancer	N (%)	
6. Age Distribution		
Adult programmes	N (%)	
Age 18–65	N (%)	
Age >65	N (%)	
Pediatric programmes	N (%)	
Age 0–1		
Age 2–18		
7. Referring Service and/or Physician	N (%)	

(Continued)

Table 11.1 (*continued*) Self-assessment of palliative care consultation service and inpatient unit metrics (10)

Domain	Measure	Action plan and potential barriers
8. Discharge Distribution		
Live discharges	N (%)	
Live discharge with hospice services	N (%)	
Inpatient deaths	N (%)	
Percentage of all hospital deaths on PCU	%	
9. Patient Billing Status, at time of:		
Admission: acute care/hospice pass-through	%/%	
Discharge: acute care/hospice pass-through	%/%	
10. Length of Stay (LOS)	Hospital admission-PCU admission, PCU admission- d/c, LOS (median and mean)	
11. Length-of-Stay Outliers (PCU LOS >14 days)	N (%)	

patient and family satisfaction with care and with physician communication (11,15,17–22). These findings reflect not only the clinical goals as listed above, but also the most common reasons for a hospital palliative care consultation: pain and other symptom management, assistance establishing goals of care, discharge or transition planning, and support in the setting of a new terminal diagnosis (23). Similarly, in a prospective evaluation of 50 cases referred to the palliative care service at a tertiary teaching hospital in Sydney, Australia, pain management was the most common reason for consultation. The palliative care team provided a median number of three recommendations per patient, including advice regarding discharge planning in 62% of the cases. Recommendations for discharge planning and transitional care area were rated as most helpful by the referring team (24).

The impact of hospital-based palliative care services as measured by patient and family outcomes is perhaps the most salient evidence of the advantages and disadvantages of receiving palliative care in the hospital setting, as opposed to home or a community-based long-term care setting. Most patients prefer to die at home, in a familiar and comfortable setting, with unhindered access to family and friends. Yet patients with serious illnesses and those near the end of life may experience symptom severity and complexity, overwhelming to an informal caregiver. While lacking the familiarity of home, the hospital may provide respite and support to over-burdened caregivers and highly-skilled symptom management and relief to suffering patients. Care of such complexity may be prohibitively difficult to organize in the home setting.

Healthcare costs and utilization

Case control and observational studies of palliative care and ethics consultation services have demonstrated reductions in costs per day and in hospital and ICU lengths of stay, presumably because of enhanced support for discussions about the goals of care and the ensuing facilitation of patient and family decisions about the types and settings of future care, resulting in less over-treatment and fewer expensive treatments at the end of life (20,25–31). This evidence has supported hospitals' efforts to invest in palliative care services.

Specifically, researchers at Massey Cancer Center in Richmond, Virginia, studied costs and charges for patients transferred to the Palliative Care Unit (29). The authors found that daily patient costs and charges decreased by 66% after transfer to the Palliative Care Unit. Using a case-control design, the same authors found an almost 60% reduction in average daily costs and charges for patients who were transferred to the Palliative Care Unit compared with those cared for elsewhere in the hospital.

Marked reductions in hospital and ICU length of stay were observed after palliative care consultation at Mount Sinai Hospital in New York, NY. For patients with a hospital length of stay greater than 14 days, those with a palliative care consultation had a length of stay reduction of 4.8 days. Patients with an ICU length of stay of greater than 14 days had a mean reduction of ICU length of stay of 10 days compared with diagnosis-related group (DRG)-matched control patients (for patients who die in the hospital after a palliative care consultation versus patients who die without one) (32).

Palliative care services provide additional fiscal benefits that are more difficult to measure: palliative care communications interventions often clarify the goals of care sufficiently so that a patient and his or her family may choose to leave the hospital for hospice or certified home health agency care at home, in a skilled nursing facility, or an inpatient hospice unit. Without the clarification of the goals of care, no rational discharge plan can be agreed on, resulting in long ICU and hospital stays and a high rate of in-hospital death.

Challenges for the future

Multiple factors prevent the full use of hospital-based palliative care, including gaps in palliative care expertise and leadership, cultural issues that prevent timely referral for palliative care services, and fiscal limitations. Frequent, repeated counselling of patients and families and education of clinical colleagues can be extremely time-consuming. The inadequacy of current strategies for compensation for clinical services of this nature has been mentioned. Improved and more consistent financial support for institutional palliative care initiatives is required to develop the number and quality of programmes needed to care for the aging population.

Education and the palliative care workforce

Palliative medicine, as a medical subspecialty, is a relatively new field and many countries still lack both sub-specialty training and certification in the field (33). For example, in the US, palliative medicine only recently received the American Board of Medical Subspecialty certification required for government support of graduate medical education. As of January 2010, there were a total of 74 active programmes offering 181 fellowship positions including 27 research slots in the US (34). While training programmes in tertiary care centres across the US and other countries aim to produce the faculty leaders for palliative medicine educational and research programmes, the number of graduates each year is small in comparison with the growing need to train future physicians to provide high quality care to a rising number of seriously ill patients. Indeed, recent estimates suggest that there is only one palliative medicine physician for every 1,200 patients with a serious or life-threatening illness in the United States. To place a specialist in palliative medicine in every hospital or community would require exponential growth in the number of trainees and training programmes. A more achievable goal is to teach every clinician the basic skills of palliative care. The Educating Physicians in End-of-life Care (EPEC) project and End-of-Life Nursing Education Consortium (ELNEC) both provide extensive training in palliative medicine and nursing to non-specialists (35). ELNEC in particular has focused on providing extensive nursing training to 67 countries outside the United States. In addition, both the Liaison Committee for Medical Education (LCME) and the Accreditation Council for Graduate Medical Education (ACGME) now require or strongly encourage programmes to provide undergraduate and postgraduate training in palliative care in order to be accredited.

Misperception of palliative care as end-of-life care only

Cultural attitudes toward disease and death are pervasive barriers to the optimal employment of hospital-based palliative care services. The current culture celebrates activity, accomplishment, and youth and denies death (36). The consumer society seems to consider not only health, but also immortality a product to which people are entitled. Advances in public health and the technologies of medicine feed this death-denying culture, and patients, families, and physicians may pursue questionably effective, burdensome therapies rather than confront the simple truth that a life may be coming to its natural end. Partly for these reasons, palliative care consultation often is deferred until the final days or hours of life. At Mount Sinai Hospital (New York, NY), 77% of patients referred to palliative care are already severely disabled or moribund at the time of consultation (37). A more rational model of care is to begin palliative care interventions to some degree at the time of diagnosis of any serious, chronic, or life-limiting illness, regardless of prognosis and whether curative treatments are likely to be beneficial. At this time, disease-modifying therapies are likely to compose the bulk of interventions. As disease progresses, however, disease-modifying therapies may become more burdensome and limited in terms of their benefits, and correspondingly palliative care interventions may come to constitute the greater share of care. The concurrent delivery of disease-modifying therapy and palliative care allows for smoother transitions in care as disease progresses and goals of care shift. Indeed, a recent randomized controlled trial of early palliative care for patients with lung cancer demonstrated improvements in quality of life, mood, and prolonged survival among patients receiving palliative care (38).

Significant deficiencies in the hospital care of dying patients remain. Studies of leading academic centres in the US and Australia have demonstrated that many patients dying in hospital do not receive timely palliative care services, experience uncontrolled symptoms, and have limited opportunity to discuss goals of care (39,40). Misperceptions surrounding palliative care and cultural reluctance to discuss death remain significant barriers to consultation.

Reimbursement for palliative care service

A major tenet of palliative care is that people are entitled to coordinated, patient-centred, and family-centred care across a wide spectrum of settings. This same principle is fundamental to the leading proposals for payment reform in the US health care debate. A major barrier to the expansion of palliative care in the US has been the lack of a national health care system and the predominance of the fee-for-service reimbursement structure. This current model of health care has contributed to the fragmentation and waste currently observed in the US health care system. Proposed alternative reimbursement structures include Accountable Care Organizations and Bundled Payments. Both structures would incentivize health care providers to collaborate in order to achieve well-coordinated, patient-centred, high quality care across care settings. This may provide opportunities for hospital-based palliative care services to partner with community providers. For example, many US hospice programmes have already forged strong, mutually beneficial partnerships with hospitals in their communities (41). Partnering with hospices can give hospitalized patients access to an untapped repository of palliative care expertise. Hospices bring interdisciplinary palliative care expertise and the ability to case manage the care of complex and seriously ill patients across multiple care settings, spiritual care services, volunteer support for patient and family caregivers, and bereavement programming and support for family members for at least one year after the patient has died. For patients in hospice, hospitals may provide acute care expertise and secondary and tertiary care specialty services. Together these institutions can meet most, if not all, of the needs of seriously ill patients over a range of illnesses, disease stages, and clinical settings. A strong link between hospitals and community hospices can also help to overcome one of the main barriers to hospice referral—the implication of abandonment by the hospital's primary medical team and the resultant patient and family feeling of a forced transfer out of the hospital. If hospice professionals and hospital staff work together and see themselves and are seen by patients as part of the same team, the discontinuities inherent in the experience of the transfer are minimized.

With either an Accountable Care Organization or Bundled Payment structure, hospitals stand to benefit financially from collaboration with hospice programmes. Hospice partnerships can facilitate hospital discharge and thereby help reduce length of stay for some of the longest stay, sickest, and most costly patients in the hospital, increasing bed capacity for new admissions. Furthermore, these reimbursement structures provide hospitals with a fixed payment independent of the services provided, so that even if a hospitalized patient cannot be discharged to another care setting, the involvement of a hospice or palliative care team can lead to marked reductions in hospital cost by decreasing pharmacy costs, number of diagnostic procedures, and use of intensive care.

Box 11.1 Important public health challenges for palliative care in hospitals

Developed countries:

◆ Aging population and rapid growth in demand for palliative care services

◆ Limited availability of palliative care clinicians and clinical training programmes

◆ Cultural barriers to timely referral for palliative care services

◆ Fiscal constraints due to inadequate reimbursement methods for palliative clinical services.

Developing countries:

◆ Limited medical and financial resources and infrastructure

◆ Restricted access to medications, in particular opiates

◆ Lack of palliative care training among local clinical care providers

◆ Cultural differences concerning patient autonomy, communication of 'bad news', and truth telling regarding prognosis.

Palliative care in the developing world

The World Health Organization has recently increased attention given to the unmet palliative care needs in developing countries (42). Only 6% of world's palliative care services are located in Asia and Africa, yet these regions are home to the majority of the world's population and areas with the highest rates of cancer and HIV/AIDS (43). Efforts to deliver palliative care are impeded by limited medical and financial resources, restricted access to medications, lack of training among local clinical care providers, and often by strong cultural differences regarding communicating 'bad news', and truth telling (44). In particular, the availability of opiates is extremely limited and, in some areas, strong cultural resistance to the use of opiates is an additional barrier (45). Readers interested in a more thorough discussion of the existing and developing palliative care services around the world are directed to Chapters 18 to 20.

Conclusion

Hospital-based palliative care teams have evolved as a natural outgrowth of the modern hospice movement. Patients with chronic, serious, or life-limiting illness often experience extraordinary levels of physical, emotional, social, and spiritual distress. The hospital-based palliative care teams are able to address the suffering of these patients, whatever their prognosis and diagnosis may be. In the US, the provision of palliative care to patients with serious illness has been impeded by a fragmented, fee-for-service health care system and a cultural imperative to deny death. Expanded palliative medicine training for clinicians and health care reform may present new opportunities to increase access to palliative care services across hospitals and the continuum of care.

References

(1) Saunders DC. Global developments and the hospice information service. *Palliat Med*. 2000; **14** (1): 1–2.

(2) Higginson IJ, Bruera E. Do we need palliative care audit in developing countries? *Palliat Med*. 2002; **16** (6): 546–7.

(3) Dunlop RJ, Hockley JM. *Hospital-Based Palliative Care Teams: The Hospital–Hospice Interface*. New York: Oxford University Press, 1998.

(4) O'Neill WM, O'Connor P, Latimer EJ. Hospital palliative care services: Three models in three countries. *J Pain Symptom Manage*. 1992; **7** (7): 406–13.

(5) Bates T, Hoy AM, Clarke DG, Laird PP. The St Thomas' hospital terminal care support team. A new concept of hospice care. *Lancet*. 1981; **1** (8231): 1201–3.

(6) Mount BM. The problem of caring for the dying in a general hospital: The palliative care unit as a possible solution. *Can Med Assoc J*. 1976; **115** (2): 119.

(7) Rocafort J, Centeno C. *EPAC Review of Palliative Care in Europe*. Milano, Italy: IAHPC Press, 2008.

(8) Wright M, Wood J, Lynch T, Clark D. Mapping levels of palliative care development: A global view. *J Pain Symptom Manage*. 2008; **35** (5): 469–85.

(9) American Hospital Association (AHA) Annual Survey Database Fiscal Year 2008.

(10) Center to Advance Palliative Care (CAPC), Consensus Metrics Self-Assessment Tools. http://www.capc.org/tools-for-palliative-care-programs/measurement/. Accessed 25/5/2011.

(11) Casarett D, Pickard A, Bailey FA, et al. Do palliative consultations improve patient outcomes? *J Am Geriatr Soc*. 2008; **56** (4): 593–9.

(12) Du Pen SL, Du Pen AR, Polissar N, et al. Implementing guidelines for cancer pain management: Results of a randomized controlled clinical trial. *Journal of Clinical Oncology*. 1999; **17** (1): 361.

(13) Higginson IJ, Finlay IG, Goodwin DM, et al. Is there evidence that palliative care teams alter end-of-life experiences of patients and their caregivers? *J Pain Symptom Manage*. 2003; **25** (2): 150–68.

(14) Zhang B, Wright AA, Huskamp HA, et al. Health care costs in the last week of life: Associations with end-of-life conversations. *Arch Intern Med*. 2009; **169** (5): 480.

(15) Manfredi PL, Morrison RS, Morris J, Goldhirsch SL, Carter JM, Meier DE. Palliative care consultations: How do they impact the care of hospitalized patients? *J Pain Symptom Manage*. 2000; 20 (3): 166–73.

(16) Jack B, Hillier V, Williams A, Oldham J. Hospital based palliative care teams improve the symptoms of cancer patients. *Palliat Med*. 2003; **17** (6): 498.

(17) Jordhoy MS, Fayers P, Loge JH, Ahlner-Elmqvist M, Kaasa S. Quality of life in palliative cancer care: Results from a cluster randomized trial. *Journal of Clinical Oncology*. 2001; **19** (18): 3884.

(18) Gade G, Venohr I, Conner D, et al. Impact of an inpatient palliative care team: A randomized controlled trial. *J Palliat Med*. 2008; **11** (2): 180–90.

(19) Ringdal GI, Jordhøy MS, Kaasa S. Family satisfaction with end-of-life care for cancer patients in a cluster randomized trial. *J Pain Symptom Manage*. 2002; **24** (1): 53–63.

(20) Lilly CM, De Meo DL, Sonna LA, et al. An intensive communication intervention for the critically ill. *Am J Med*. 2000; **109** (6): 469–75.

(21) Bass DM, Noelker LS, Rechlin LR. The moderating influence of service use on negative caregiving consequences. *The Journals of Gerontology: Series B.* 1996; **51** (3): S121.

(22) Teno JM, Clarridge BR, Casey V, et al. Family perspectives on end-of-life care at the last place of care. *JAMA.* 2004; **291** (1): 88–93.

(23) Pan CX, Morrison RS, Meier DE, et al. How prevalent are hospital-based palliative care programs? Status report and future directions. *J Palliat Med.* 2001; **4** (3): 315–24.

(24) Virik K, Glare P. Profile and evaluation of a palliative medicine consultation service within a tertiary teaching hospital in Sydney, Australia. *J Pain Symptom Manage.* 2002; **23** (1): 17–25.

(25) Schapiro R, Byock I, Parker S, Twohig JS. Living and dying well with cancer: Successfully integrating palliative care and cancer treatment. *J Pain Symptom Manage.* 2003; 25: 19–28.

(26) Penrod JD, Deb P, Luhrs C, et al. Cost and utilization outcomes of patients receiving hospital-based palliative care consultation. *J Palliat Med.* 2006; **9** (4): 855–60.

(27) Raftery JP, Addington-Hall JM, MacDonald LD, et al. A randomized controlled trial of the cost-effectiveness of a district co-ordinating service for terminally ill cancer patients. *Palliat Med.* 1996; **10** (2): 151.

(28) Schneiderman LJ, Gilmer T, Teetzel HD, et al. Effect of ethics consultations on nonbeneficial life-sustaining treatments in the intensive care setting: A randomized controlled trial. *JAMA.* 2003; **290** (9): 1166.

(29) Smith TJ, Coyne P, Cassel B, Penberthy L, Hopson A, Hager MA. A high-volume specialist palliative care unit and team may reduce in-hospital end-of-life care costs. *J Palliat Med.* 2003; **6** (5): 699–705.

(30) Back AL, Li YF, Sales AE. Impact of palliative care case management on resource use by patients dying of cancer at a Veterans Affairs medical center. *J Palliat Med.* 2005; **8** (1): 26–35.

(31) Campbell ML, Guzman JA. Impact of a proactive approach to improve end-of-life care in a medical ICU. *Chest.* 2003; **123** (1): 266.

(32) Morrison RS. Palliative care length of stay savings as compared to non-palliative care, DRG-matched hospital deaths. In: Meier DE, Spragens LH, Sutton S (eds), *A Guide to Building a Hospital-Based Palliative Care Program.* New York: Center to Advance Palliative Care, 2004.

(33) Kaasa S, Jordhoy MS, Haugen DF. Palliative care in Norway: A national public health model. *J Pain Symptom Manage.* 2007; **33** (5): 599–604.

(34) Fellowship program directory. http://www.aahpm.org/fellowship/default/fellowshipdirectory. html. Accessed 10 Jan 2011.

(35) The EPEC project http://www.epec.net/EPEC/Webpages/index.cfm. Accessed 25/1/2011.

(36) Becker E. *The Denial of Death.* New York, NY: Free Press, 1997.

(37) The Mount Sinai School of Medicine, Brookdale Department of Geriatrics and Palliative Medicine, Lillian and Benjamin Hertzberg Palliative Care Institute, Clinical Consultation Database.

(38) Temel JS, Greer JA, Muzikansky A, et al. Early palliative care for patients with metastatic non-small-cell lung cancer. *N Engl J Med* **363**: 733–42, 2010.

(39) Le BHC, Watt JN. Care of the dying in Australia's busiest hospital: Benefits of palliative care consultation and methods to enhance access. *J Palliat Med.* 2010; **13** (7): 855–60.

(40) Walling AM, Asch SM, Lorenz KA, et al. The quality of care provided to hospitalized patients at the end of life. *Arch Intern Med.* 2010; **170** (12): 1057–63.

(41) Beresford L. *Hospital–Hospice Partnerships in Palliative Care: Creating a Continuum of Service.* Alexandria, VA: National and Palliative Care Organization, 2001.

(42) Sepúlveda C, Marlin A, Yoshida T, Ullrich A. Palliative care—the World Health Organization's global perspective. *J Pain Symptom Manage.* 2002; **24** (2): 91–6.

(43) Webster R, Lacey J, Quine S. Palliative care: A public health priority in developing countries. *J Public Health Policy*. 2007; **28** (1): 28–39.

(44) Harding R, Higginson IJ. Palliative care in sub-Saharan Africa. *The Lancet*. 2005; **365** (9475): 1971–7.

(45) Crane K. Palliative care gains ground in developing countries. *J Natl Cancer Inst*. 2010; **102** (21): 1613.

Part V

Inequalities at the end of life: Under-served groups

Chapter 12

Non-cancer patients as an under-served group

Julia Addington-Hall and Katherine Hunt

Initial cancer focus

In the beginning

Dame Cicely Saunders dated the beginning of what she called 'the modern hospice movement' to the opening of St Christopher's Hospice in 1967 (1). Clark argues that it is more accurate to see the opening of St Christopher's as a 'crucial *outcome* of ideas and strategies developed over the preceding decade, in which can be located the essential characteristics of the subsequent hospice movement' (2). One key decision made during this period was that the hospice would admit only terminally ill cancer patients, although it would also have a separate wing for elderly and chronically ill patients. This need not have been the case.

Dame Cicely had gained much of her experience in caring for the dying and had refined her vision for hospice care when working at two existing homes for the dying in London: St Luke's House, founded in 1893, where she learnt about the effectiveness of regular administration of analgesia and St Joseph's Hospice, founded in 1905, where she was impressed by individual care (3). These homes were part of a limited number opened in the nineteenth or early twentieth century, usually by religious orders, to provide for the first time institutional care for the terminally ill, in this case the 'respectable' poor, usually dying from pulmonary TB, who were unable to receive adequate nursing care in over-crowded and poverty-stricken home conditions (4). These homes continued to be needed into the mid-twentieth century, as the new NHS made no provision for terminal care (3). Influential reports in the 1950s identified substantial deficiencies in the medical, social and economic welfare of, for the first time, terminally ill cancer patients (5) and of all terminally ill patients (6). The Marie Curie Foundation responded to the first report by opening a series of homes specifically for terminally ill cancer patients, as well as its night nursing service. Growing arguments for terminal care to be a priority for the NHS focused on all causes, however, not just cancer (3). Similarly, the focus of the first empirical research on the experiences of dying patients was on terminal illness per se, not specifically cancer (7;8). Both studies reported more distress in patients who did not have cancer than in cancer patients: Exton Smith found chronic conditions to be associated with more distress than cancer in older patients (7), whilst Hinton found pain to be higher in cancer patients but overall physical distress more prevalent and more severe in patients with heart or renal failure (8).

The evidence therefore indicated that patients dying from conditions other than cancer experienced at least as much distress as terminally cancer patients, if not more. To provide care for people dying from all causes would have been consistent with past practice. Why then was the decision made to focus the embryonic hospice movement on cancer, with its continuing consequences for the shape of hospice and palliative care provision world-wide? A definitive answer to this awaits an appropriate analysis of archives of the hospice movement. However, in 1960 Dame Cicely indicated that it was patients between the ages of 40 and 60 with cancers of the cervix or with breast secondaries whom she regarded as having particularly difficult pain problems (3). The decision is, therefore, presumably based in part on her clinical experience. It is also clear that Dame Cicely, together with her colleagues and supporters, wanted to create a new way of caring for the dying, one which combined excellent terminal care with research into pain, symptom control and terminal care in general and with education for the whole multi-professional team. A focus on cancer was necessary to achieve these aims; without focus it would be impossible to make any real scientific advances in understanding the causes of suffering or in develop-ing effective solutions. The focus on cancer made sense because of the advances which were being made at that time in the understanding of pain, with the recent publication of Melzack and Wall's gate theory. There was, therefore, the strong likelihood of major advances in pain control for terminally ill cancer patients. A cancer focus also helped limit demand on the new services, and served to distinguish terminal care from the emerging discipline of geriatric medicine. In addition, cancer had now replaced infectious diseases as the leading cause of premature death, and was the archetypal death of modern society, characterized by isolation, social death, pain and physical suffering. Then, as now, the social construction of cancer and aging differ in ways which, if one is starting a new fund-raising venture and seeking to change attitudes to terminal care, probably favour the former.

The next decades

As the principles and practice of modern hospice and palliative care expanded across the UK and beyond, some services decided that patients dying with neurological conditions, particularly MND (or ALS), experienced such severe suffering and had such high unmet needs in the last months of life that they too should receive care from hospice services. The rapid growth in the number of people affected by AIDS/HIV in the USA, Europe and the UK in the 1980s also challenged the focus of hospices on cancer, with an articulate, well-informed client-group in the gay community questioning why they should be excluded from services when they too were suffering severe symptoms, in need of social, psychological, and spiritual support, and dying. Initially, major voices within the hospice movement favoured the instigation of separate hospices for people with AIDS/HIV. Whilst this may have been a reflection of the stigma associated with the condition at the time, it is also congruent with the stated hope of hospice pioneers that what they were doing in cancer, others would take on and achieve in other terminal conditions. A number of hospices specifically for AIDS/HIV did open in industrialized countries; some are still in operation but increasingly in these countries hospice and palliative care for people with AIDS/HIV has been provided alongside that for other conditions.

Population-based commissioning

A major change in health policy in England and Wales in 1990 led to a separation of those providing health care from those purchasing (or later, commissioning) it. For the first time, health authorities (later Primary Care Trusts, with a change to GP commissioning groups proposed as we write) were given responsibility for assessing and then purchasing health care for a defined population. In palliative care, as in other health care conditions, this led to a growth of interest in epidemiologically-based needs assessment, and the development (at least in theory) of services based on population needs, rather than local custom, patient or clinician demand, historical funding distributions or centralized decision-making.

Up to this point, much hospice and palliative care research, like clinical practice, had been focused on cancer, making it difficult for those attempting to look at palliative care need across the whole population to look much beyond the number of deaths from different causes in different populations. However, the Regional Study of Care for the Dying (the RSCD) in the UK and the SUPPORT study in the USA, both of which began publishing their findings in the mid-1990s, demonstrated that cancer patients were not alone at the end of life in experiencing severe pain and other physical symptoms, in needing better psychological support, in having unmet needs for social and practical support, and in needing better communication from health professionals. The SUPPORT study demonstrated that hospitalized patients in the last three days of life with heart failure and COPD had physical and emotional symptoms that were hard to tolerate, and that rates of pain were similar in cancer and non-cancer patients (9). Similarly, the RSCD reported that patients who died from heart disease commonly experienced a wide range of symptoms such as dyspnoea, low mood, pain, and nausea, and 1 in 6 had symptoms as severe as patients dying of cancer and managed by palliative care services (10). The RSCD also found that those who died from COPD had symptoms not only associated with respiratory problems, but also experienced low mood and symptoms more typically associated with cancer, such as pain (11). Moreover, although those who died from stroke and dementia had higher levels of functional problems, they still suffered from a cluster of symptoms more commonly associated with cancer such as pain and loss of appetite (12). These findings, along with others published in the same decade, provided evidence to those seeking to purchase, commission or provide services on the basis of need that palliative care in the last months of life was not restricted to people with cancer. They therefore challenged the status quo because in the UK at that time, 96 per cent of patients who received care from hospice or specialist palliative care services had cancer (13). However, most hospices and services reported that they would accept referrals for patients with non-malignant disease (13) and an expert report to the Department of Health in 1992 recommended that all patients should have access to palliative care services (14).

The 2000s

The initial focus of hospice and palliative care services has been increasingly challenged. In the UK, the policy framework for commissioning cancer palliative care services from the Department of Health made it clear that palliative care should be provided on the basis of need, not diagnosis, and this has been reinforced by the country's first End of Life Strategy (2008) which outlined a comprehensive framework to promote high quality end-of-life care for all adults (end-of-life care in this context is defined as 'care that helps all those with advanced, progressive, incurable illness to live as well as possible until they die . . . it includes management of pain and other symptoms and provision of psycho-logical, social, spiritual and practical support' (15)). This was in fact preceded by a series of disease-specific strategies such as the National Service Frameworks for Coronary Heart Disease (16) and Older People (17) which also highlighted the need for targeted and spe-cialized end-of-life care for these patients. In reality, hospice and specialist palliative care service provision has struggled to keep up with the rhetoric of government policy, and still almost all patients who access hospice and palliative care services in the UK have cancer.

Evidence of inequalities?

Evidence that people with conditions other than cancer have physical, psychological, social, or spiritual needs at the end of life similar to those of cancer patients is not sufficient in itself to justify claims that it is unjust or an example of inequality to exclude non-cancer patients from these services. In order to be certain that there are indeed inequities in access to hospice and palliative care across diagnostic groups we must demonstrate firstly that patients in each group have comparable needs, secondly that these needs are within the remit of palliative care, thirdly, that these needs are not already being adequately met, fourthly that palliative care is an effective and acceptable intervention for these needs, and finally that palliative care is available (or available in greater quantities) for one group than for others.

The first issue is ascertaining whether groups have comparable needs. This has been assessed in a number of studies by comparing scores of different groups on, for example, symptom rating, psychological measurement or palliative outcome scales. These studies have played an important role in extending our understanding of palliative care needs beyond cancer. They rest, however, on the assumption that all patients (or all relatives in after-death studies) have similar notions of, for example, severity in mind when answering symptom questions. This is called into question by the fact that symptom severity ratings are amongst the least reliable in proxy–patient comparisons (18;19). Comparisons of problem severity (but not presence) between conditions therefore should be treated with suspicion.

The second issue is the difficulty in ascertaining which needs lie within the remit of palliative care. A number of approaches have been used, including deriving questions from defini-tions of palliative care and developing questionnaires based on professional opinion, in order to ascertain the prevalence of problems seen as within the remit of palliative care such as pain and other symptoms, psychological symptoms and family concerns. There is a danger that these may lead to the presumption that every person with one of these problems needs palliative care, overlooking the role of other health and social professionals already involved who also adopt (or try to adopt) a holistic view of care (for example, nursing, primary or geriatric care). This may, of course, in part reflect a more widespread confusion when discussing palliative care needs between whether these are needs which require input from professionals with a specialist training in palliative care (specialist palliative care needs) or whether they are needs which any health professional should be able to address (general palliative care needs). Another approach, adopted in the RSCD, is to apply to non-cancer patients the criteria used to distinguish cancer patients who receive palliative care from those who do not: this may provide more useful information on the proportion of non-cancer patients who might be expected to need palliative care, but it is still predicated on the role of palliative care in cancer, rather than on an understanding of what it can do beyond cancer (20).

According to the NHS definition of need for health care ('the ability to benefit from health care' (21)), it is not enough to demonstrate or express a need for a service, it is also necessary to demonstrate that benefit would arise from that service. In the 1990s, there was little enough robust evidence that hospice and specialist palliative care services benefited cancer patients, and none that they benefited non-cancer patients. The evidence-base as regards cancer has expanded, but the evidence for benefits beyond cancer remains limited. In the absence of such evidence, whilst there are clearly differentials in access to hospice and specialist palliative care services, care should be taken not to presume that a combination of evidence of needs apparently within the remit of palliative care, and differences in access to palliative care, automatically equate to inequalities in access. Given the widespread growth in provision of hospice and palliative care services beyond cancer in recent years and the continuing research and clinical interest in the issue, it is highly unlikely that the current situation is one of equality. It should not be presumed, however, that a 'fair' situation would be one in which the proportion of cancer patients receiving hospice and palliative care reflects precisely the proportion of cancer deaths. It is possible that cancer patients may always have particularly high levels of need for palliative care compared with most (if not all) other diagnostic groups; this is, as yet, an untested proposition.

The debate in this chapter so far has been about 'non-cancer'. This is itself adding to the lack of clarity about the role of hospice and palliative care beyond cancer and the reason for this is, of course, that 'non-cancer' exists as a term only in relation to cancer; it places three quarters of people who die into one group linked only by what they do not have, rather than by any unifying characteristics. The next section, therefore, discusses how the debate about the provision of palliative care beyond cancer has been clarified by the introduction and development of three main 'dying trajectories'. It uses these to illustrate some of the main barriers to, and facilitators of, expanding palliative care services beyond cancer.

Beyond cancer

The dying trajectories referred to here refer to archetypical patterns of change in performance function in the weeks or months before death initially theoretically derived by Lynn et al. (22), and later by Lunney et al. (23) tested in EPESE study data. These differentiate between three patterns: the cancer or terminal illness trajectory, characterized by good performance status followed by rapid decline and death, the organ failure trajectory, characterized by a number of sudden rapid dips and recoveries to a somewhat lower starting point with a final similar dip from which there is no recovery, and the frailty trajectory, characterized by much lower functioning throughout, with small oscillations on a gradual decline towards death. These trajectories are theoretical constructs rather than empirically-derived pathways which all, or even most, patients can be expected to follow. Nevertheless, like other theoretically derived trajectories, they are useful in aiding analysis of complex social situations.

Most hospice and palliative care services were, at least initially, designed around the cancer trajectory: they provided intensive support for a limited period, ending with the patient's death (or following bereavement care). Referral to these services was predicated upon knowing the patient's prognosis, either because of the requirement of the funders (as with the MEDICARE hospice benefit in the USA), in order to manage demand, or to ensure the patient was suitable to receive care. This effectively excluded patients on, for example, the organ failure trajectory whose prognosis was much less certain. There remains a lack of good prognostic indicators in, for example, congestive heart failure (CHF) and COPD. The need for patients to have a clear prognosis before referral to hospice and palliative care services remains a significant barrier to referral in the UK. A number of investigators are investigating this by researching better methods of prognostication. There is also, however, an apparent reluctance on the part of patients, health professionals, and the wider society to talk about death and dying outside cancer, which limits discussions about prognosis beyond even the limits imposed by the lack of prognostic certainty. This is being addressed by a nationwide drive to increase willingness across society to talk about death and dying and by increased communication training for health professionals. Experience in the USA suggests that prognostic uncertainty is not an absolute barrier to referral to hospice, with CHF and COPD patients making up a small proportion of referrals, but that these referrals are received very close to death, limiting the impact that the hospice can have on their care.

The difficulty in diagnosing dying in the organ failure trajectories, leading either to exclusion from hospice and palliative care or to referral very close to death, suggests the need for a different approach to addressing palliative care needs in these conditions, one that does not rely on an accurate prognostic estimate to be made or active treatment to be stopped before action is taken to address palliative care issues. This is comparable with the WHO definition of palliative care, which suggests that it is applicable 'early in the course of illness, in conjunction with other therapies that are intended to prolong life' (24) and which has increasing resonance within cancer palliative care where several countries recognize that reliance on prognostic indicators can lead to late referrals. The need to develop palliative care models appropriate for organ failure trajectories has been addressed in different ways in different health care settings. In the USA, where hospice care is predominately community-based and primarily focused on the last days of life, palliative medicine has developed as a specialty focused on the care of seriously ill patients in hospital (25), which, according to the American Academy of Hospice and Palliative

Medicine (26) provides specialist expertise for those with 'active, progressive, far advanced disease for whom the prognosis is limited and the focus of care is quality of life'. In the UK, the emphasis has been on specialists in palliative care working in partnership with those already providing care for these patients (for example, heart failure nurses, cardiologists and GPs) to support them in meeting patients' palliative care needs, providing specialist care themselves only to the most complex cases. In each case, the emphasis is on working together with other specialties to meet the patient's palliative care needs, regardless of prognosis. In the USA this is augmented by access to hospice for those patients who are clearly dying; these patients can increasingly access community palliative care services in the UK.

The frailty trajectory presents different challenges, mainly in the difficulty associated with identifying the terminal phase. Frailty is associated with decline across multiple systems and frequent, often avoidable, hospital admissions. Further, frail elderly people present with atypical signs and symptoms of disease, which is perhaps a result of the catalogue of symptoms associated with multiple morbidity and subclinical disease (27–29), but has the effect of further complicating prognostication.

Many patients whose last months resemble this trajectory have dementia and will have declined physically and cognitively over an extended period. The estimated prevalence of dementia in the UK is 683,597 and because the number affected increases considerably with age (12.2% prevalence in those aged between 80 and 84 years but a 32.5% prevalence in those aged over 95 years), a rapidly ageing population means that the prevalence is forecast to increase to almost one million by 2021 (30). This demands a shift in the way that patients with dementia are cared for at the end of life, yet assumptions about the illness itself, an insufficiently educated healthcare workforce, and the inability of dementia patients to communicate need lie at the heart of barriers to access.

There are significant variations both between and within countries in how patients with dementia are treated, for example in relation to the usual treatment of pneumonia, the placement of feeding tubes, and the use of DNR orders, perhaps because although dementia is a terminal illness, it has not traditionally been seen as one. As with general age-related decline, prognostication of the end-stage of dementia is challenging and acts as a barrier to the provision of palliative care. However, in contrast to general age-related decline, difficulties in communicating symptom severity and care needs are a further barrier to accessing palliative care. Indeed, patients with dementia are much less likely to receive adequate pain relief than those with other conditions (31). Patients with dementia do not have equal access to palliative care services (32;33) yet they have been shown to suffer from many of the symptoms experienced by patients dying from other causes eg cancer such as pain, loss of appetite and depression (12;34). Acute illness (often in the form of bacterial infections) is common in dementia patients and often leads to hospitalization. The dementia illness trajectory is viewed as a variant of the frailty trajectory in that it is punctuated by declines caused by episodes of acute illness (35) which eventually result in death.

The further barrier to the provision of palliative care in dementia patients stems from a common failure to view dementia as a long term condition that has a terminal phase. This is evidenced by healthcare professionals and families having difficulty in assigning dementia as the cause of death. Thus, death certificates frequently cite acute infections such as pneumonia as the cause of death, rather than dementia as the underlying cause (33). It is likely that a lack of skills and education among healthcare staff as well as families contributes to the paucity of palliative care provision for older people with dementia (34). However, a recently renewed research and policy focus on end-of-life care for dementia patients marks a shift in management of the illness and a positive step towards ensuring a 'good death' for those unable to articulate their needs.

Conclusion

End-of-life care for those with non-cancer conditions remains a public health challenge. With the demographic shift towards a more aged population and the forecasted increases in long-term conditions, the numbers of people following frailty and organ failure trajectories is growing rapidly. Dying trajectories, although mainly theoretical constructs, appear helpful in encouraging imaginative solutions to improving end of life care beyond cancer. One reason for this is that they encourage us to look beyond the 'non-cancer' label, which does little to illuminate the needs of the majority who die from other causes, or to promote the development of appropriate services.

References

(1) Saunders, C (1996) Hospice. *Mortality*, **1**: 317–22.

(2) Clark, D (1998) Originating a movement: Cicily Saunders and the development of St Christopher's Hospice, 1957–1967. *Mortality*, **3** (1): 43–63.

(3) Clark, D (1999) Cradle to the grave? Terminal care in the United Kingdom, 1948–67. *Mortality*, **4** (3): 225–47.

(4) Humphreys, C (2001) 'Waiting for the last summons': The establishment of the first hospices in England 1878–1914. *Mortality*, **6** (2): 146–66.

(5) Gough Thomas, J (1962) Day and night nursing for cancer patients. *District Nursing*, Nov.: 174–5.

(6) Glyn Hughes, HL (1962) *Peace at the last. A survey of terminal care in the United Kingdom*. London: The Calouste Gulbenkian Foundation.

(7) Exton Smith, AN (1961) Terminal illness in the aged. *The Lancet*, **5**: 305–8.

(8) Hinton J (1963) The physical and mental distress of the dying. *Quarterly Journal of Medicine*, New Series, XXXII: 1–20.

(9) Lynn, J, Teno, J, Phillips, RS, Wu, A, Desbiens, N, Harrold, J, Claessens, MT, Wenger, N, Kreling, B, and Connors, AF (1997) Perceptions of family members of the dying experience of older and seriously ill patients. *Annals of Internal Medicine*, **126**: 97–106.

(10) McCarthy, M, Lay, M, and Addington-Hall, J (1996) Dying from heart disease. *Journal of the Royal College of Physicians of London*, **30** (4): 325–8.

(11) Edmonds, EP, Karlson, S, Khan, S, and Addington-Hall, J (2001) A comparison of the palliative care needs of patients dying from chronic respiratory diseases and lung cancer. *Palliative Medicine*,**15** (4): 287–95.

(12) McCarthy, M, Addington-Hall, J, and Altmann, D (1997) The experience of dying with dementia: A retrospective study. *International Journal of Geriatric Psychiatry*, **12**: 404–9.

(13) Eve, A, Smith, AM, and Tebbit, P (1997) Hospice and palliative care in the UK 1994–1995 including a summary of trends 1990–1995. *Palliative Medicine*, **11**: 31–43.

(14) Standing Medical Advisory Committee and Standing Nursing and Midwifery Advisory Committee (1992). *The Principles and Practice of Palliative Care*. London: Standing Medical Advisory Committee and Standing Nursing and Midwifery Advisory Committee.

(15) Department of Health, UK (2008) *End of Life Care Strategy—Promoting High Quality Care for all adults at the end of life*. London: HMSO.

(16) Department of Health, UK (2000) *National Service Framework: Coronary Heart Disease*. London: HMSO.

(17) Department of Health, UK (2001) *National Service Framework: Older People*. London: HMSO.

(18) McPherson, C and Addington-Hall, J (2003) Judging the quality of care at the end of life: Can proxies provide reliable information? *Social Science and Medicine*, **56**: 95–109.

(19) McPherson, C and Addington-Hall, J (2004) How do proxies' perceptions of patients' pain, anxiety, and depression change during the bereavement period? *Journal of Palliative Care*, **20**: 12–19.

(20) Addington-Hall, J, Fakhoury, W, and McCarthy, M (1998) Specialist palliative care in non-malignant disease. *Palliative Medicine*, **12**: 417–27.

(21) Stevens, A and Raftery, J (1994) *Health Care Needs Assessment: The Epidemiologically Based Needs Reviews*. Oxford: Radcliffe Medical Press.

(22) Lynn, J, Harrell, F, Cohn, F, Wagner, D, and Connors, A (1997) Prognoses of seriously ill hospitalised patients on the days before death: Implications for patient care and public policy. *New Horizons*, **5** (1): 56–61.

(23) Lunney, J, Lynn, J, Foley, D, Lipson, S, and Guralnik, J (2003) Patterns of functional decline at the end of life. *JAMA*, **18**: 2387–92.

(24) World Health Organization. WHO Definition of Palliative Care, available at www.who.int/cance/ palliative/definition/en/. Accessed 19/2/2011.

(25) Byock, I (1998) Hospice and palliative care: a parting of the ways or a path to the future? *Journal of Palliative Medicine*, **1**: 165–76.

(26) American Academy of Hospice and Palliative Medicine (1999) *Hospice and palliative medicine: Core curriculum and review syllabus*. Dubuque, Iowa: Kendall/Hunt.

(27) Fried, LP, Tangen, C, Walston, J, Newman, AB, Hirsch, C, Gottdiener, J, Seeman, T, Tracy, R, Kop, WJ, Burke, G, and McBurnie, MA (2001) Frailty in older adults: Evidence for a phenotype. *Journal of Gerontology: Medical Sciences*, **56A** (3): M146–56.

(28) Morley, JE, Mitchell Perry III, H, and Miller, DK (2002) Something about frailty. *Journal of Gerontology: Medical Sciences*, **57A** (11): M698–M704.

(29) Rockwood, K (2005) What would make a definition of frailty useful? *Age and Ageing*, **34**: 432–4.

(30) Alzheimer's Society (2007) *Dementia UK: A Report Into The Prevalence and Cost of Dementia. Summary of key findings, 2007*. London: Alzheimer's Society.

(31) Teno, JM (2001) Persistent pain in nursing home residents. *JAMA*, **285**: 2081.

(32) Audit Commission (2002) *Forget Me Not: Developing Mental Health Services for Older People in England*. London: Audit Commission.

(33) Sachs, G, Shega, J, and Cox-Hayley, D (2004) Barriers to excellent end of life care for patients with dementia. *Journal of General and Internal Medicine*, **19**: 1057–63.

(34) Ouldred, E and Bryant, B (2008) Dementia care. Part 3: end of life care for people with advanced dementia. *British Journal of Nursing*, **17** (5): 308–14.

(35) Shega, J, Levin, A, and Hougham, G (2003) Palliative Excellence in Alzheimer Care Efforts (PEACE): a program description. *Journal of Palliative Medicine*, **6**: 315–20.

Chapter 13

Palliative care for the older adult

Kevin Brazil

Introduction

The societal shift towards an older population has implications for how palliative care should be provided. This chapter will identify some considerations that policy-makers and health care providers should regard in the provision of palliative care for the older adult.

Challenges of an ageing population

Many countries have experienced dramatic improvements in population life expectancy. In Europe, the proportion of people over the age of 65 represents 15% of the population in most European Union countries (1). The proportion of older persons, and particularly those over 80, has increased significantly in recent decades presenting profound economic and social consequences for most, if not all, countries (2).

Improved standards of living and medical advances in the prevention and control of formerly fatal infectious diseases have made it possible for an increasing number of persons to reach an age at which they become more vulnerable to chronic diseases. A rise in the prevalence of chronic diseases such as heart disease, arthritis, and diabetes has been reported among older adults in most industrial countries (3,4). The development of a chronic disease is complex, occurring across the lifespan and influenced by numerous factors including personal income, education, employment, and the environment. Often individuals with chronic disease will have multiple chronic conditions (5).

The financial situation of the older adult can compound the challenge of living with a chronic health condition. Older adults are usually not employed and are dependent on a fixed income and any saved assets. Poverty rates vary dramatically across the European Union with older adults facing the highest poverty risk rate in Latvia (51%) and lowest in Hungary (4%) (6). In Canada it has been reported that 6.8% of older adults live below the poverty line with 19% having an income that hovers near it. Those individuals whose income is close to the poverty line experience difficulty accessing the benefits of income-tested programmes and are forced to get by with extremely small budgets (7). The inflation of rent, taxes, and increased cost of utilities can influence how older adults manage and at times force the individual to make choices between purchases required for management of a chronic health condition and daily living expenses.

It has been reported that older adults with chronic health conditions are high users of health and social care resources (8–10). Older adults have been reported to have more frequent visits to physicians, to be hospitalized more frequently, and to have longer lengths of hospital stays compared with younger adults (5,8,9). Further, older adults usually have multiple chronic conditions, which require using several different services and seeing many different providers, and this makes the continuity and coordination of care a significant issue for this population (11,12).

Problems of ageism

Underlying the issues regarding the provision of care to the older adult is the concern of ageism (13). Ageism is described as the presence of a belief held by a health care provider that conditions such as depression, pain, and other disorders are a normal part of aging and that the older individual will not benefit from treatment. This attitude can discriminate or otherwise disadvantage an older adult in the nature of the care provided. Research evidence has revealed that there is a prevailing bias that health care is delivered at odds with the best interests of the older adult (14). Among health care professionals, ageism can manifest itself in the belief that poor health is an inevitable consequence of aging. Healthcare professionals can make assumptions about older patients based on age rather than functional status. As in other forms of prejudice and discrimination, ageism is a product of culture, an attitude or belief that is endemic in society that may manifest itself in the delivery of health care. The evidence suggests that older adults are less likely to be identified for proven medical interventions thus often leading to inappropriate or incomplete treatment (15). Research evidence has also revealed that older adults may be ignored by physicians or may suffer inappropriate aggressive treatment (14). Both extremes reveal a lack of understanding of how to manage and treat the complex health needs of the older adult. Fortunately, poor health is not an inevitable consequence of aging and many interventions currently exist that could reduce much of the disability and illness of older adults. Unfortunately, many health care providers have limited training in the care and management of older adults, reinforcing the presence of ageism in the way care is provided. Without proper training, health care professionals are not able to address the many factors that influence the health of older adults.

Care at home for older people

A unique aspect of care for the older adult is the significance of the home as a place of care. In most countries, older adults live at home where the last years of life are spent in the care of family members (16). The support provided by family caregivers can range from a few hours per week to continuous care. In Canada it has been reported that informal caregivers provide about 80 percent of all home care to older adults living in the community. Further, one in four of those providing care are over the age of 65 (17). While informal caregivers have reported the benefits of these responsibilities, the wide range of negative consequences to caregivers themselves is well documented (18).

Understanding the relationship the older adult has with the health care system places in context the discussion on palliative care for the older adult. Most deaths in developed countries occur in people over the age of 65. With an aging population, the pattern of disease that people suffer and die from changes with more people dying as a result of chronic diseases. In fact, it can be difficult to identify any one disease as a single cause of death, as many older adults suffer from multiple chronic illnesses (19). An appreciation of the broader issues that influence the quality of life and care of the older adult offers insight into how the provision of palliative care may best be positioned in order to support the older adult.

Challenges in the provision of palliative care for the older adult

Broadly defined, palliative care is a holistic approach to care for individuals with progressive and advanced disease with limited prospects for long-term survival (20). Despite the fact that death occurs predominantly in older adults the current practice of palliative care in developed countries has been criticized as oriented towards a younger population diagnosed with cancer. The dying process is different for older compared with younger adults. A younger adult may die from one disease and the period of care is typically a matter of months. Palliative care for the older adult may concern a primary disease such as cancer (the majority of new cancers are found in persons over the age of 60 years) accompanied with multiple co-morbidities that may include hypertension, diabetes, or arthritis (19). The burden of illness is greater for the older palliative patient who may present to the physician conditions associated with aging such as dementia, incontinence and sensory deficits that require attention in conjunction with common terminal symptoms such as pain, nausea, and shortness of breath (21).

Dying with pain is a major concern for older patients. Unfortunately pain is a symptom that is often under-assessed and under-treated (16). The prevalence of significant pain in older adults has been estimated to be as high as 25% to 56% (22). Pain assessment and management is different for older adults compared with younger adults. Older adults have a tendency to under-report pain where cognitive impairment, impaired sensory function, denial and avoidance all contribute to under-reporting. Multiple concurrent conditions and multiple sources of pain along with the incidence of side effects and complications associated with treatment of pain also makes the assessment and management of pain more difficult in the older adult. In palliative care of patients with dementia, pain assessment and treatment are difficult when the patient is unable to report their pain and health care providers are challenged in assessing the presence and magnitude of pain. Dementia is a unique challenge in providing palliative care to older adults. As a terminal illness, it affects 4% of people over the age of 70, increasing to 13% of those over the age of 80 with many of them dying in nursing homes (16).

Aside from the management of physical symptoms, older adults experience a longer period of functional dependence and a greater need of informal care in the later stages of life (23). In truth, home care relies on family care. As stated earlier, informal caregivers provide the majority of care to the dependent older adult. Unfortunately, the majority of family caregivers lack the experience and knowledge in coping with the intensity of caring for a terminally ill individual (24,25). This lack of knowledge and inadequate experience of caregiving, along with the overwhelming and numerous tasks of the caregiver, poses a potential threat not only to the care recipient, but also to the caregiver who may experience significant physical, emotional, and financial strain (26).

An aspect of providing palliative care to the older adult is the diversity of settings where palliation may occur which range from the home, assisted living facilities, hospices, and hospitals to nursing homes. A transition across these settings is not unusual for an individual, raising concern about the quality of coordination and continuity of care across these settings. The variety of settings where palliation for the older adult may occur adds another consideration to the health care provider who must be familiar with these settings in order to assist families and patients to make informed decisions about meeting the needs of the older adult. Nursing homes are increasingly becoming the site of death for older adults. It has been reported that up to 20% of individuals over the age of 65 in the United States die in nursing homes with the projection that by 2020 40% of Americans will die there (27). The available evidence indicates that the quality of care provided to dying residents of nursing homes is often inadequate (28–30). Pain management is a notable area (31). Often the fear of opiate abuse and lack of knowledge of proper drug prescribing underlie why pain is under-treated (32). In addition to inadequate pain management, advance care planning is often not attempted or not completed comprehensively in nursing homes (33). Inappropriate and unnecessary hospitalization is also a concern that has been identified by both nursing home staff and families of residents (34). Furthermore, educational gaps in the training of staff coupled with communication problems between health care providers, family members, and residents represent major barriers to quality palliative care (35–38).

The issue of prognosis is another significant issue in providing palliative care to the older person. The difficulty in assessing prognosis in non-cancer conditions has been one of the major barriers to implementing palliative care. Another obstacle to providing palliative care to the older person has been termed 'prognostic paralysis' when a physician is unable to determine prognosis and initiate discussions on advance care planning and palliative care (39). In some instances physicians may also be reluctant to diagnose an individual as palliative if any hope of improvement exists, which is difficult to predict in chronic disease. In both cases, the consequence can be the denial of access to timely palliative care.

The provision of palliative care to the older adult presents unique challenges ranging from social and medical considerations to understanding the diverse care settings where palliation occurs. The strong presence of family members in caring for the older adult challenges health care providers to broaden the scope of their concern to include the family as a partner in shared care as well as to safeguard their well being. The present level to which these elements are addressed by the health care system show that we have a long way to go to provide quality palliative care to the older adult.

Reforming the provision of palliative care

There is a strong body of evidence suggesting that the current health care system does not adequately respond to the needs of older adults (9,40). Health care in developed countries is organized around an acute, episodic model of care that no longer meets the needs of many individuals, especially older adults who typically have multiple chronic conditions. The provision of palliative care in this context typically results in care being initiated either too late or not at all. A study on palliative care referral rates conducted in Nova Scotia, Canada, revealed that individuals of 65 years and older were less likely to be referred than individuals under age 65, demonstrating that access to palliative care declines with age (41).

Recognizing the failure of the current model of health care in meeting the needs of the older adult has resulted in calls for an alternative paradigm for care (9,40). As part of this reform, there is a need to revisit how palliative care is integrated with life-prolonging care. A significant barrier in this regard is the misunderstanding by many health care providers that providing palliative care implies the withdrawal of active treatment (42). To counter this perception the World Health Organization's definition of palliative care encourages the application of palliative care early in the course of an illness and in conjunction with other therapies.

The integration of palliative care with life-prolonging care is important to ensure optimal care for the older adult; Morrison and Meir (43) have described this integration as a 'simultaneous' model of palliative care. This approach suggests that palliative care would be delivered at the same time as life prolonging treatments. Temel et al. (44) reported from their research that early integration of palliative care with standard cancer care can improve survival time and quality of life and mood among patients with lung cancer. The early integration of palliative care with life-prolonging care could remove the distinction between the two encouraging the view that care is simply responding to patient need and preference.

Systemic change is required to facilitate the integration of palliative care with life-prolonging care. An essential first step is philosophical, adopting the view that end-of-life care may span years not just weeks or months and that care is determined by patient preference and need and not by diagnosis or setting. Building on this philosophy in reforming care requires a systems-integrated approach targeting the individual health care provider, considering new ways of how service is delivered and addressing broad structure and policy elements. Illustrative examples of the types of efforts that may be pursued in each of these categories follow. Education is a key strategy at the level of the individual provider where the principles and practices of palliative care become an integral feature of care for the older adult. In the case of service delivery, strategies are required to promote inter-professional engagement, which offers the opportunity to bring together diverse specialties. This model of practice would promote closer relations between palliative care specialists and other specialties facilitating earlier referral to palliative care services and fostering new collaborative/shared approaches in the care of the older adult who has a life limiting illness. Structural considerations should include consideration of the development of advanced patient information systems that would facilitate continuity and coordination of care across settings of care.

It is clear that the prevailing model of palliative care is not suited to the older adult. Fortunately, there is a growing recognition that reform of how care is delivered is necessary. This requires a sustained effort that is most successful when pursued at a national health policy level. The importance of this issue is sharpened by the knowledge that many countries are experiencing a shift in the historical balance between young and old. The implications of this shift include a reduced workforce, due to an aging population, having serious consequences for the financing of health care systems.

Summary of key points

- ◆ A societal shift towards an older population has implications for how palliative care is viewed and provided
- ◆ Underlying the provision of healthcare is the concern of ageism, where the delivery of care provided is at odds with the best interests of the older adult
- ◆ The current practice of palliative care has been critiqued as oriented towards a younger population with a diagnosis of cancer
- ◆ Care needs of the older adult at the end of life present unique challenges ranging from social and medical considerations to understanding the diverse settings of care where palliation occurs.

References

(1) OECD Factbook. Economic, environmental and social statistics, population and migration, elderly population, ageing societies. 2009 [cited 14 Dec 2010]. Available from: http://puck.sourceoecd.org/vl=31265302/cl=11/nw=1/rpsv/factbook2009/01/02/01/index.htm.

(2) Christensen K, Doblhammer G, Rau R, Vaupel JW. Ageing populations: The challenges ahead. *Lancet*. 2009; **374** (9696): 1106–1208.

(3) Crimmins EM, Saito Y. Change in the prevalence of diseases among older Americans: 1984–1994. Demographic Research. 2000 [cited 14 Dec 2010]. Available from: http://www.demographic-research.org/Volumes/Vol3/9/3-9.pdf.

(4) Lafortune G, Balestat G. Trends in severe disability among elderly people: Assessing the evidence in 12 OECD countries and the future implications. OECD Health Working Papers, No. 26. 2007 [cited 14 Dec 2010]. Available from: http://www.oecd.org/dataoecd/13/8/38343783.pdf.

(5) Health Council of Canada. Why health care renewal matters: Learning from Canadians with chronic health conditions. 2007 [cited 14 Dec 2010]. Available from: http://www.healthcouncilcanada.ca/docs/rpts/2007/outcomes2/Outcomes2FINAL.pdf.

(6) Zaidi A. Poverty risks for older people in EU countries—An update. Policy brief January (11) 2010. European Centre. 2010 [cited 14 Dec 2010]. Available at: http://www.euro.centre.org/data/‾1264603415_56681.pdf.

(7) National Advisory Council on Aging, Government of Canada. Seniors on the margins. Aging in poverty in Canada. 2005 [cited 14 Dec 2010]. Available from: http://dsp-psd.pwgsc.gc.ca/Collection/H88-5-3-2005E.pdf.

(8) Rice DP, Estes CL. Health of the elderly: Policy issues and challenges. *Health Affairs*. 1984; **3** (4): 25–49.

(9) Rechel B, Doyle Y, Grundy E, McKee M. How can health systems respond to population ageing? World Health Organization. 2009 [cited 14 Dec]. Available from: http://www.euro.who.int/__data/assets/pdf_file/0004/64966/E92560.pdf.

(10) Denton FT, Spencer BG. Chronic health conditions: Changing prevalence in an aging population and some implications for the delivery of health care services. *Can J Aging*. 2010; **29** (1): 11–21.

(11) Wagner EH, Austin BT, Davis C, Hindmarch M, Schaefer J, Bonomi J. Improving chronic illness care: Translating evidence into action. *Health Affairs*. 2001; **20** (6): 64–78.

(12) MacAdam M. Frameworks of integrated care for the elderly: A systematic review. Canadian Policy Research Networks. 2008 [cited 14 Dec 2010]. Available from: http://www.cprn.org/doc.cfm?doc=-1890&l=en.

(13) Butler RH. *Why Survive? Being Old in America*. Baltimore: Johns Hopkins University Press, 2003.

(14) Alliance for Aging Research. Ageism, how healthcare fails the elderly. 2003 [cited 14 Dec 2010]. Available from: http://www.agingresearch.org/content/article/detail/694/.

(15) Centers for Disease Control and Prevention. Healthy aging: Preventing disease and improving quality of life among older Americans. 2003 [cited 14 Dec 2010]. Available from: http://www.subnet.nga.org/ci/assets/HealthyAging.pdf.

(16) Davies E, Higginson IJ. Better palliative care for older people. World Health Organization. 2004 [cited 14 Dec 2010]. Available from: http://www.euro.who.int/__data/assets/pdf_file/0009/98235/E82933.pdf.

(17) Special Senate Committee on Aging. Senate Canada. Canada's aging population: Seizing the opportunity. 2009 [cited 14 Dec]. Available from: http://www.parl.gc.ca/40/2/parlbus/commbus/senate/com-e/agei-e/rep-e/AgingFinalReport-e.pdf.

(18) Gaugler JE, Kane RA, Langlois J. Assessment of family caregivers of older adults. In RL Kane and RA Kane (eds), *Assessing Older Persons: Measures, Meaning, and Practical Applications*. Oxford: Oxford University Press, 2000, 320–59.

(19) Goldstein NE, Morrison RS. The intersection between geriatrics and palliative care: A call for a new research agenda. *J Am Geriatr Soc*. 2005; **53** (9): 1593–8.

(20) World Health Organization. WHO definition of palliative care. 2009 [cited 14 Dec 2010]. Available from: http://www.who.int/cancer/palliative/definition/en/.

(21) Kapo J, Morrison LJ, Solomon L. Palliative care for the older adult. *J Palliat Med*. 2007; **1**: 185–209.

(22) Ferrell BA, Whiteman JE. Pain. In RS Morrison and DE Meier (eds), *Geriatric Palliative Care*. Oxford: Oxford University Press, 2003, 205–29.

(23) Emanuel EJ, Fairclough DL, Slutsman J, Alpert H, Baldwin D, Emanuel LL. Assistance from family members, friends, paid care givers, and volunteers in the care of terminally ill patients. *N Engl J Med*. 1999; **341**: 956–63.

(24) Ross MM, MacLean MJ, Cain R, Sellick S, Fisher R. End of life care: The experience of seniors and informal caregivers. *Can J Aging*. 2002; **21** (1): 137–46.

(25) Sankar A. Images of home death and the elderly patient. *Generations*. 1993; **7** (2): 59–63.

(26) Brazil K, Bédard M, Willison K, Hode M. Caregiving and its impact on families of the terminally ill. *Aging Ment Health*. 2003; **7** (5): 376–82.

(27) Carter JM, Chichin E. Palliative care in the nursing home. In RS Morrison and DE Meier (eds), *Geriatric Palliative Care*. Oxford: Oxford University Press, 2003, 357–75.

(28) Miller SC, Teno JM, Mor V. Hospice and palliative care in nursing homes. *Clin Geriatr Med*. 2004; **20** (4): 717–34.

(29) Ersek M, Wilson SA. The challenges and opportunities in providing end-of-life care in nursing homes. *J Palliat Med*. 2003; **6** (1): 45–57.

(30) Oliver DP, Porock D, Zweig S. End-of-life care in U.S. nursing homes: A review of the evidence. *J Am Med Dir Assoc*. 2004; **5** (3): 147–55.

(31) Teno JM, Weitzen S, Wetle T, Mor V. Persistent pain in nursing home residents. *JAMA*. 2001; **285** (16): 2081.

(32) Hanson LC, Henderson M. Care of the dying in long-term care settings. *Clin Geriatr Med*. 2000; **16** (2): 225–37.

(33) Travis SS, Loving G, McClanahan L, Bernard M. Hospitalization patterns and palliation in the last year of life among residents in long-term care. *Gerontologist*. 2001; **41** (2): 153–60.

(34) Travis SS, Bernard M, Dixon S, McAuley WJ, Loving G, McClanahan L. Obstacles to palliation and end-of-life care in a long-term care facility. *Gerontologist.* 2002; **42** (3): 342–9.

(35) Hanson LC, Danis M, Garrett J. What is wrong with end-of-life care? Opinions of bereaved family members. *J Am Geriatr Soc.* 1997; **45** (11): 1339–44.

(36) Hanson LC, Henderson M, Menon M. As individual as death itself: A focus group study of terminal care in nursing homes. *J Palliat Med.* 2002; **5** (1): 117–25.

(37) Patterson C, Molloy W, Jubelius R, Guyatt GH, Bedard M. Provisional educational needs of health care providers in palliative care in three nursing homes in Ontario. *J Palliat Care.* 1997; **13** (3): 13–17.

(38) Teno JM, Clarridge BR, Casey V, Welch LC, Wetle T, Shield R, et al. Family perspectives on end-of-life care at the last place of care. *JAMA.* 2004; **291** (1): 88–93.

(39) Murray SA, Boyd K, Sheikh A. Palliative care in chronic illness. *BMJ.* 2005; **330**: 611–12.

(40) World Health Organization. Innovative care for chronic conditions. 2002 [cited 14 Dec 2010]. Available from: http://www.who.int/diabetesactiononline/about/iccc_exec_summary_eng.pdf.

(41) Burge J, Johnston G, Lawson B, Dewar R, Cumings I. Population-based trends in referral of the elderly to a comprehensive palliative care programme. *Palliat Med.* 2002; **16**: 255–6.

(42) Gwyther L. Just palliative care? Integrated models of care. *J Pain Symptom Manage.* 2009; **36** (5): 517–19.

(43) Morrison RS, Meier DE (eds). *Geriatric Palliative Care.* New York: Oxford University Press, 2003.

(44) Temel JS, Greer JA, Muzikansky A, Gallagher ER, Admane S, Jackson VA, et al. Early palliative care for patients with metastatic non-small-cell lung cancer. *N Engl J Med.* 2010; **363**: 733–42.

Chapter 14

A public health framework for paediatric palliative and hospice care

Kari Hexem and Chris Feudtner

Introduction

Alex is a six-year-old with progressive neurologic deterioration due to an untreatable mitochondrial disorder. Alex first became symptomatic at six months of age, and since has experienced worsening seizure disorder and mounting frailty due to impaired coughing and swallowing, with consequent respiratory compromise.

Although childhood death in the UK, the United States, and Europe is an infrequent event, the provision of paediatric health care before death, specifically or more generally in the setting of grave life-threatening illness, is none the less a public health issue, demanding not only an individualized plan of clinical care but also a population-level approach (see textbox). In this chapter, we outline a public health framework for paediatric palliative and hospice care to facilitate the focus on key public health concerns and to better understand how they apply in paediatric palliative and hospice care. Throughout the chapter, we use the fictionalized case of Alex to illustrate aspects of these tasks.

Key tenets of improving paediatric palliative care

1. Collaborate, Communicate, and Support Decision-Making

2. Minimize Distressing Symptoms

3. Provide Emotional and Spiritual Support

4. Maximize Other Quality of Life Enhancers

5. Visualize and Address the Full Population at Need

6. Provide a Continuum of Care across Multiple Sites

7. Appreciate and Manage Trade-offs Adroitly

8. Operate in Accord with an Evidence Base to Maximize Safety and Effectiveness

9. Practice the Art of Individualization

See Feudtner 2004 'Perspectives on Quality at the End of Life'(1) for further description of these tenets.

---

1. **Assessing patterns of health and disease in populations**

Alex's mitochondrial disorder has a population prevalence of 2 in 100,000 live births. While it usually affects infants, it has been known occasionally to present in older children, teenagers, and adults. Alex may remain stable for months at a time, then experience an acute crisis and subsequently recover, making it difficult to predict accurately when he will die.

To determine the public health impact of children in need of paediatric palliative care services, it is necessary first to discern the number and causes of deaths in childhood within a population, identify changes over time within a population, and compare death and disease prevalence among populations.

In the United States, where we have conducted our population-level research, the 2005 infant mortality rate was 6.89 infant deaths per 1,000 live births, which has been stable since 2002 after a steady decline for more than 40 years (2). The five most common causes of deaths in these children were accidents (42.4%), homicide (10.9%), cancer (8.4%), suicide (7.4%), and congenital malformations, deformations, and chromosomal abnormalities (4.6%) (2).

This cohort of children who die can be divided into two subgroups: children who die very rapidly from recent-onset conditions such as extreme prematurity, fulminant infections, or trauma; and those whose death is attributable to an underlying complex chronic condition (CCC) that reduces limited life expectancy.

Children with serious CCCs, who would be likely to benefit from palliative care services, may also be described in terms of age distribution and disease categories. In our own research, we have found that over 20% of childhood deaths in the United States were attributed to an underlying CCC (3). Slightly more than half (57%) of these deaths were in children less than 1 year of age. Cardiovascular (32%) and congenital/genetic (26%) conditions accounted for the majority of deaths in children less than one year of age, while in older children cancer (43%) and neuromuscular (23%) conditions were more common causes of death. Over this observation period, the number of deaths attributable to CCCs has declined, in accordance with overall declines in the total number and rate of paediatric deaths (4).

2. **Promoting wellness**

When Alex smiles and waves his hands he seems happy. Unfortunately, Alex frequently appears to be in pain. His mother has been suffering from bad headaches. Because Alex's parents spend most of their free time caring for Alex, the parents sometimes wonder how this affects Alex's older sister.

Public health has always focused on an 'upstream' approach to medical care. In accordance with this line of thinking, paediatric palliative care aims to promote wellness in children and families receiving these services by employing a multidisciplinary approach to three main components of care: pain management, quality of life enhancement, and decision-making support.

Pain and quality of life are major concerns for families caring for a child with a complex chronic condition. In semi-structured interviews with parents of children in a US intensive care unit, 64% of parents said they would consider withdrawing life-sustaining therapies if their child were suffering and 51% said they would base their decision on quality of life considerations (5). Most of the studies on pain and quality of life concerns in paediatric palliative care originate from oncology (6). Of note, though, since children at different ages and with different diseases have different experiences with pain and quality of life, further research is necessary to broaden categories of pain and quality of life concerns in paediatric palliative care, as well as to identify age and disease specific concerns.

Parents and siblings may also have a diminished quality of life when a child is very ill. For example, in a 2008 UK study on the impact of paediatric tracheostomy, 28 caregivers reported adverse effects on their sleep, relationship, social life, and ability to work (7). A 2002 meta-analysis on the effect on siblings of children with chronic illness suggested modest negative psychological effects on siblings, while recommending more 'methodologically sound studies' be conducted (8). Understanding the impact of the child's illness on their immediate family is important both for the overall well-being of the family and for planning sustainable long-term care trajectories.

In order to manage pain optimally and to improve quality of life for both the children and their families, paediatric palliative care emphasizes decision-making support. Decision-making support helps parents to identify their main goals for their child and family, address conflicts, and make a plan for the future (9,10). One important component in creating decision-making tools is the understanding of how parents approach decision-making. A quantitative study of parents of children receiving palliative care which found that both parental affect and level of hopeful thinking were important in predicting which families instituted a limit of intervention order for their child provides an excellent example of how to ground decision-making support in empirical research (11).

3. Understanding the social determinants of health

Ever since Alex's mother left her job to focus on Alex's health and complex medical care, the family has struggled to manage within a tighter budget. Although Alex's parents have been fighting more since Alex's recent hospitalization, and they worry about how Alex's siblings are doing, they none the less feel as if Alex's disease has brought them closer as a family.

When developing a care plan to address the needs of a child in a particular family, awareness of the social and economic conditions in which families live is crucial. Social and financial resources are likely to influence one another. Social resources available to families include, but are not limited to, a well-functioning family unit (12,13), the ability of individual parents to manage their own mental and physical health (14), and access to additional sources of support (15). Economic resources include parental employment and the family's financial stability (16–19), and the availability of high-quality health care coverage (20).

Families who are part of a racial or ethnic minority, are very poor, or live in a rural or otherwise resource-poor geographical area, are likely to experience greater resource constraints. For example, in a 1993 study comparing black and white parents of chronically ill children in a Southern US hospital, group differences were observed in the size of intimate networks, levels of support provided, and type of support (15).

4. Considering nested levels of influence and impact

*After contracting what appears to be a viral illness, Alex was hospitalized last week. After long delib-
eration, the family has decided to institute a DNR order for Alex, but there have been some difficulties
making sure the DNR order will be followed if Alex goes back to school.*

Multiple nested levels of influence and impact exist for each child receiving palliative care
services. The level of employers, schools, and the health care system (Level III), and the
level of government and policy (Level IV) both influence how palliative care is coordinated for a particular child within a particular family. The difficulties surrounding DNR
orders within US public schools is an excellent example of the impact of both of these
higher levels, and their effects on the child and family (21).

5. Improving quality while promoting equity

*When Alex was diagnosed, his family moved closer to a major children's hospital with a palliative care
team. With the support of this team in coordination with community-based hospice and home nursing
services, Alex lives at home. His parents feel that over the years, while his condition has worsened, the
care he receives keeps improving.*

A final key tenet of public health is the simultaneous improvement of quality and promotion
of justice. One important example of an area in which paediatric palliative care has combined these dual goals is with regard to the location of a child's care and place of death.
Most families would prefer to have their child die in the home, and in keeping with this
goal, trends over time have led to increasing numbers of home deaths in children, even as
most deaths continue to occur in hospitals (3).

Which children are more likely to die in hospitals? Infants are much more likely to die
in the hospital than older children. In 2003, 32.2% of children 10–19 years and 30.7% of
children of one to nine years of age died in the home, while only 7.3% of infants did (3).
Racial and ethnic minorities, compared with white patients, were more likely to die in
hospital (3). Although a recent retrospective study of parents of deceased children with
cancer has suggested that parental participation in planning the location of death may be
more important to parents than the location of death itself (22), the comparatively smaller
number of home deaths in racial and socio-economic minorities suggests a need for further
research to identify potential disparities that may exist.

Conclusion

Our knowledge base regarding each of these tasks has glaring gaps, and research that fills in
these gaps will be an important next step. In particular, delineating the resources and tasks
facing parents, and clarifying how the multilevel factors influence each other, will help policy
makers determine how best to create legislation and regulations to benefit these families.

Sadly but unavoidably, some children die. While minimizing the underlying causes of childhood mortality and extreme morbidity is an essential pursuit, society has an obligation to care
for children living with terminal conditions. Providing an effective public health infrastructure
that supports these children and their families is a paramount goal for paediatric palliative care.

References

(1) Feudtner C. Perspectives on quality at the end of life. *Arch Pediatr Adolesc Med.* May 2004; **158** (5): 415–18.

(2) Hamilton BE, Minino AM, Martin JA, Kochanek KD, Strobino DM, Guyer B. Annual summary of vital statistics: 2005. *Pediatrics.* Feb 2007; **119** (2): 345–60.

(3) Feudtner C, Feinstein JA, Satchell M, Zhao H, Kang TI. Shifting place of death among children with complex chronic conditions in the United States, 1989–2003. *JAMA.* 27 Jun 2007; **297** (24): 2725–32.

(4) Guyer B, Freedman MA, Strobino DM, Sondik EJ. Annual summary of vital statistics: trends in the health of Americans during the 20th century. *Pediatrics.* Dec 2000; **106** (6): 1307–17.

(5) Michelson KN, Koogler T, Sullivan C, Ortega Mdel P, Hall E, Frader J. Parental views on withdrawing life-sustaining therapies in critically ill children. *Arch Pediatr Adolesc Med.* Nov 2009; **163** (11): 986–92.

(6) Hechler T, Blankenburg M, Friedrichsdorf SJ, et al. Parents' perspective on symptoms, quality of life, characteristics of death and end-of-life decisions for children dying from cancer. *Klin Padiatr.* May–Jun 2008; **220** (3): 166–74.

(7) Hopkins C, Whetstone S, Foster T, Blaney S, Morrison G. The impact of paediatric tracheostomy on both patient and parent. *Int J Pediatr Otorhinolaryngol.* Jan 2009; **73** (1): 15–20.

(8) Sharpe D, Rossiter L. Siblings of children with a chronic illness: A meta-analysis. *J Pediatr Psychol.* Dec 2002; **27** (8): 699–710.

(9) Feudtner C. Collaborative communication in pediatric palliative care: A foundation for problem-solving and decision-making. *Pediatr Clin North Am.* Oct 2007; **54** (5): 583–607, ix.

(10) Pousset G, Bilsen J, Cohen J, Chambaere K, Deliens L, Mortier F. Medical end-of-life decisions in children in Flanders, Belgium: A population-based postmortem survey. *Arch Pediatr Adolesc Med.* Jun 2010; **164** (6): 547–53.

(11) Feudtner C, Carroll KW, Hexem KR, Silberman J, Kang TI, Kazak AE. Parental hopeful patterns of thinking, emotions, and pediatric palliative care decision making: A prospective cohort study. *Arch Pediatr Adolesc Med.* Sep 2010; **164** (9): 831–9.

(12) Kazak AE. Families of chronically ill children: A systems and social-ecological model of adaptation and challenge. *J Consult Clin Psychol.* 1989 Feb 1989; **57** (1): 25–30.

(13) Cappelli M, McGarth PJ, Daniels T, Manion I, Schillinger J. Marital quality of parents of children with spina bifida: a case-comparison study. *J Dev Behav Pediatr.* 1994 Oct 1994; **15** (5): 320–6.

(14) Heyman MB, Harmatz P, Acree M, et al. Economic and psychologic costs for maternal caregivers of gastrostomy-dependent children. *J Pediatr.* 2004 Oct 2004; **145** (4): 511–16.

(15) Williams HA. A comparison of social support and social networks of black parents and white parents with chronically ill children. *Soc Sci Med.* Dec 1993; **37** (12): 1509–20.

(16) Thyen U, Kuhlthau K, Perrin JM. Employment, childcare, and mental health of mothers caring for children assisted by technology. *Pediatrics.* Jun 1999; **103** (6): 1235–42.

(17) Einam M, Cuskelly M. Paid employment of mothers and fathers of an adult child with multiple disabilities. *J Intellect Disabil Res.* Feb 2002; **46** (Pt 2): 158–67.

(18) Schuster MA, Chung PJ, Elliott MN, Garfield CF, Vestal KD, Klein DJ. Perceived effects of leave from work and the role of paid leave among parents of children with special health care needs. *Am J Public Health.* Apr 2009; **99** (4): 698–705.

(19) Osberg JS, Kahn P, Rowe K, Brooke MM. Pediatric trauma: Impact on work and family finances. *Pediatrics.* Nov 1996; **98** (5): 890–7.

(20) Carroll JM, Torkildson C, Winsness JS. Issues related to providing quality pediatric palliative care in the community. *Pediatr Clin North Am.* Oct 2007; **54** (5): 813–27, xiii.

(21) Hone-Warren M. Exploration of school administrator attitudes regarding do not resuscitate policies in the school setting. *J Sch Nurs.* 2007 Apr; **23** (2): 98–103.

(22) Dussel V, Kreicbergs U, Hilden JM, et al. Looking beyond where children die: determinants and effects of planning a child's location of death. *J Pain Symptom Manage.* Jan 2009; **37** (1): 33–43.

Chapter 15

End-of-life care for patients with intellectual disabilities

Irene Tuffrey-Wijne, Annemieke Wagemans, and Leopold Curfs

Introduction

People with intellectual disabilities are among the most vulnerable in society. The provision of end-of-life care for people with intellectual disabilities is becoming an issue of increasing concern. This is an ageing population. Comprehensive and up-to-date morbidity and mortality data are lacking, mostly due to methodological problems (including the lack of a data base of people with intellectual disabilities in many countries). However, it is evident that with increased longevity among those with intellectual disabilities there is also a rising incidence of life-limiting illnesses such as cancer (1) or dementia (2). How are the end-of-life care needs of this group being met? Are they able to access appropriate palliative care services when they need it? The challenge facing those with intellectual disabilities in achieving equal access to palliative or end-of-life care services is the focus of this chapter.

People with intellectual disabilities

People with intellectual disabilities have a range of limitations. There are three aspects to the definition of intellectual disability: (a) significant limitations in intellectual functioning, together with (b) significant limitations in adaptive behaviour as expressed in conceptual, social, and practical skills, which (c) originate before the age of 18 (3).

An estimated 1–3% of the world population have intellectual disabilities (4). The number is rising, due partly to reduced mortality among older adults. By 2021, the number of people over the age of 50 with intellectual disabilities in England is expected to have increased by 53% (5). Despite these estimates, life expectancy remains lower than for that of the rest of the population. A mortality study in 1998 found that adults with intellectual disabilities were 58 times more likely to die before the age of 50 years than people in the general population (6).

Equity of treatment and care?

It is recognized that these shocking figures result not only from health problems relating to the underlying causes of intellectual disability, but also to the inequality of access to health services. In the UK, there has been a range of reports that have consistently high-lighted the poor quality of care for people with intellectual disabilities in both primary and acute secondary health care (7). A report into access to health care for people with learning disabilities (8) found 'appalling examples of discrimination, abuse and neglect across the range of health services [. . .] People with learning disabilities appear to receive less effective care than they are entitled to receive.'

That such discrimination exists is evident in worrying reports of people with intellectual disability being denied potentially curative cancer treatments, even when the illness is diagnosed in time. McEnhill (9) describes two cases where the decision not to give cancer treatment to people with intellectual disabilities was based on an assumption that the person could not consent to treatment; these assumptions were shown to be unfounded.

Although there is a dearth of empirical data on access to palliative care services, the available evidence suggests that referral rates to palliative care services are low (10; 11).

The challenges: reasons for poor access to palliative care services

What could be the underlying reasons for inequitable health care at the end of life? There are a range of possible contributing factors: some are inherent in the presence of intellectual disability, whilst others are part of the systems and structures of health care services.

Communication

Difficulties with communication have been consistently reported as a major obstacle in supporting people with intellectual disabilities around end-of-life care issues (12). Problems may arise due to a lack of comprehension and a lack of verbal skills, affecting assessment and the provision of psychosocial support (13). In our questionnaire survey of 959 palliative care staff in London, containing both open and closed questions (response rate 57%), one specialist palliative care nurse summed it up: 'If people aren't communicating in a normal conventional way, then there's always the danger that you're missing something. I'd be particularly concerned about psychological needs and understanding of disease and prognosis, and how one would get that information across' (11).

One likely effect of communication difficulties is a lack of timely referrals to secondary health care services.

Late referrals

One obvious reason for non-referral is late or missed diagnosis. Late presentation of the illness can result in advanced disease with severe symptomatology (12). Apart from com-munication problems (where the patient does not report symptoms clearly), there may be 'diagnostic overshadowing', where symptoms are attributed to the learning disability itself, rather than to an underlying physical illness. There may also be preventable illness as a result of inadequate screening. There is evidence of low uptake of cancer screening by people with intellectual disabilities, partly because they are less likely than the general population to be invited for screening procedures like cervical smears or mammograms (14;15).

Lack of knowledge and training

Many health service staff, including palliative care staff, have very limited knowledge about intellectual disability. The above-mentioned survey of palliative care staff in London found that two-thirds had never received any training on intellectually disability, either before or after qualifying (11). In the absences of training, there is often ignorance and fear among health care staff, reinforcing negative attitudes and values towards people with intellectual disabilities and their carers (8).

Lack of partnership working

Partnership working and communication between different agencies providing care is often highlighted in the literature as key to the provision of good end-of-life care for people with intellectual disabilities, although in practice such partnership working is often lacking (12). People with intellectual disabilities are often highly dependent on their family and paid carers (16). Although listening to the person with intellectual disabilities is paramount, family and other carers also need to be included as equal partners in care; their opinions, understanding, and assessments are important.

Capacity and consent

Many, although by no means all, people with intellectual disabilities have impaired capacity to consent to treatment and care. This clearly affects the delivery of services, and is an important issue. The law on capacity and consent to treatment varies in different countries. In England, it is the duty of health care professionals to assess capacity, and to ensure that all possible steps have been taken to enable understanding. This includes a requirement that any information is given in a format the patient can understand. However, it is likely that many health professionals lack the skills and knowledge to undertake this task. In our experience, uncertainty among health care staff about capacity to consent to treatment, and about how to proceed if such consent cannot easily be obtained, is a major obstacle in the provision of appropriate treatment and care. The real-life scenario below illustrates this. This is an issue of growing importance, as increasing numbers of people with intellectual disabilities require access to mainstream health services and face a diagnosis that warrants treatment decisions. Further research is clearly needed about assumptions made by health care professionals about the capacity of people with intellectual disabilities to understand information about diagnosis, prognosis and treatment options, and about the extent to which such assumptions influence health care decisions.

Case study: Agnes Kramer

Agnes Kramer was a 67-year-old woman with mild intellectual disabilities, who lived with her brother and his family in the Netherlands, following the death of their mother. She attended a local day centre and managed well at home, occupying herself with knitting and doing the laundry. She had been complaining increasingly about a painful hip; when, a few months later, she started to lose weight as well, she was admitted to hospital for investigations. Unfortunately, the pain in her hip was not caused by an infection as was initially thought, but by secondary cancer. Ms Kramer had had an operation for breast cancer several years earlier.

The results of the tests were discussed with her family but not with Ms Kramer herself–the hospital team did not think she would be able to understand. She was transferred to a residential care centre for people with intellectual disabilities in order to get stronger. The hospital referral letter stated: 'Because of her intellectual disabilities, this lady is not eligible for chemotherapy. Adequate pain relief please.' When staff at the centre talked to the family, it seemed they had not understood that Ms Kramer's prognosis was poor and that her cancer would not be treated. Further conversations with the family were needed to explain what was happening; this was made more difficult by complicated relationships between Ms Kramer's various siblings. Further possibilities for chemotherapy treatment were investigated by the centre, but Ms Kramer deteriorated rapidly. She died a month later. Nobody ever discussed her prognosis with her—her family was highly protective and did not want anyone to talk to her about dying, even though the staff believed it would be better to do so.

Ms Kramer's final months were characterized not only by the consequences of the late presentation of her cancer recurrence, but also by a lack of discussion about the decision to forego treatment. It appears that this non-treatment decision was based not only on Ms Kramer's medical situation, but also on a (quite possibly erroneous) decision by doctors that she would not be able to make treatment decisions, or cope with chemotherapy. It may well be that, after careful discussion with Ms Kramer and her family, the decision to give only palliative treatment would still stand; however, the lack of such discussion, and the refusal of the family to discuss her situation with her, deprived Ms Kramer from the opportunity to make her wishes known. This is not only poor practice: in some countries, including England and Wales, it is even against the law not to involve someone like Agnes, who is likely to be able to make choices if the options are explained clearly and simply, in decisions around treatment and care.

Conclusion

The specific needs of people with intellectual disabilities at the end of life are getting more attention; one example of such interest is the emergence of the Palliative Care for People with Learning Disabilities Network (www.pcpld.org), where professionals from any specialty can share experiences and resources. However, there are still huge inequalities, and possibly even discrimination. Some improvements can and should be made by individual services and practitioners, in particular in ensuring that they make 'reasonable adjustments' in order to meet the needs of people with intellectual disabilities. Such adjustments include the need to modify communication (for example, using simple sentences and pictures), allowing extra time, including the family and other carers as partners in care, finding creative ways to meet individual needs, and liaising with other service providers. This alone is not enough: there also needs to be a commitment at regional and national level to provide policies and guidelines for services around inclusion of people with intellectual disabilities, and to support training initiatives.

How good services are at providing appropriate end-of-life care for this highly vulnerable group is certainly a measure of how well they address inequalities overall.

References

(1) Hogg J, Tuffrey-Wijne I. Cancer and intellectual disabilities: A review of some key contextual issues. *Journal of Applied Research in Intellectual Disabilities* 2008; **21** (6): 509–18.

(2) Visser F, Aldenkamp A, van Huffelen A, Kuilman M, Overweg J, van Wijk J. Prospective study of the prevalence of Alzheimer-type dementia in insitutionalized individuals with Down Syndrome. *American Journal on Mental Retardation* 1997; **101** (4): 400–12.

(3) Schalock R, Borthwick-Duffy S, Bradley V, Buntinx W, Coulter D, Craig E, et al. *Intellectual Disability: Definition, Classification, and System of Supports*, 11th edn. Washington: AAIDD, 2010.

(4) Mash E, Wolfe D. *Abnormal Child Psychology*, 3rd edn. Belmont: Thomson Wadsworth, 2004.

(5) Emerson E, Hatton C. *People with Learning Disabilities in England*. Lancaster: Centre for Disability Research, 2008.

(6) Hollins S, Attard MT, von Fraunhofer N, McGuigan S, Sedgwick P. Mortality in people with learning disability: Risks, causes, and death certification findings in London. *Developmental Medicine & Child Neurology* 1998; **40** (1): 50–6.

(7) Disability Rights Commission. Equal Treatment: Closing the Gap—A Formal Investigation Into Physical Health Inequalities Experienced by People with Learning Disabilities and/or Mental Health Problems. London: Disability Rights Commission, 2006.

(8) Michael J. *Healthcare for All: Report of the Independent Inquiry into Access to Healthcare for People with Learning Disabilities*. London: Aldrick Press, 2008.

(9) McEnhill L. Disability. In D Oliviere and B Monroe B (eds), *Death, Dying and Social Differences*. Oxford: Oxford University Press, 2004, 97–118.

(10) Speet M, Francke A, Courtens A, Curfs L. *Zorg rondom het levenseinde van mensen met een verstandelijke beperking: een inventariserend onderzoek* ('End-of-life care for people with intellectual disabilities: A scoping study'). Utrecht: Nivel, 2006.

(11) Tuffrey-Wijne I, Whelton R, Curfs L, Hollins S. Palliative care provision for people with intellectual disabilities: a questionnaire survey of specialist palliative care professionals in London. *Palliative Medicine* 2008; **22** (3): 281–90.

(12) Tuffrey-Wijne I, Hogg J, Curfs L. End-of-life and palliative care for people with intellectual disabilities who have cancer or other life-limiting illness: A review of the literature and available resources. *Journal of Applied Research in Intellectual Disability* 2007; **20** (4): 331–44.

(13) Tuffrey-Wijne I, McEnhill L. Communication difficulties and intellectual disability in end-of-life care. *International Journal of Palliative Nursing* 2008; **14** (4): 192–7.

(14) Davies N, Duff M. Breast cancer screening for older women with intellectual disability living in community group home. *Journal of Intellectual Disability Research* 2001; **45** (3): 253–7.

(15) Sullivan SG, Hussain R, Slack-Smith LM, Bittles AH. Breast cancer and the uptake of mammography screening services by women with intellectual disabilities. *Preventative Medicine* 2003; **37**: 507–12.

(16) Tuffrey-Wijne I. Exploring the lived experiences of people with learning disabilities who are dying of cancer. *Nursing Times* 2010; **106** (19): 15–18.

Chapter 16

End-of-life care for people who live in rural or remote areas versus those who live in urban areas

Donna M. Wilson and Deepthi Mohankumar

Introduction

The purpose of this chapter is to highlight groups that are under-served and otherwise disadvantaged at the end of life. The focus will be primarily on people who live in rural or remote areas. Despite some important benefits to living and dying outside metropolitan areas, rural/remote persons are often disadvantaged as they reach the end of life, and in many different ways. Although it is impossible to highlight all global issues, this chapter summarizes relevant current research and emphasizes key aspects of rural/remote inequity for attention. Some comparative points about urban under-served groups are also made, as it would be unfair to categorize all people who live in or near cities as having better end-of-life care chances than rural/remote persons.

The need to understand and address rural/remote inequities

Inequity is essentially a lack of fairness, with some individuals or groups less privileged than others. Health inequities are concerning because health is fundamentally important to all people and health inequities are often avoidable (1). Health inequities or disparities, as outlined by the National Centre on Minority Health and Health Disparities (2) in the United States, are *'differences in the incidence, prevalence, mortality, burden of diseases and other adverse health conditions or outcomes that exist among specific population groups [...] Health disparities can affect populations groups based on gender, age, ethnicity, socioeconomic status, geography, sexual orientation, disability or special health care needs and occur among groups who have persistently experienced historical trauma, social disadvantage or discrimination, and systematically experience worse health or greater health risks than more advantaged social groups.'* Despite global health advances, disparities in the burden of death and illnesses affecting disadvantaged populations continue to exist, but especially among rural/remote peoples worldwide (3–5).

Rural/remote communities are often characterized by their distance from urban areas or population density. For instance, 'rural' people are defined by Statistics Canada as individuals living in towns and municipalities outside the commuting zone of larger urban centres with populations of 10,000 or more (6). Another common definition is an

OECD one which categorizes rural communities as those with fewer than 150 inhabitants per square kilometre (6). Although some rural people live in the countryside on farms or ranches, many live in towns or villages; some live in remote areas such as hunting lodges. This chapter combines rural and remote peoples into one population group, despite differences across and among them.

Rural/remote versus urban differences in health and health care

Although rural/remote areas are often thought of as healthy places to live, rural/remote populations are typically not as healthy as urban ones (4). A recent report on the health of rural/remote Canadians revealed lower levels of health across virtually all measures, and with personal health risk-taking (i.e. lack of seatbelt use and smoking rates) at much higher levels (3). As Canada has a publicly-funded health care system, these health differences result in higher health care utilization rates for rural/remote Canadians (7). In countries without accessible publicly funded health care, great disparity between health care needs and health care utilization is evident (4).

According to the World Health Organization (5) many preventable health risks are now evident worldwide, e.g. obesity and the complications associated with it like type-2 diabetes and inactivity leading to heart disease and stroke (5). Obesity is particularly prevalent among rural/remote populations in developed and developing countries (8). With accident or injury rates also high (9), avoidable disabilities and sudden or unexpected deaths are common. However, as rural/remote people typically have a significant burden of morbidity from higher chronic illness rates (3–5), their end-of-life care and support needs are often more pronounced and prolonged than those of urban peoples.

Although higher poverty rates, lower education levels, and other socio-demographic differences help explain greater rural/remote health inequity (4), health care quality and access issues are also important. Rural/remote persons often have few local health care services, and some lack local access to even the most basic services (10,11). People living in rural/remote areas must usually travel to urban centres for health care, as local health care services have remained undeveloped or have shifted to urban areas. Health care specialists and modern diagnostic and treatment options are typically centred in cities now. This consolidation greatly disadvantages rural/remote terminally-ill persons. Not only are they typically less healthy and wealthy, but they must often repeatedly travel greater distances for health care over the course of a terminal illness. This travelling is too burdensome for some, with the result that they do not obtain the care they need.

Some rural/remote communities are active, however, in ensuring local end-of-life support (12–14). Hospital beds for respite and end-stage dying are in greater supply in some Canadian rural/remote areas than urban areas, e.g. in towns where leaders have actively advocated for hospitals to open or remain open (15). Transportation to and from cities for health care is also provided at little or no cost to rural/urban individuals in some communities. It is also important to note that rural/remote populations may be more accepting of death and dying, perhaps in keeping with their closer connections to nature, with this attitude impacting how death and dying are understood and addressed. A study of 'good' rural/remote deaths found death and dying are common and openly addressed in rural/remote communities, with community connectedness and group responsibility for community members being significant 'good death' factors (15). Another study found more openness among rural/remote health care providers and patients about the transition from curative to palliative care (16). This acceptance may help ensure services exist locally (15). Rural/remote people, for instance, may initiate a hospital visiting and home or farm maintenance programme to help community members. Funds may be raised to build and operate a hospice.

Rural/remote trends

Two important interrelated trends are also increasing end-of-life inequity among rural/remote populations: urbanization and rural/remote population changes. In developing and developed countries, there is marked migration from rural/remote areas to cities, with new immigrants also typically settling into cities; only 20% of Canadians and 17% of Americans now live in rural/remote areas (3,17). Most rural/remote areas globally have had a decline in real population numbers, and mainly as a result of younger residents seeking education and work in metropolitan areas (18). This youth migration reduces local family support networks, and travelling home to help ill or dying persons may be prohibitively time consuming and expensive (19,20). Urbanization has also contributed to the consolidation of health care in cities, as hospitals and other expensive health care services are more justifiable there.

Rural/remote population changes comprise another important trend. Rural/remote population aging, one of the most important changes, is mainly occurring because of the movement of younger persons to cities (21). Some rural/remote areas are also attractive for retirement. Over time, rural/remote areas tend to develop higher proportions of very old single women, as females typically live longer than males (21). Older women are at great risk of unmet care needs as they often outlive their spouses and have children who relocate. Not only do rural/remote areas need to provide more aged care, but they also need to prepare for more death and dying, as death is largely an event of old age. In addition, as new immigrants settle into cities, rural/remote areas are increasingly populated by the descendants of original settlers, often farmers, ranchers, and small business operators. These people differ from urbanites in a number of ways, including working into later life; having to seek health care in cities is a problem as it takes them away from their livelihoods (22).

Rural/remote areas are also prime locations for Aboriginal persons (22). Aboriginal persons have typically been disadvantaged through long-standing poverty and cultural discrimination. They have distinct historically-based health and health care preferences that are little understood by policy-makers and health care professionals. Aboriginal and other rural/remote persons who are used to living in sparsely populated areas experience considerable anxiety when travelling to and within cities for health care, in part because this care is from strangers (15).

End-of-life supports are important, as most deaths today are not sudden and unexpected. Terminal illnesses are usually characterized by declining health, sudden transitions in health, and changing care needs. A literature review revealed the problem that rural/remote terminally-ill persons spend a considerable amount of time outside their communities, with death occurring at times in distant city hospitals (23). Not only do rural/remote people want to die in their homes or home communities, but deaths in cities could mean few if any family members are present (15).

Dying people are among the most vulnerable in any society, and so it is concerning that rural/remote people have some additional barriers that reduce their chances of achieving 'good' deaths (15). As suggested by Gomes and Higginson (24), there is urgency in understanding rural/remote factors that influence achieving a 'good' death. Future research will be particularly important for helping to bring to the forefront differences in rural/remote versus urban palliative care expectations and preferences (14). Regardless of the current minimal amount of evidence to assist planning for 'good' rural/remote deaths, cultural sensitivity and individualized care are imperative (15,23).

Metropolitan issues

People living in metropolitan areas, particularly those in substandard inner city housing and the homeless, face similar end-of-life challenges (25). Urban poverty is linked to ill health and reduced health care access, with new immigrants often poor, and thus at high risk of illnesses and inadequate health care (18). Poor urbanites are disadvantaged in many ways, such as through having to spend disproportionately more for trips to obtain health care. Poor urbanites also have less ability to take time off work to care for ill and dying family members, and they are more greatly impacted when paying for the medications and supplies that are required for terminal illnesses and home-based deaths. This point is important, as home deaths are preferred now in both urban and rural/remote areas, but with families often receiving little assistance to fulfil this preference. Although poverty has been raised as a major barrier to good urban deaths (25); any urbanite with race/ethnic, language, cultural, or other barriers can be at a disadvantage when needing end-of-life care.

Conclusion

Many rural/remote populations and some urban sub-populations have inequities that disadvantage them when ill, with end-of-life inequities highly concerning. It is important for researchers to increase understanding of these inequities, so that services for terminally-ill persons and their families better meet the needs of under-served populations. At the same time, researchers and others must remain cognizant of the fact that all dying people are vulnerable to unmet care and support needs, and thus at risk of avoidable 'bad' deaths.

References

(1) Pan American Health Organization. Health inequities. 2004. Available from: http://www.paho.org/english/dd/ais/be_v25n4-inequity_journal_health.htm.

(2) National Centre on Minority Health and Health Disparities. NIH health disparities strategic plan and budget [Internet]. No date. Available from: http://ncmhd.nih.gov/about_ncmhd/index2.aqsp.

(3) Canadian Institute for Health Information. How healthy are rural Canadians? An analysis of their health status and health determinants. Ottawa: CIHI; 2006.

(4) Hartley D. Rural health disparities, population health and rural culture. *Am J Public Health*, 2004; **94** (10): 1675–8.

(5) World Health Organization. Global health risks. Mortality and burden of disease attributed to selected major risks. Geneva: Author; 2009.

(6) du Plessis V, Beshiri R, Bollman RD, Clemenson H. Definitions of 'rural'. Ottawa: Statistics Canada, Agricultural Division; 2002. Catalogue no. 21-006-MIE–No. 061.

(7) Sanchez M, Vellanky S, Herring J, Liang J, Jia H. CIHI survey: Variations in Canadian rates of hospitalization for ambulatory care sensitive conditions. *Healthcare Quarterly* 2008; **11** (4): 20–2.

(8) Abubakari AR, Lauder W, Jones C, Kirk A, Agyemang C, Bhopal RS. Prevalence and time trends in diabetes and physical inactivity among adult West African populations: The epidemic has arrived. *Public Health* 2009; **123** (9): 602–14.

(9) Wang SY, Li YH, Chi GB, Xiao SY, Ozanne-Smith J, Stevenson M, Phillips MR. Injury-related fatalities in China: An under-recognised public-health problem. *Lancet* 2008; **372** (9651): 1765–73.

(10) Ansari Z, Laditka JN, Laditka SB. Access to health care and hospitalization for ambulatory care sensitive conditions. *Med Care Res Rev* 2006; **63** (6): 719–41.

(11) World Health Organization. The World Health Report 2008—Primary Health Care (Now More Than Ever). Geneva: Author; 2008.

(12) Kelley ML. Developing rural communities' capacity for palliative care: A conceptual model. *J Palliat Care* 2007; **23** (3): 143–53.

(13) McGrath P, Hollewa H, McGrath Z. Practical problems for aboriginal palliative care service provision in rural and remote areas: Equipment, power and travel issues. *Collegian: J Royal College Nurs Australia* 2007; **14** (3): 21–6.

(14) Wilson DM, Justice C, Sheps S, Thomas R, Reid P, Leibovici K. Planning and providing end-of-life care in rural areas. *J Rural Health* 2006; **22** (2): 174–81.

(15) Wilson DM, Fillion L, Thomas R, Justice C, Bhardwaj P, Veillette A. The 'good' rural death: A report of an ethnographic study in Alberta, Canada. *J Palliat Care* 2009; **25** (1): 21–9.

(16) Van Vorst RF, Crane LA, Barton PL, Kutner JS, Kallail KJ, Westfall JM. Barriers to quality care for dying patients in rural communities. *J Rural Health* 2006; **22** (3): 248–53.

(17) United States Department of Agriculture. State Fact Sheets: United States. 2010. Retrieved from http://www.ers.usda.gov/statefacts/us.htm.

(18) Galea S, Freudenberg N, Vlahov D. Cities and population health. *Soc Sci Med* 2005; **60** (5): 1017–33.

(19) Dennett A, Stilwell J. Population turnover and churn: Enhancing understanding of internal migration in Britain through measures of stability. *Popul Trends* 2008; **134**: 24–41.

(20) Hoi le V, Phuc HD, Dung TV, Chuc NT, Lindholm L. Remaining life expectancy among older people in a rural area of Vietnam: Trends and socioeconomic inequalities during a period of multiple transitions. *BMC Public Health* 2009; **9**: 471.

(21) United Nations. World population ageing: 1950–2050. No date. Available from: http://www.un.org/esa/population/publications/worldageing19502050/.

(22) Clemenson H, Bollman R. Structure and change in Canada's rural demography: An update to 2006. Ottawa: Statistics Canada, Rural and Small Town Canada Analysis Bulletin 2008; **7** (7), catalogue no. 21-006-XWE2007007.

(23) Thomas R, Wilson DM, Justice C, Birch S, Sheps S. A literature review of preferences for end-of-life care in developed countries by individuals with different cultural affiliations and ethnicity. *J Hospice & Palliat Nurs* 2008; **10** (3): 142–63.

(24) Gomes B, Higginson IJ. Where people die (1974–2030): Past trends, future projections and implications for care. *Palliat Med* 2008; **22**: 33–41.

(25) Houttekier D, Cohen J, Bilsen J, Addington-Hall J, Onwuteaka-Philipsen B, Deliens L. Place of death in metropolitan regions: Metropolitan versus non-metropolitan variation in place of death in Belgium, the Netherlands and England. *Health and Place* 2010; **16** (1): 132–9.

Chapter 17

Social inequalities at the end of life

Jonathan Koffman

Taking a human rights-based approach to palliative and end-of-life care

Palliative care now encompasses a wide range of specialist services, but began in the UK in the 1960s with the development of the modern hospice movement by Dame Cicely Saunders when she founded St Christopher's Hospice in Sydenham, London. The number of hospices and specialist palliative care services has increased rapidly since that time. In 1980, there were fewer than 80 in-patient hospices and 100 home support teams in the UK and the Republic of Ireland. By 2010 this had increased to 220 in-patient hospices comprising approximately 2,500 beds, 417 home care and extended home care support teams, and 282 day care centres along with more than 307 hospital support teams (1). Whilst the actual supply of specialist palliative care plays a role in determining which patients with progressive disease and their families receive care, concerns have been raised about other factors influencing the accessibility of care at the end of life for all those who might benefit from it.

This chapter appraises the evidence, principally from the UK and the USA, to determine in which ways the 'socially excluded'—the poor, black, and minority ethnic (BME) groups, asylum seekers and refugees, the homeless, those within the penal system, and drug users—fare with respect to accessing specialist palliative care and related services during advanced disease and at the end of life. Other socially excluded populations, older people, and those with intellectual disabilities are examined in detail elsewhere in this book. However, this list of those who could be deemed 'socially disenfranchised' is not exhaustive; among other groups are travelling communities and those who abuse alcohol. To date, however, little attention and therefore published research has focused on either their met or unmet palliative care needs, testimony to their social distance from the mainstream. This chapter then makes suggestions how those involved in public health policy and the delivery of palliative care and related services can extend care to include these disadvantaged groups.

What is social exclusion and what are its causes?

The concept of equality of access to health care is a central objective of many health care systems throughout the world and has been an important pillar of the United Kingdom National Health Service since its inception in 1948. In the early 1970s, Julian Tudor Hart coined the phrase 'inverse care law' to describe the observation that those who were in the greatest apparent need of care often had the worst access to it (2). Although this is not true of the whole health system, a growing body of evidence has accumulated demonstrating that socially disenfranchised sections of society fare poorly with regard to secondary and tertiary medical care, including people with advanced disease and their families. At the very end of the previous century, commitment to tackle health inequalities has been harnessed under the wing of 'social exclusion' (3) which includes poverty and low income but is broader, addressing some of the wider causes and consequences of social deprivation.

Social exclusion is something that can happen to anyone though people from certain backgrounds and experiences are more likely to suffer; older people are particularly at risk. People from black and minority ethnic communities are disproportionately exposed to risk of social exclusion; they are more likely than others to live in deprived areas and in over-crowded housing, more likely to be poor and unemployed—regardless of age, sex, qualifications, and place of residence—and more likely to report ill health than white people (4). None of these risk categories are mutually exclusive and may operate in combination with others at any time.

Who are the 'excluded' at the end-of-life?

Palliative care, free-at-the-point-of-delivery from the NHS and the independent charitable sector, has become more prominent within the UK and other countries in the developed world. Nevertheless, it has still been slow to reach certain patients and population groups who could benefit from it. Below I examine the available evidence on access to palliative care by poor and other disenfranchised population groups.

The poor

> Poverty means going short materially, socially and emotionally. It means spending less on food, on heating, and on clothing than someone on average income . . . Above all, poverty takes away the tools to build the blocks of the future and steals away the opportunity to have a life unmarked by sickness, a decent education, a secure home and a long retirement. ((5), p. 3)

Britain leads western Europe in its poverty, with twice as many poor households as Belgium, Denmark, Italy, Holland, or Sweden (6). While overall personal income rose substantially in the 1980s and 1990s, the gap between the richest and the poorest has grown dramatically (7). Evidence from studies suggests that poverty influences the overall experience of those at the end of life in a number of ways.

Firstly, dying can be an expensive business, involving frequent trips to hospital, hospital clinics, GPs, pharmacies, in addition to purchasing aids, loss of income, and loss of future income for any dependant. The legacy of poverty also extends beyond death causing financial worries which have been shown to lead to psychological distress (8).

Secondly, studies have shown that between 50% and 70% of patients would prefer to be cared for at home for as long as possible, and to die at home given the choice (9). However, there is growing evidence that place of death is closely related to socio-economic status; those living in poor areas are less likely to die at home, whereas the probability of death in hospital appears to increase as area deprivation increases (10).

Thirdly, the delivery of specialist palliative care services is accessed more often by those occupying higher social-economic groups. If services are available to those in poorer groups, in order to achieve the same outcomes of care nearly twice as many resources are required by service providers compared with areas where deprivation is lower (11).

Fourthly, poverty can significantly contribute to shaping people's knowledge and expectations of palliative care and related services. This may have consequences for the up-take of services at the end of life and during bereavement. Recent research conducted among oncology patients identified that those living in materially and socially deprived areas were more that eight times less likely to understand what palliative care was than those living in more affluent areas. Moreover, knowledge of Macmillan nurses and their contribution towards the care of people with advanced cancer was seven times less likely, even after taking other factors into consideration (12).

The homeless mentally ill

It is well known that the environments of homelessness are extremely hazardous and contribute to higher levels of physical and mental health morbidity and mortality. The homeless lack customary and regular access to conventional housing and include people living in shelters, on streets, in abandoned buildings, in subways, or in other places not intended as dwellings (13). As many as a third may suffer from serious and persistent mental illness (SPMI) problems (14). Providing palliative and end-of-life care to a homeless seriously mentally ill person is particularly challenging because continuity and follow-up are extremely difficult if the patient is not living in a stable environment. For persons with SPMI living on the streets with a terminal illness, their bleak life circumstances may also contribute to their rapid decline. Hopelessness may be associated with the early stages of severe physical illness; there is a correlation between adverse life events and the onset of serious illness and death (15). Moreover, many homeless people are cut off from their families of origin; providing home hospice care in which family members may offer con-siderable help becomes highly challenging if not impossible.

People with dementia

Dementia is a term used to describe various different brain disorders that have in common a loss of brain function that is usually progressive and eventually severe. In recent years dementia has become a major concern for all developed countries and the number of people with this condition has increased steadily. Dementia can legitimately be seen as a terminal illness (16). Families typically describe poor advance care planning and inadequate symptom control, with distress associated with pain, pressure sores, constipation, restlessness and shortness of breath. It is exceptional for these patients to spend their last days in a hospice, and any involvement of formal palliative care services is still unusual (17). Research has indicated that older people with dementia dying on an acute medical ward in a London hospital were less likely to be referred to palliative care teams than patients who are cognitively intact, and were prescribed fewer palliative medications. Further, few patients had their spiritual needs assessed or addressed while they were dying (18).

People from black and minority ethnic groups

Ethnicity is difficult to define, but most definitions reflect self-identification with cultural traditions that provide both a meaningful social identity and boundaries between groups (19).

Although there is a significant lack of data about people from minority ethnic communities, the available data from the UK, USA, and Australia confirm that some BME groups experience high levels of social and economic disadvantage. People from minority ethnic communities also suffer the consequences of overt and inadvertent racial discrimination—individual and institutional—and an inadequate recognition and understanding of other complexities they may experience, for example barriers like language, cultural, and religious differences (20;21). They also experience 'social invisibility' where routinely collected data from a number of sources is partially or completely inadequate. For example, death registration certificates only record country of origin or country of birth, not ethnicity. Hospital minimum data set (MDS) information and cancer registration data frequently omit self-assigned ethnicity; classifications of ethnic difference may be outdated or applied incorrectly (22;23).

Health system level factors such as poor access to health care services have been reported among BME groups in the United Kingdom, USA, and Australia (24–28). This is also an issue for end of life care where the impact of ageing on BME groups now means larger numbers of older members within these communities will require health services for advanced disease. A limited number of descriptive reports exist and have identified poor access to appropriate care at the end of life for these communities. Low rates of cancer were seen as one explanation for low uptake of service provision (29), but the figures were likely to have been inaccurate because of inadequate ethnic monitoring (30).

Recent studies have alluded to inadequate knowledge about end-of-life care among BME communities living in the USA and UK (12;31) . Participants in Born et al.'s study of African Americans and Latinos revealed 'an overwhelming lack of awareness of hospice, and what it had to offer' (32). Randhawa and Owens' focus groups of Sikh women living in Luton in the UK were aware of hospice, but none were familiar with the term 'palliative care' or of Macmillan nursing care (33). The International Observatory on End-of-Life Care that monitors the global development of hospice and palliative care services around the world reports that palliative care and related services suggest this may be attributed to the lack of comparable services in under-developed and medium developed countries compared with Europe and English-speaking countries (34); immigrants may not have had exposure to or knowledge of palliative care services provided by hospices or other health care institutions in their home countries.

Refugees and asylum seekers

Estimating the total number of refugees and asylum seekers worldwide is extremely difficult as definitions differ widely. In the UK, refugees are defined as those granted permission to stay in the UK under the terms of the 1951 Refugee Convention because of a well-founded fear of persecution due to race, religion, nationality, political opinion, or membership of a social group (35). Asylum seekers are those who have submitted an application for protection under the Geneva Convention and are waiting for the claim to be decided by the Home Office. There were around 25,670 applications for asylum in the UK in 2008, a 10% increase on the previous year; many are located in London (36). It is extremely difficult to obtain demographic information on refugees and asylum seekers at the local level in the UK, making development of services accessible to these groups difficult (37).

Although refugees and asylum seekers are often grouped together they are not necessarily a homogenous group, and have varying experiences and needs (38). Many refugees have health problems, for example parasitic or nutritional diseases (39), and diseases such as hepatitis, tuberculosis, and HIV and AIDS, which frequently overlap with problems of social deprivation. Their health problems are also amplified by family separation, hostility and racism from the host population, poverty, and social isolation.

Individuals from sub-Saharan Africa, many of whom may be refugees and asylum seekers, make up the second largest group of people affected by HIV in the UK (40). They are more likely to be socially disadvantaged and isolated, much less aware of the healthcare to which they are entitled, and more likely to present only when symptomatic. Experience has demonstrated that this patient group continues to require palliative care despite the advances made with highly active anti-retroviral therapy (HAART) because they tend to present late with AIDS-related illnesses and have higher rates of tuberculosis, both of which are linked to a poorer prognosis. For many patients who do not have a GP and are reluctant to register with one, lack of a stable home environment and reluctance to access local services may mean that dying at home is not an option (41).

Drug users

There is very little literature on how drug users utilize specialist palliative care services. Most research has looked at how pain is managed among patients with cancer or AIDS, comparing pain reports and adequacy of analgesic therapy in patients with AIDS with and without a history of substance abuse (42–44). A single exploratory study in the USA explored the experiences of hospices providing care to intravenous HIV/AIDs drug users (43). The survey revealed that the provision of community palliative care was frequently problematic because of poor living conditions, many of which were considered unsafe to visit. Differences have also been found in psychological distress and adequacy of pain treatment. Patients with substance abuse also had higher levels of depression and psychological distress, fewer sources of support, and significantly lower quality of life, and were less likely to receive adequate pain medication (42).

It has been suggested that drug users require a modified health care system which understands and considers their particular problems and that the initiation and maintenance of contact may require a variety of initiatives (45). Morrison and Ruben (46) similarly argue that services need to deliver care to these groups in imaginative and innovative ways which are not judgmental and encourage contact without reinforcing traditional stereotypes. Without appropriate services, they argue, high levels of mortality amongst drug users will continue.

Prisoners

As of July 2010 there were an estimated 85,400 prisoners in England and Wales of whom 13,134 were serving indeterminate sentences (47). Historically, prison healthcare has been organized outside the National Health Service. This has given rise to questions about equity, standards, professional isolation and whether the Prison Service has the capacity to carry out its healthcare function (48).

To date, very little United Kingdom literature has focused on the palliative care needs of prisoners and what has is largely descriptive or relates to single case histories. More research has taken place in the USA where a number of palliative care programmes have been developed for prisoners, for example the Louisiana State Penitentiary at Angola (49). This is largely because in Louisiana sentencing laws are tougher than in any other State and the courts hand out a large number of life sentences where parole is rarely granted. As a result an estimated 85% of Angola's 5,200 inmates will grow old and die in prison (49).

There are a number of problems in introducing palliative care into prisons, not least the mutual distrust between staff and prisoners. Effective symptom control, particularly adequate pain control, can be difficult under these circumstances, and drugs to manage pain control may be used for illicit purposes. In addition, visiting by family and friends can be restricted, not least because the prison may be located at some distance from them.

The magnitude of the problem: implications for palliative care policy and service development

Since the introduction of the National Health Service in the UK, and in other countries where social welfare has become commonplace, health care has been widely extended across many sections of the population. However, universal access to care and treatment has remained elusive at the end of life.

Palliative care provided by the modern hospice movement, despite laudable aspirations to extend the right to care as widely as possible, has been shown to be inequitable on a number of fronts. This chapter has explored evidence that population and patients groups silent in life remain so during death. If we view the public health of the end of life as 'the science and art of preventing suffering and promoting quality of life of the terminally ill and their families through the organized efforts of society' (50) there are many potential solutions to the problems outlined in this chapter. However, none will be successful in isolation. Firstly, the knowledge and attitudes of health and social care professionals about which populations are socially excluded and how to engage with them, must be improved. This concern can be addressed, in part, through the conduct of a comprehensive needs assessment be it epidemiological, comparative, or corporate including the meaningful collation and interpretation of experiences and views from a variety of sources (51) including the views of patients and informal carers and providers of care, as well as purchasers and planners.

Second, there is an urgent need to raise public awareness of palliative care services and to provide public education about the care provided, to reduce any misconceptions that may be influencing access to services (12). Innovative approaches to disseminating relevant information about patient and care related issues and local palliative care services could contribute to raising awareness of relevant services. NHS Direct, the national nurse-led telephone helpline, represents an example (52). However, current evidence indicates it has been underused by older people, ethnic minorities, and other disadvantaged groups (53). Widening the user base of the helpline requires a deeper understanding of appropriate and acceptable methods of sharing information.

Lastly, some consider the charitable sector to be uniquely suited to supporting new ideas that extend care to the point where they can be accepted and integrated into society, becoming the social norm rather than the exception. In the USA, the Robert Wood Johnson Foundation has been successful in pump-priming pilot projects that have increased awareness of, and access to, palliative care among socially deprived communities (54) and, despite differences in the funding arrangements of care, in recent years the UK has followed suit. At a UK level, *Help the Hospices* is working with representatives from local hospices and other key organizations on a Widening Access Project (WAP) aiming to work with local adult and children's hospices to reduce the barriers to hospice and palliative care that people face as a result of social exclusion.

References

(1) Help the Hospices. Hospice and Palliative Care Directory: United Kingdom and Ireland 2009–2010. London: Help the Hospices, 2010.

(2) Hart JT. The inverse care law. *Lancet* 1971; **1**: (7696): 405–12.

(3) Barratt H. Website of the week: The health of the excluded. *BMJ* 2001; **323**: 240.

(4) Acheson D. *Independent Inquiry into Inequalities in Health Report*. London: The Stationery Office, 1998.

(5) Oppenheim C. *Poverty: The Facts*. London: Child Poverty Action Group, 1990.

(6) Shaw M, Davey Smith G, Dorling D. Health inequalities and New Labour: how the promises compare with real progress. *BMJ* 2005; **330**: 1016–21.

(7) Office for National Statistics. Social Trends. London: HMSO, 2000.

(8) Koffman J, Donaldson N, Hotopf M, Higginson IJ. Does ethnicity matter? Bereavement outcomes in two ethnic groups living in the United Kingdom. *Palliative and Supportive Care* 2005; **3**: 183–90.

(9) Gomes B, Higginson IJ. Home or hospital: Choices at the end of life. *J R Soc Med* 2004; **97** (9): 413–14.

(10) Beccaro M, Costantini M, ISDOC Study Group. Inequity in the provision of and access to palliative care for cancer patients. Results from the Italian survey of the dying of cancer (ISDOC). *BMC Public Health* 2007; **7** (66).

(11) Clark C. Social deprivation increases workload in palliative care of terminally ill patients. *BMJ* 1997; **314**: 1202.

(12) Koffman J, Burke G, Dias A, Ravel B, Byrne J, Gonzales J, et al. Demographic factors and awareness of palliative care and related services. *Palliative Medicine* 2007; **21** (2): 145–53.

(13) Kushel MB, Miaskowski C. End-of-life care for homeless patients: 'She says she is there to help me in any situation'. *JAMA* 2006; **296**: 2959–66.

(14) Hughes A. The poor and underserved. In BR Ferrell and N. Coyle (eds) *Textbook of Palliative Nursing*. New York: Oxford University Press, 2001, 461–6.

(15) Sims A. Why the excess mortality from psychiatric illness? *BMJ* 1987; **294**: 986–7.

(16) Addington-Hall JM. *Positive Partnerships: Palliative Care for Adults with Severe Mental Health Problems*. London: National Council for Hospices and Specialist Palliative Care Services, 2000.

(17) Bayer A. Death with dementia: The need for better care. *Age and Ageing* 2006; **35** (2): 101–2.

(18) Sampson EL, Gould V, Lee D, Blanchard MR. Differences in care received by patients with and without dementia who died during acute hospital admission: A retrospective case note study. *Age and Ageing* 2006; **35**: 187–9.

(19) Koffman J, Crawley L. Cultural aspects of palliative medicine. In G Hanks, N Cherny, M Falloon, S Kaasa, and R Portenoy (eds), *Oxford Textbook of Palliative Medicine*, 4th edn. Oxford: Oxford University Press, 2008.

(20) Anonymous. Personal view: Trying to overcome racism in the NHS. *BMJ* 2000; **320**: 357.

(21) Coker N. Understanding race and racism. In N Coker (ed.), *Racism in Medicine: An Agenda for Change*. London: King's Fund Publishing, 2001, 1–22.

(22) Koffman J, Higginson IJ. Minority ethnic groups and *Our healthier nation*. *Journal of Public Health Medicine* 2000; **22** (2): 245.

(23) Thames Cancer Registry. *Cancer in South East England 2004: Cancer Incidence, Prevalence, Survival and Treatment of Residents of South East England*. London: Thames Cancer Registry, King's College London, 2006.

(24) Blendon RJ, Schoen C, DesRoches CM, Osborn R, Scoles KL, Zapert K. Inequities in health care: A five-country survey. *Health Affairs* 2002; **21** (3): 182–91.

(25) Department of Health. *Inequalities in Health: Report of an Independent Inquiry Chaired by Sir Donald Acheson*. London: The Stationary Office, 1998.

(26) Dyer O. Disparities in health widen between rich and poor in England. *BMJ* 2005; **331**: 419.

(27) Harding S, Maxwell R. Difference in mortality of migrants. In F Drever and M Whitehead (eds), *Health Inequalities: Decennial supplement Series DS no.15*. London: The Stationary Office, 1997.

(28) O'Neill J, Marconi K. Access to palliative care in the USA: Why emphasize vulnerable groups? *Journal of the Royal Society of Medicine* 2001; **94**: 452–4.

(29) Hill D, Penso D. Opening doors: Improving access to hospice and specialist palliative care services by members of the black and ethnic minority communities. London: National Council for Hospice and Specialist Palliative Care Services; 1995. Occasional Paper 7.

(30) Aspinall PJ. Ethnic groups and *Our healthier nation*: whither the information base? *Journal of Public Health Medicine* 1999; **21**: 125–32.

(31) Higginson IJ, Koffman J. Public health and palliative care. *Clinics in Geriatric Medicine* 2005; **21**: 41–5.

(32) Born W, Allen Greiner K, Sylvia E, Butler J, Ahluwalia J. Knowledge, attitudes, and beliefs about end-of-life care among inner-city African Americans and Latinos. *Journal of Palliative Medicine* 2004; **7** (2): 247–56.

(33) Randhawa G, Owens A. The meanings of cancer and perceptions of cancer services among South Asians in Luton, UK. *British Journal of Cancer* 2004; **91**: 62–8.

(34) International Observatory on End of Life Care. Global Development. 2006.

(35) Office of the High Commissioner for Human Rights. *Convention Relating to the Status of Refugees*. Geneva: Office of the High Commissioner for Human Rights, 1951.

(36) Home Office. *Monthly Assylum Statistics May 2010*. London: Home Office, 2010.

(37) Bardsley M, Hamm J, Lowdell C, Morgan M. Developing health assessment for black and minority ethnic groups: Analysing routine health information. London: Health of Londoners Project, 2000.

(38) Burnett A, Fassil Y. Meeting the Health Needs of Refugees and Asylum Seekers in the UK: An Information and Resource Pack for Health Workers. London: Department of Health' 2002.

(39) Jones D, Gill PS. Refugees and primary care: Tackling the inequalities. *BMJ* 1998; **317**: 1444–6.

(40) Brogan G, George R. HIV/AIDS: Symptoms and the impact of new treatments. *Palliat Med* 1999; **1** (4): 104–10.

(41) Easterbrook P, Meadway J. The changing epidemiology of HIV infection: New challenges for HIV palliative care. *J R Soc Med* 2001; **94** (442): 448.

(42) Breitbart W, Rosenfeld B, Passik M, Kaim M. A comparison of pain report and adequacy of analgesic therapy in ambulatory AIDS patients with and without a history of substance abuse. *Pain* 1997; **72**: 235–43.

(43) Cox C. Hospice care for injection drug using AIDS patients. *The Hospice Journal* 1999; **14** (1): 13–24.

(44) Morgan B. Knowing how to play the game: Hospitalized substance abusers' strategies for obtaining pain relief. *Pain Management Nursing* 2006; **7** (1): 31–41.

(45) Brettle RP. Injection drug use-related HIV infection. In MW Adler (ed.), *ABC of AIDS*, 5th edn. London: BMJ Publishing, 2001.

(46) Morrison CL, Ruben SM. The development of healthcare services for drug misusers and prostitutes. *Postgrad Med J* 1995; **71**: 593–7.

(47) Ministry of Justice. Ministry of Justice Statistics Bulletin: Population in custody monthly tables June 2010 England and Wales. London: Ministry of Justice, 2010.

(48) Joint Prison Service & National Health Service Executive Working Group. *The Future Organisation of Prison Health Care*. London: Department of Health, 1999.

(49) Project for Dying in America. Dying in prison: a growing problem emerges from behind bars. *PDIA Newsletter* **3**, 1–3. 1998. Project for Dying in America. Ref Type: Magazine Article.

(50) Deliens L. Public health (research) at the end of life. *Progress in Palliative Care* 2007; **15** (2): 103–7.

(51) Koffman J, Harding R, Higginson IJ. Palliative care: The magnitude of the problem. In G Mitchell (ed.), *Palliative Care: A Patient Centred Approach*. London: Routledge, 2008, 7–34.

(52) Department of Health. *The New NHS: Modern, Dependable*. Cmd 3807. London: Stationary Office, 1997.

(53) George S. NHS Direct audited. *BMJ* 2002; **324**: 558–9.

(54) Gibson R. Palliative care for the poor and disenfranchised: A view from the Robert Wood Johnson Foundation. *J R Soc Med* 2001; **94**: 486–9.

Part VI

End-of-life care policies

Chapter 18

Design, implementation, and evaluation of palliative care programmes and services with a public health WHO perspective

Xavier Gómez-Batiste, Jose Espinosa,
M. Pau González-Olmedo, Marisa Martínez-Muñoz,
Cristina Lasmarias, Anna Novellas, Elba Beas,
Josep Porta-Sales, Jordi Trelis, Candela Calle,
and Jan Stjernsward

Introduction

As illustrated in Chapter 1, health care systems face the challenge of responding to demographic and epidemiological changes. In most countries, 60% to 75% of the population will die from a chronic disease characterized by a limited prognosis, a progressive evolution and frequent crises of needs. Such diseases cause suffering and are associated with high demand and use of health and social resources.

Modern palliative care started with British hospices in the 1960s. A very adequate model of care and organization to look after terminal patients and their families was developed. In the 1980s this model was extended to different levels of the health care system.

From the 1990s onwards the WHO has been proposing palliative care as a key element of health care systems, inserted into mainstream planning and organization. Accordingly, WHO Public Health Palliative Care Programmes were implemented. These programmes were defined as the systematic application of several measures to improve the care of advanced and terminal patients and their families at a population level either at the sector, regional or national level.

In this chapter, the principles, aims, and elements of WHO Public Health Programmes are described.

Palliative Care Public Health Programmes (PCPHPs)
Definitions and concepts

Palliative Care Public Health Programmes (PCPHPs) are defined as the systematic measures taken with the aim of improving the quality of care for advanced and terminal patients and their families in a population-based context (either at national, regional, or district levels). Their main aims are coverage for all, equity, and quality of palliative care. Most PCPHPs are led by the Health Administration in cooperation with organizations and professionals. The WHO Demonstration Projects (or pilot projects to implement National Plans in a specific context) were designed in the 1990s to elaborate a systematic approach and evaluation with the aims of generating evidence (1–3) and following the recommendations of international bodies (4,5).

Vision, values, aims, and elements of PCPHP (6,7)

The vision of a PCPHP consists of developing a comprehensive system to look after patients with advanced and terminal conditions to promote their adequate care and quality of life.

The principles and values of PCPHPs are based on the consideration of quality end-of-life care (EOLC) as a Human right (8) (Box 18.1), and the support of people in vulnerable conditions with respect for their values and preferences.

The aims consist of the development of a system of care inserted into the health care system.

The elements of PCPHPs are listed in the Box 18.2 (7).

Context analysis and needs assessment, and clear definition of the characteristics of the target population

To implement a PCPHP efficiently, targeting it to the actual needs of a population, a context analysis is done. The context analysis can include demographic, social, geographic aspects, and data about the organization, funding, and capacity of existing health care services. In countries having existing palliative care services, a qualitative analysis can be useful to assess the situation.

Box 18.1 Principles of PCPHPs

- Model of care: based on patients' and families' needs
- Model of organization: based on a competent interdisciplinary team, with clinical ethics, case management, and advance care planning
- Based on population needs and adapted to demography and settings in the health care system
- Community oriented
- Good care as a human right
- Coverage, equity, access, and quality to every patient in need of it
- Quality: effectiveness, efficiency, satisfaction, continuity, sustainability
- Systematic evaluation of results, accountability, evidence
- Social interaction

Box 18.2 Components of PCPHPs

- Clear leadership
- Needs and context assessment
- Clear model of care and intervention and definition of the target patients
- General measures in conventional services (especially primary care)
- Specialist services in settings
- Sectorized networks with coordination, continuing, and emergency care
- Education and training at all levels
- Research planning
- Availability and accessibility of opioids and essential drugs
- Legislation, standards, budget and models of funding and purchasing
- Evaluation and improvement of quality
- Evaluation of results, indicators
- Action plans at short, mid, and long term
- Social implication: volunteers, social involvement in the cultural, social, and ethical debates around the end of life

In most developed countries with an ageing population (more than 15% over 65) an average mortality rate of 9/1,000 per year can be assumed, of which 60–75% die from a chronic advanced progressive illness (9,10). The proportion of cancer vs non-cancer within this group is around 1:1.5 or 1:2.

Estimation of prevalence is relevant as most chronic conditions other than cancer can have a longer advanced period in need of palliative measures (11–13). Prevalence of patients with advanced cancer averages at about 0.1–0.2% and of non-cancer chronic advanced diseases at 1.2–1.4%.

Once the mortality and prevalence are estimated, the proportion of target patients in need of palliative care specialist interventions can also be estimated at around 60% for cancer and 30–60% for non-cancer.

In countries with low income and fragile health care systems, many patients are diagnosed at an advanced phases of disease, and a community approach could be the best choice, as has been shown in Kerala (12). In Latin America, most countries have a fragmented health care system and palliative care needs to be adapted to the different organizations (14). In former Soviet Union countries, palliative care and geriatric care can be useful cornerstones of reforms of the health care system (15). In Middle and South African countries, the AIDS epidemic is the most relevant need (16), whereas in developed countries the ageing population and cancer are the most frequent needs.

In order to define the target patients and assess the need for palliative measures in individual patients and in settings of conventional health care services, the adapted version of the

Gold Standards Framework (GSF) (17) could help to determine the prevalence of advanced patients. Population-based surveys can also provide a good insight (18).

General palliative care measures in conventional health care services

The WHO Collaborating Centre for Public Health Palliative Care Programmes at the Catalan Institute of Oncology (WHOCC-ICO) has proposed a number of measures to improve the care of patients in conventional services having a high prevalence of advanced-terminal patients with any condition. Some of the recommendations are shown in Table 18.1. This implementation of general measures does not exclude the need for specialist services to care for patients with more complex palliative needs (19).

Table 18.1 Proposed measures in conventional services: primary care, oncology, geriatrics, nursing homes (WHOCC-ICO, 2009). Gómez-Batiste X, et al. *How to design and implement Palliative Care Public Health Services: Foundation measures* available at: http://www.iconcologia.net/catala/qualy/centre_projectes.htm

Aim	Primary Care	Hospital Care
Improving the capacity of professionals	Basic and intermediate training in Palliative Care	
Identification of patients in need (Gold Standards Framework) Registries	Identification of patients in need Use of GSF Clinical charts with registries (symptom checklist, etc.), assessment tools, etc.	
Internal and external reference professionals	Specific reference professionals (doctors, nurses, others) with advanced training and dedication to palliative care	
Improving accessibility to patients and families	Promotion of home care Phone support programmes Access to rapid consultation Direct access to palliative care beds information Free access of families to hospital	
Improving continuing care and emergency care	Advance care planning, continuing care, 24-hour phone access, preventive attitude, tailored emergency care, direct access to PC beds	
Specific times and places for patients and families	Specific times for advanced patients and families	Specific outpatients times for advanced patients and families Advanced terminal patients grouped in units
Improving family care	Education and support for careers Prevention and treatment of complicated bereavement	
Promotion of teamwork	Team meetings Team support and prevention of burnout	
Promotion of privacy and dignity	Individual bedrooms	
Assessing and improving the quality of care	Policies: pain, last days, etc. EoL inserted into the quality assessment	
Coordination and integrated care with Specialist Palliative Care Services	Criteria of intervention and shared care with PCSs Nurses able to demand services	

Implementation of palliative care services

The WHO prescribes several steps in the implementation of specialist palliative care services (20). Initially, the main goal is to set up a solid core and diversified nucleus of services and professional leaders who could offer results in the short term and spread knowledge. Support teams in cancer centres or in the community are good examples. At this phase, feasibility due to local conditions (leadership, institutional support) is the most relevant factor for success. In a more advanced phase, the aims will consist of spreading and diversifying types of services and then achieving coverage.

Specialist palliative care services can be defined as interdisciplinary teams with advanced training, devoted to advanced and terminal patients and their families, which practise the model and process of care and are clearly identified by patients, families, and other services. There are different levels and types of services: support teams (in hospital, at home or both), palliative care units (beds), outpatient clinics, day hospitals, and hospices. These services and activities can be undergone in any setting within the health care system. A comprehensive palliative care network is a system of palliative care services offering all the services in a district and acting in an integrated way. Reference palliative care services produce advanced training and research and are usually located in university hospitals. We use the term *transitional measures* when there is a specific implementation of a trained professional in a conventional service not fulfilling the criteria of a specialist team, but devoted to palliative care. Good examples are specialist nurses (e.g. the Macmillan Nurses in the UK) or individual reference doctors in oncology or primary care services. These measures are frequently the first step in the development of a service.

The WHOCC-ICO recommended standards of specialist services are listed in the Box 18.3.

Every palliative Care service must have a Strategic Plan (21) (Figure 18.1). During the initial phases, the most relevant factors are the adequate leadership, the selection and specialist training of the team and the internal and external consensus. The training ought to include the clinical aspects, for all members, and the organizational (leadership, quality, business planning) aspects, for leaders.

Box 18.3 Standards of specialist services in developed countries

- 1 Support Team accessible in all institutional settings
- 1 Home Care Support Team/100,000–150,000 inhabitants
- 1 Hospital Support Team + Outpatient's clinic in Hospitals
- 80–100 palliative care beds/million inhabitants (20–30% in Acute care, 40–50% in Mid-stay, and 30–40% in Nursing Homes)
- Reference services with Hospital Support team, Palliative Care Unit, research and education in University Hospitals and Cancer centres
- Sectorized models (metropolitan, urban, rural)

Gómez Batiste X, Espinosa J, Marisa Martínez-Muñoz, Jordi Trelis, and Candela Calle. *How to design and implement Palliative Care Public Health Programmes: Foundation measures* available at: http://www.iconcologia.net/catala/qualy/centre_projectes.htm

Funding and purchasing palliative care (22,23)

Elaborating a global budget for palliative care is strongly advisable. Palliative care funding and/or purchasing must be included in the general health care models in each country. There are several ways of funding/purchasing services, whether based on structure, activity, results or combinations of all, to encourage quality, education, and research.

Palliative care services are believed to be very efficient in developed countries, due to their impact on the reduction of hospital stays, emergencies, and costs in the last months of life by means of avoiding over-treatment. Published data on the costs and savings of a regional palliative care programme (22) show that, at the regional level, the palliative care network is self-financed, because it saves more resources than it costs.

Training strategies (24)

Training is one of the cornerstones of any plan. Levels of clinical training must be defined: high or specialist for full time professionals, intermediate for professionals dealing with high proportions of palliative patients in their specialist training, and basic for all professionals. Additionally, it is very important to train leaders in organizational leadership and team leadership as well. There are several phases of a strategy for training. Initially, the main objective is to build up a core nucleus of leaders and pioneering experiences. Once this is established, they can be referents for the training of other specialist and conventional services. The final aim should be to achieve full appropriate coverage of all the levels needed in every setting.

Accessibility and availability of opioids and other necessary drugs

Useful basic drugs for palliative care, including opioids (25), are well-defined. Strong opioids are needed for treating severe cancer pain, and oral morphine is the drug of choice, because of its effectiveness and low cost, combined with other measures (26–29).

There are two main levels of barriers to adequate pain management, medical and regulatory. The medical barriers are due to the lack of training and persistent myths about opioids (dependency, enhancing death, worsening of respiratory failure), and must be addressed by education and training. The regulatory barriers are related to the links with illegal narcotics traffic.

A comprehensive approach to guaranteeing the accessibility of opioids for cancer pain must include the regulatory aspects, the training of professionals, and the funding to guarantee availability irrespective of the economic status of patients (30,31).

In the meantime, until legislation is available, some measures can be implemented to facilitate access, at least for palliative care services. There are other barriers to the availability and use of opioids, more related to ignorance and prejudice, which need to be addressed by training, policies, and protocols.

There are examples of successful policies for improving access and availability of opioids in developing countries (32–34).

Legislation, standards, models of financing, and purchasing services

There are multiple referents for and examples of legislation, standards, and models for financing palliative care, including laws, decrees, and orders, at all levels. In Catalonia a very short decree regulates the funding and purchasing of palliative care, as well as the standards and definitions of services, and a Spanish Ministerial Order regulates the availability of opioids. Additionally, Catalonia has introduced access to good palliative care in the Catalan Estatut (Statute of Autonomy) (35). In most Spanish regions, there are specific regional plans for palliative care.

Evaluation of results and quality improvement of Palliative Care Programs

The evaluation of results of a PCPHP must be done systematically and regularly. There are two methods for evaluation: quantitative and qualitative. For both, it is fundamental to define beforehand the definition of terms of indicators and the sources of data.

To make a quantitative evaluation of a programme, several quality indicators can be used, those of structure, process, or results. Key results of a PCPHP (36) are the total figures of *specialist services* the patients attended and the *direct coverage* (% of patients looked after by specialist services), the *geographical coverage* (% of districts having available palliative care services), the *accessibility*, the *opioid consumption* (In DDD). As for the services, the outputs (length of stay, length of intervention, characteristics of patients, mortality, etc.), their quality (37), their *clinical results* (effectiveness) (38) and cost/efficiency (39), the global costs (22), the satisfaction of patients and families, the number of professionals trained, and the coverage for the levels of training can be measured.

The qualitative evaluation of the services of PCPHPs can be done in several ways. A systematic methodology has been developed for the evaluation and improvement of the quality of palliative care in conventional or specialist services, and for Public Health Programmes. This methodology is based on a SWOT (Strong Points, Weaknesses or Areas for Improvement, Harms and Opportunities) analysis, followed by the definition of objectives, actions and timeframes for every dimension by means of building up a systematic quality improvement plan.

Expected results of Public Health Programmes

There are several examples of results obtained through PCPHPs in different scenarios (see: (3, 40–43)).

In Catalonia, the WHO Demonstration Project of palliative care implementation was designed in 1989 and rapidly implemented. It has produced four quantitative evalua-tions, i.e. one every five years (44), and three qualitative evaluations. Their experience of international cooperation with 36 countries has been recognized by the WHOCC-ICO (45). Its main aim is to spread the Public Health WHO perspectives for palliative care by supporting organizations and ministries in the design, implementation, and evaluation of programmes, as well as to generate experience and evidence. There are three more

WHO Collaborating Centres devoted to palliative care: the Cicely Saunders Institute at King's College in London, the Sobell House Centre in Oxford, with long and prestigious experience in clinical training, and the Pain Policy Centre in Wisconsin. The role of WHO Collaborating centres is to give support to the WHO and other organizations in the development of palliative care and the generation and dissemination of experience and evidence.

Conclusions and recommendations

In order to face the challenge posed by 60–75% of the population dying from chronic progressive diseases, palliative care must be one of the priority elements of any public health system, since access to good palliative care at the end of life is considered as a basic human right. There are solid examples of how PCPHPs have achieved results in different regions or countries, with common aims of coverage, equity, and quality, and which have developed elements including needs assessment, the implementation of specialist services, measures in conventional services, legislation and standards, opioid availability, funding, training, research and evaluation of results. There are valid indicators for monitoring the evolution of programmes.

The WHO has adopted a strong role in the promotion and spreading of palliative care as a main issue in health care systems. There is solid evidence of its global and individual effectiveness, efficiency, cost efficiency and its satisfactory results and defined indicators and standards of quality. Furthermore, palliative care adds value to a health care system, as the comprehensive approach, the interdisciplinary approach, the model of care, the ethical decision-making, and the value of helping people in difficult situations all serve to improve the quality of the whole health care system.

Palliative care as an indicator of dignity and a basic human right

The development of palliative care is an excellent indicator of the respect of any society or/ and organization for the dignity of persons in the vulnerable end-of-life situation, and access to good palliative care must be considered as a human right for any person in need of it (46), in every place, at any time.

References

(1) Gómez-Batiste X, Fontanals MD, Roca J, Stjernswärd J, Trias X. Palliative care in Catalonia 1990–95. *Palliat Med*. 1992; **6**: 321–7.

(2) Kumar SK. Kerala, India: A regional community-based palliative care model. *J Pain Symptom Manage* 2007; **33** (5): 623–7.

(3) Fainsinger RL, Brenneis C, Fassbender K. Edmonton, Canada: A regional model of palliative care development. *J Pain Symptom Manage* 2007; **33** (5): 634–9.

(4) Palliative Care: The Solid Facts. Copenhagen. WHO regional Office for Europe. 2004. http://www.euro.who.int/publications. Accessed June 2010.

(5) Xavier Gómez-Batiste and Silvia Paz. Public palliative care: Review of key developments and implementation issues. *Current Opinion in Supportive and Palliative Care* 2007, **1**: 213–17.

(6) Stjernsward J, Gómez-Batiste X. Palliative Medicine—The global perspective: Closing the know-do gap. In: Walsh D (ed.), *Palliative Medicine*. Philadelphia: Elsevier, 2008, 2–8.

(7) Gómez-Batiste X, Porta-Sales J, Paz S, Stjernsward J, and Rocafort J. Program development: Palliative medicine and public health services. In: Walsh D (ed.), *Palliative Medicine*. Philadelphia: Elsevier, 2008, 198–202.

(8) Estrategia Cuidados Paliativos del Sistema Nacional de Salud. Ministerio Sanidad y Consumo, Madrid 2007. Available at www.estrategiaencuidadospaliativos.es. Accesed June 2010.

(9) McNamara B, Rosenwax LK, Holman CD. A method for defining and estimating the palliative care population. *J Pain Symptom Manage* 2006; **32**: 5–12.

(10) Xavier Gómez-Batiste, Jose Espinosa, Josep Porta, y Enric Benito. Modelos de atención, organización y mejora de calidad para la atención de enfermos avanzados terminales y sus familias: la aportación de los cuidados paliativos. *Med Clin* (Barcelona). 2010; **135** (2): 83–9.

(11) Sanz Ortiz J, Gómez Batiste X, Gómez Sancho M, Núñez Olarte JM. Cuidados Paliativos. Recomendaciones de la Sociedad Española de Cuidados Paliativos. Madrid: Ministerio de Sanidad y Consumo, 1993.

(12) Franks PJ, Salisbury C, Bosanquet N, et al. The level of need for palliative care: A systematic review of the literature. *Palliat Med.* 2000; **14**: 93–104.

(13) Addington-Hall J, McCarthy M. Regional study of care for the dying: Methods and sample characteristics. *Palliat Med.* 1995 Jan; **9** (1): 27–35.

(14) Wenk R, Bertolino M. Palliative care development in south America: A focus in Argentina. *Journal of Pain and Symptom Management* 2007; **33** (5): 645–50.

(15) Muszbek K. Enhancing Hungarian palliative care delivery. *Journal of Pain and Symptom Management* 2007; **33** (5): 605–9.

(16) Jagwe J, Merriman A. Uganda: Delivering analgesia in Rural Africa: Opioid availability and nurse prescribing. *Journal of Pain and Symptom Management* 2007; **33** (5): 547–51.

(17) Available at www.goldstandardsframework.nhs.uk. Accessed June 2010.

(18) Gomez-Batiste X, et al. Morir de cáncer en Catalunya: estudio poblacional del último mes de vida de enfermos de cáncer. *Med Pal* 2001; **8** (3): 134–7.

(19) Palliative Care Australia. A guide to palliative care Service development: A population-based approach 2003. www.pallcare.org.

(20) X.Gómez-Batiste. Programas Públicos de Cuidados Paliativos. En: Organización de servicios y programas de Cuidados Paliativos. Eds: Xavier Gómez-Batiste, Josep Porta, Albert Tuca, Jan Stjernsward. Madrid: ARAN, 2005, 153–78.

(21) X.Gómez-Batiste. Modelos de organización en cuidados paliativos. En: Organización de servicios y programas de Cuidados Paliativos. Eds: Xavier Gómez-Batiste, Josep Porta, Albert Tuca, Jan Stjernsward. Madrid: ARAN, 2005, 55–80.

(22) Paz-Ruiz S, Gómez-Batiste X, Espinosa J, Porta-Sales J, and Esperalba J. The costs and savings of a regional palliative care program: The Catalan experience at 18 years. *J Pain Symptom Manage* 2009; **38** (1): 87–96.

(23) Callaway M, Foley K, De Lima L, Connor SR, Dix O, Lynch T, Wright M, Clark D. Funding for palliative care programs in developing countries. *Journal of Pain and Symptom Management* 2007; **33** (5): 509–13.

(24) X Gómez-Batiste, D Sánchez, L Guanter, et al. Area de Capacitación Específica (ACE) y Diploma de Acreditación Avanzada (DAA) en Medicina Paliativa. Documento SECPAL. *Jornadas de Formación SECPAL*, pp. 7-34. Madrid: ARAN, 2005.

(25) De Lima L, Krakauer E, Lorenz K, Praill D, MacDonald N, Doyle D. Ensuring palliative medicine availability: The development of the IAHPC list of essential medicines for palliative care. *J Pain Symptom Manage.* 2007; **33** (5): 521–6.

(26) Hanks GW, de Conno F, Cherny N, Hanna M, et al. Morphine and alternative opioids in cancer pain: The EAPC recommendations. *British Journal of Cancer* (2001); **84** (5): 587–93.

(27) World Health Organization, Cancer pain relief and palliative care: Report of the WHO expert committee on cancer pain relief and active supportive care (Technical Report Series 804). Geneva: World Health Organization, 1990.

(28) Joranson DE, Ryan KM. Ensuring opioid availability: Methods and resources. *J Pain Symptom Manage.* 2007; **33** (5): 527–32.

(29) World Health Organization, Achieving balance in national opioids control policy: Guidelines for assessment, World Health Organization, Geneva (2000). Available from http://www.painpolicy. wisc.edu/publicat. Accessed December 2010.

(30) Aaron M. Gilson Chapter 14: Laws and policies affecting pain management . In *Bonica's Management of Pain*, 4th edn, 2010, pp. 165–83. Available in http://www.painpolicy.wisc.edu/publicat. Accessed December 2010.

(31) David E. Joranson, Karen M. Ryan, Martha A. Maurer. Opioid policy, availability, and access in developing and nonindustrialized countries. In *Bonica's Management of Pain,* 4th edn, 2010, pp. 194–208. Available in http://www.painpolicy.wisc.edu/publicat. Accessed December 2010.

(32) Mosoiu D, Mungiu OC, Gigore B, Landon A. Romania: Changing the regulatory environment. *J Pain Symptom Manage.* 2007; **33** (5): 610–14.

(33) D. Mosoiu, K.M. Ryan, D.E. Joranson, and J.P. Garthwaite, Reforming drug control policy for palliative care in Romania, *Lancet* 367 (2006) (9528): 2110–17. Available from http://www.painpolicy. wisc.edu/publicat. Accessed December 2010.

(34) D.E. Joranson, M.R. Rajagopal, and A.M. Gilson. Improving access to opioid analgesics for palliative care in India. *J Pain Symptom Manage* 2002; **24** (2): 152–9. Available from http://www.painpolicy. wisc.edu/publicat/. Accessed December 2010.

(35) Parlament of Catalonia. Organic Law 6/2006 of 19 July, on the Reform of the Statute of Autonomy of Catalonia. Article 20.1. Available at www.gencat.cat/parlament. Accessed September 2010.

(36) Gómez-Batiste X, Ferris F, et al. Ensure quality public health programmes. A Spanish Model. *Eur J Palliat Care* 2008; **15** (4): 195–9.

(37) Gómez-Batiste X, Ferris F, et al. Ensure good quality palliative care. A Spanish Model. *Eur J Palliat Care* 2008; **15** (3): 142–7.

(38) Gómez-Batiste X, Porta J, Tuca A, Pérez FJ, Pascual A, Espinosa, J, et al. Symptom control effectiveness in advanced cancer patients cared by Spanish palliative care teams: A nation-wide study. 5th EAPC Research Forum, Trondheim (Norway), May 2008. Abstract ID 350.

(39) X Gómez-Batiste, Albert Tuca, Esther Corrales, et al. Resource consumption and costs of palliative care services in Spain: A multi-center prospective study. *J Pain Symptom Manage.* 2006; **31** (6): 522–32.

(40) S Kaasa, M Jorhoy, D Haugen. Palliative care in Norway: A national public health model. *J Pain Symptom Manage.* 2007; **33** (5): 599–604.

(41) Davaasuren O, Stjernswärd J, Callaway M, Tsetsegdary G, Hagan R, Govind S, et al. Mongolia: Establishing a national palliative care program. *J Pain Symptom Manage.* 2007; **33** (5): 568–72.

(42) Stjernswärd J, Ferris F, Khleif S, Jamous W, Treish I, Milhem M, et al. Jordan palliative care initiative: A WHO demonstration project. *J Pain Symptom Manage.* 2007; **33** (5): 628–33.

(43) Herrera E, Rocafort J, De Lima L, Bruera E, García-Peña F, Fernández-Vara G. Regional palliative care program in Extremadura: An effective public health care model in a sparsely populated region. *J Pain Symptom Manage.* 2007; **33** (5): 591–8.

(44) Xavier Gómez-Batiste, Josep Porta-Sales, Antonio Pascual, Maria Nabal, Jose Espinosa, Silvia Paz, Cristina Minguell, Dulce Rodríguez, Joaquim Esperalba, Jan Stjernsward, and Marina Geli. Catalonia WHO Palliative Care Demonstration Project at 15 Years (2005). *J Pain Symptom Manage.* 2007; **33** (5): 584–90.

(45) Available at http://www.iconcologia.net/Qualy. Accessed December 2010.

(46) Brennan F. Palliative care as an international human right. *J Pain Symptom Manage.* 2007; **33**: 494–9.

Chapter 19

Public health policy regarding end-of-life care in sub-Saharan Africa

Julia Downing and Richard Harding

Introduction

Over one billion people live in Africa, i.e. 14% of the world's population (1). The continent has diverse characteristics, populations, languages, cultures, health care systems, access to medications, policies, and resources. The differences between countries in sub-Saharan Africa (SSA) and the remaining African countries are great, and this chapter will focus mainly on palliative care in countries in SSA which consists of 45 countries (Figure 19.1) and has just over 10% of the world's population.

There is wide disparity across SSA in terms of health systems and the resources available for health care. The average per capita government expenditure on health across Africa in 2007 was $34. Where government spending on health care is low and individuals are also unable to pay for private health care, a public health challenge is posed across the region (2). Health care is often provided through multiple systems including the public sector, insurance-based services, and the private sector. Whilst the exact methods of service delivery vary, public health services are often free of charge and based around a system of specialist, regional, district and home-based care, relying on comprehensive and effective referral systems. These services are supplemented and supported by services provided by the private sector and also non-governmental and/or faith-based organizations. In many countries in SSA, challenges to the delivery of health care are the inequalities and the differential access to services, with many poorer households excluded from accessing affordable and quality health care (3).

In the absence of well-resourced public health care, and poor and patchy access to palliative care (4), the provision of care often falls to the family, who may themselves be HIV infected, and care may be being provided by children. Care of family members with progressive diseases involves significant cost to the family e.g. in terms of transport, loss of earnings, loss of the ability to provide for the family through growing food, and the loss of school fees and the time to attend school.

The need for palliative care

The burden of progressive disease in SSA is great, with both communicable (primarily HIV) and non-communicable (primarily cancer) diseases. The average life expectancy in

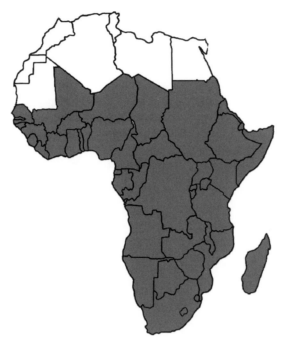

Fig. 19.1 Map of sub-Saharan Africa.

Africa in 2008 was just 53 years, 23 years less than in the Americas, with people in Zimbabwe having the lowest life expectancy in the World at just 42 years (2).

SSA continues to be heavily affected by HIV. The prevalence rate of HIV in SSA in 2008 was 5.2%—by 2009 there were an estimated 22.2 million people living with HIV and AIDS in SSA. Of these, 1.8 million were children with 390,000 new infections in children in 2008 alone (5). In Swaziland, nearly 1 in 5 infections were in children (6). Thus SSA accounted for 67% of infections worldwide, 72% of AIDS-related deaths, 68% of new infections amongst adults, and 91% of new infections among children (5).

Out of the 12.7 million new cases of cancer worldwide in 2008, 551,200 were in SSA with 421,000 cancer-related deaths (7)—25% of these cancers were related to infectious diseases compared with less than 10% in developed countries (8). The five most common cancers in the region are cervix, breast, liver, Kaposi's sarcoma, and prostate. It is anticipated that the number of new cases of cancer worldwide will increase to 15 million by 2020 and that SSA will bear the burden of the increase in incidence, morbidity, and mortality (9). Between 70% and 80% of people with cancer in Africa are diagnosed with late stage disease (10) and this, alongside a lack of accessibility to treatment (9), means accessibility to life-saving treatment is often not possible (11), thus underlining the need for palliative care services for the multi-dimensioned problems experienced.

Whilst HIV and cancer are key factors in the need for the provision of quality palliative care services across SSA, individuals with other chronic diseases such as heart disease, kidney disease, chronic obstructive airways disease, diabetes etc also benefit from palliative care.

Table 19.1 Distribution of causes of death in Uganda 2002 (13)

Causes of death	Number of deaths x 1,000
Infectious and parasitic diseases	888,6
Respiratory infections	160,4
Maternal conditions	32,2
Perinatal conditions	64,5
Nutritional deficiencies	17,5
Malignant neoplasms	49,8
Other neoplasms	1,1
Diabetes mellitus	9,0
Endocrine disorders	3,0
Neuropsychiatric conditions	10,6
Sense organ diseases	–
Cardiovascular diseases	126,6
Respiratory diseases	31,8
Digestive diseases	19,0
Genito-urinary diseases	11,4
Skin diseases	4,9
Musculoskeletal diseases	0,3
Congenital anomalies	6,6
Oral conditions	–
Unintentional injuries	66,8
Intentional injuries	49,3

This is particularly important as there is an increase in chronic life-limiting conditions in the region (12). (See Table 19.1 and Figure 19.2.)

Public health priorities for palliative care

In identifying the public health priorities for palliative care in SSA it is important to focus on the entire population, on the community as a whole, and not on individual patients or diseases. Due to the burden of disease in SSA, the majority of people in SSA will be impacted by a public health approach to palliative care.

The public health priorities for palliative care in the region are great, i.e.: HIV and AIDS, cancer, children, training for health professionals, creating a positive environment in order to retain personnel, policies for palliative care, improving access to medications and treatment and increasing the number, scope and quality of services so that those in need are able to access palliative care (which is a human right (14)), wherever they may live.

The HIV epidemic has increased the number of people needing palliative care, and has made health providers consider how palliative care is delivered throughout the disease spectrum from diagnosis through to death and into bereavement. Integration of palliative

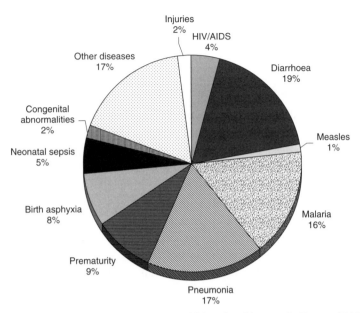

Fig. 19.2 Distribution of causes of death among children in Africa aged <5 years (%)(2).

care into all aspects of the health system is necessary; at the hospital, at the clinics, in the community, and at home. Different models of care provision have been developed and adapted (11). Data has revealed serious problems in public health HIV palliative care, with poor drug availability and frequent stock outs (15).

Statements such as the Cape Town Declaration (16), the Budapest Commitment (17), and the ICPCN Charter for Palliative Care in Children (18) all call for palliative care to be seen as a human right (14), thus raising its profile as a public health priority in the region. The provision of antiretroviral therapy (ART) and palliative care go hand-in-hand and one does not exclude the other (19), therefore advocacy for the provision of palliative care at all levels of the health care system is an integral part of advocacy for ART.

Access to cancer treatment also poses a challenge in many countries. Chemotherapy, whilst available in some centres, is often not available outside of main referral hospitals, and stock outs occur regularly. Radiotherapy is not available in all countries—the population served by each megavoltage machine in the region in 1999 ranged from 0.6 million to 70 million per machine. Sixty nine radiotherapy centres were identified in only 40 cities and 22 countries in Africa (20), whereas in the United Kingdom alone, the number of megavoltage machines in clinical use for radiotherapy increased from 184 in 1997 to 203 in 2002 (21). Whilst several new radiotherapy centres have been opened since then, there are still not enough to serve the population concerned. Diagnosis, treatment and palliation are an integral part of cancer control programmes, and it is important that palliative care is included alongside treatment and diagnosis (22).

Almost half of child deaths occur in Africa (2). The provision of high quality, appropriate and effective palliative care for children is a global concern. Particularly in light of the fact that 41% of the population in Africa is under the age of 15, and under-5 mortality in SSA is 14.5%, 7.8% higher than the global average of 6.7%, with 4.6 million child deaths in SSA in 2007 (23). Therefore, the humane and effective care of children needing palliative care within SSA is a public health priority (24).

The development of palliative care

The development of palliative care services in SSA has grown exponentially over the past ten years due to the recognition of the need for palliative care and the adoption of palliative care as a public health need. Island Hospice in Harare, Zimbabwe, the first palliative care service in the region when it was established in 1979 (25),was followed by services in South Africa, Kenya, and Uganda. A survey of hospice and palliative care services in Africa published in 2007 (26) found that only four of the countries having palliative care could be classified as approaching some form of integration with health providers, and 21 out of 47 countries (44.7%) surveyed had no identified hospice or palliative care activity. Therefore, for the majority of those living in SSA, palliative care is inaccessible, with services often being provided from isolated centres of excellence rather than integrated into existing health systems (4).

A milestone was reached in November 2002 when the Cape Town Declaration was signed. It stated that palliative care is the right of every adult and child with life-limiting illness and should be incorporated into national health care systems in order to make it accessible and affordable for all who need it (16). It was at that meeting that the African Palliative Care Association (APCA) was conceived. Since then, the APCA has been involved, alongside national palliative care associations, in leading the development of palliative care in the region. There has also been an increase in national palliative care associations in the region and those already in existence have become strengthened. Work has been undertaken in many different areas including implementation, advocacy, education and training, research, M&E, and the development of standards of care for the provision of palliative care at different levels (27).

An important part of the development of palliative care in the region has been the development and sharing of different models of care including home-based care, facility-based care, inpatient and day care services, outreach services such as roadside and mobile clinics, hospital-based palliative care teams, and specialist palliative care services (11, 28). Whilst there are generic models of palliative care across the region, these need to be adapted according to the need, culture and environment. Thus palliative care is being provided through different models in order to increase accessibility to care for all who need it. Uganda, along with South Africa, is often seen as a model for palliative care development, with palliative care included in the National Health Plan and demonstrating the public health approach to palliative care development (28).

Palliative care policy

The availability of appropriate government policy on palliative care (including a national palliative care policy, an essential medicines policy, and education policies) is the cornerstone of effective palliative care implementation. National palliative care policies will help to maintain standards of care and ensure that palliative care is promoted and made accessible to the greatest number of people possible. Alongside a national palliative care policy, policies regarding the use of strong analgesics such as opioids are vital for accessibility and the availability of appropriate medications (15).

Most countries have a national health policy in place, though for many this does not include palliative care. Inclusion of palliative care in the national health policy is vital; it allows for the identification and setting of priorities, helps identify the resources needed to support these priorities, provides a basis for resource mobilization, enhances collaboration between all relevant stakeholders, ensures that there is a framework for standards that can underpin palliative care, and enables appropriate planning for palliative care within the country. Policies, whether national policies or for essential medicines, cannot exist in isolation. They must be linked to advocacy, research, education, and implementation of palliative care services (29).

The WHO encourages African governments to institute a policy on essential medicines for adults and children that includes palliative care medicines, and is supported by appropriate policy to ensure that these medicines are accessible (3). Currently, legislation in many countries restricts the use of opioids and other strong analgesics, and restricts their prescribing to doctors. A survey of palliative care providers in 12 African countries (15) found the common factors hampering opioid supply included:

- *Availability*: e.g. central stores not stocking adequately, overly restrictive control;
- *Polices and Legislation*: e.g. punitive and prohibitive regulations;
- *Education*: e.g. existing clinicians unaware of how to assess and treat pain;
- *Practical issues*: e.g. storage requirements, not enough prescribers.

Whilst these barriers pose a great challenge to accessing pain medication, the absence of national policies and lack of government understanding about the importance of pain medication exacerbates them. The example of the Ugandan public health strategy focusing on roll-out of opioids into health districts offers important lessons of a successful multi-sectoral programme to enhance access to opioids though detailed consultation, training, and policy development (28, 29).

Palliative care training

Providing training and education is the foundation of quality care for patients and their families and therefore a key public health priority in the region. Training should target a diverse audience, including policy makers, health care workers, and the general public, in order to increase awareness, skills and knowledge of palliative care,. Through training it is possible to break down barriers to palliative care provision (30), and key to this is the training of national leaders who are responsible for education, and the integration of palliative care into the national training programmes for all health care providers (3).

The lack of palliative care education of those providing care is a major challenge. Training needs to be provided for all those involved including health professionals, lay carers (e.g. community volunteers), teachers, and religious and community leaders. It needs to be provided across the continuum of care and at both the pre-registration and post-registration levels, available to both specialists and generalists (31). The burden of disease is such that all health care professionals will care for people who need palliative care, and therefore require training.

In order to ensure the quality of the palliative care education provided, it is important to know what knowledge, skills, and attitudes are required of the individuals that one is training in order to can provide quality care. Thus, alongside the development of standards of care (31) APCA has developed core competencies for palliative care in Africa (32).

Funding palliative care

Sustainability and funding for palliative care services across SSA continue to pose a challenge. Unless palliative care is included in the national policy, as it is in Uganda, there is little or no allocation of public funds or institutional resources and it is not included in national level work plans and budgets. If palliative care in SSA is seen as an integral and essential part of the provision of health care, then this integration will help with sustainability and financing of the services provided. However, with limited funding available for health care across the region, governments often have not had either the economic ability or the political will to implement palliative care. Therefore services have been provided by non-governmental organisations reliant on donor funding and fundraising from external sources (33).

Recently there has been an increase in funding available for palliative care and several initiatives are underway to promote its development in Africa. An evidence base for the African palliative care context is also beginning to emerge (34), with an analysis of models of service delivery and an appraisal of the literature relating to services in sub-Saharan Africa, thus helping to secure funding and demonstrating the impact and effectiveness of palliative care services.

However, whilst more funds for palliative care have become available, these are often restricted to activities in specific countries, or to care for people with specific diseases, e.g. HIV, or to a specific age group, e.g. adults and not children. Whilst from a donor perspective this is understandable, this can cause challenges for organizations seeking to provide palliative care for all those who need it.

Issues around the sustainability of services along with financial problems are common to most palliative care programmes within SSA. Where possible they need to identify sources of funds to support their operational costs. There are also major issues regarding care for the bereaved and orphaned (33).

Conclusion

There is an overwhelming need for quality palliative care services across SSA. Centres of excellence exist and enormous advocacy gains have been made. Lessons have been learnt in terms of coverage, lobbying and advocacy, and innovative low cost integrated palliative care in an unpredictable trajectory that can be useful for other regions of the world. However, palliative care remains a public health priority within the region and practitioners need to continue to be innovative, adapting and developing appropriate models of care that best meet the public health needs for all.

Summary of key challenges for the development of palliative care in SSA(11)

- ◆ the need for palliative care in the region vs. the number of service providers
- ◆ limitations of existing service models
- ◆ delayed health-seeking behaviour
- ◆ a lack of trained health professionals and a reliance on community health workers
- ◆ limited availability of drugs and other resources
- ◆ extending coverage and ensuring quality
- ◆ lack of recognition of the importance of palliative care
- ◆ logistics and infrastructure
- ◆ high burden of disease
- ◆ role overload and conflict, particularly for nurses
- ◆ developing services that are sustainable
- ◆ lack of research and evidence to show the value added of palliative care in Africa.

References

(1) World Atlas. *Africa*. Available at: http://www.worldatlas.com/webimage/countrys/af.htm (accessed 18 June 2010).

(2) World Health Organization (2010) *World Health Statistics 2010*. Geneva: WHO.

(3) Mwangi-Powell, FN, Ddungu, H., Downing, J., Kiyange, F., Powell, R.A., and Baguma, A. (2010) Palliative care in Africa. In BR Ferrell and N Coyle (eds), *The Oxford Textbook of Palliative Nursing*. Oxford: Oxford University Press.

(4) Harding, R., and Higginson, I.J. (2005) Palliative care in sub-Saharan Africa: An appraisal. *Lancet*, **365**, 1971–7.

(5) UNAIDS (2009) *AIDS Epidemic Update*. Geneva: UNAIDS.

(6) Mngadi, S., Fraser, N., Mkhatshwa, H., et al. (2009) *Swaziland: HIV Prevention Response and Modes of Transmission Analysis*. Mbabane: National Emergency Response Council on HIV/AIDS.

(7) GLOBOCAN (2008) (IARC) *Section of Cancer Information (16/6/2010)*.

(8) Rastogi, T., Hildesheim, A., and Sinha, R. (2004) Opportunities for cancer epidemiology in developing countries. *National Reviews Cancer*, **4**, 909–17.

(9) Kanavos, P. (2006) The rising burden of cancer in the developing world. *Annals of Oncology*, **17** (Suppl 8), 15–23.

(10) Hamad, H.M.A. (2006) Cancer initiatives in Sudan. *Annals of Oncology*, **17**(Suppl 8), 32–6.

(11) Downing, J., Powell, R.A., and Mwangi-Powell, F. (2010) Home-based palliative care in sub-Saharan Africa. *Home Healthcare Nurse*, **28** (5) (May), 298–307.

(12) Mathers, C.D., and Longar, D. (2006) Projections of global mortality and burden of disease from 2002 to 2030. *PLoS Medicine*, **3** (11), 2011–30.

(13) World Health Organization (2004) *Cause of death statistics*. Geneva: WHO.

(14) Gwyther, L., Brennan, F., and Harding, R. (2009) Advancing palliative care as a human right. *Journal of Pain and Symptom Management,* **38** (5), 767–74.

(15) Harding, R., Powell, R.A., Kiyange, F., Mwangi-Powell, F., and Downing, J. (2010) Provision of pain and symptom-relieving drugs for HIV/AIDS in Sub-Saharan Africa. *Journal of Pain and Symptom Management,* **40** (3), 405–15.

(16) Mpanga Sebuyira, L., Mwangi-Powell, F., Pereira, J., and Spence C. (2003) The Cape Town Palliative Care Declaration: Home-grown solutions for sub-Saharan Africa. *Journal of Palliative Medicine,* **6**, 341–3.

(17) European Association for Palliative Care (2007) *The Budapest Commitments.* Available at: http://www.eapcnet.org/congresses/Budapest2007/Buda- pest2007Commitments.htm. (Accessed 11 November 2009.)

(18) International Children's Palliative Care Network. The ICPCN Charter of Rights for Life limited and life-threatened children. http://www.icpcn.org.uk/page.asp?section=000100010014&sectionTitle=-Charter. (Accessed 21 June 2010.)

(19) Harding, R., Molloy, T., Easterbrook, P.E., Frame, K., and Higginson, I.J. (2006) Is antiretroviral therapy associated with symptom prevalence and burden? *International Journal of STD & AIDS,* **17**, 400–5.

(20) Levin, C., El Gueddari, B., and Meghzifene, A. (1999) Radiation therapy in Africa: Distribution and equipment. *Radiother Oncol,* **52**, 79–84.

(21) Board of the Faculty of Clinical Oncology, The Royal College of Radiologists (2003) *Equipment, Workload and Staffing for Radiotherapy in the UK 1997–2002.* London: Royal College of Radiologists.

(22) World Health Organization (2002) *National Cancer Control Programmes: Policies and Managerial Guidelines.* Geneva: WHO.

(23) United Nations (2009) *The Millennium Development Goals Report 2009.* New York: United Nations.

(24) Harding, R., Sherr, L., and Albertyn, R. (2010) *The Status of Paediatric Palliative Care in Sub-Saharan Africa: An Appraisal.* London: Diana Princess of Wales Memorial Fund.

(25) Wright, M., and Clark, D. (2006) *Hospice and Palliative Care in Africa: A Review of Developments and Challenges.* Oxford: Oxford University Press.

(26) Clark, D., Wright, M., Hunt, J., and Lynch, T. (2007) Hospice and palliative care development in Africa: A multi-method review of services and experiences. *Journal of Pain and Symptom Management,* **33**, 698–710.

(27) APCA (2010) *Standards for Palliative Care in Africa.* Kampala: APCA.

(28) Merriman, A., and Harding, R. (2010) Pain control in the African context: The Ugandan introduction of affordable morphine to relieve suffering at the end of life. *BioMedCentral Philosophy, Ethics, and Humanities in Medicine,* **5** (10), 1–6.

(29) Logie, D., and Harding, R. (2005) An evaluation of a morphine public health programme for cancer and AIDS pain relief in Sub-Saharan Africa. *BioMedCentral Public Health,* **5** (82).

(30) Downing, J. (2009) The development of the Nankya model of palliative care development. *International Journal of Palliative Nursing,* **14** (9), 459–64.

(31) Downing, J., Finch, L., Garanganga, E., et al. (2006) Role of the nurse in resource-limited settings. In L. Gwyther, A. Merriman, L. Mpanga Sebuyira, and H. Schietinger (eds), *A Clinical Guide to Supportive and Palliative Care for HIV/AIDS in Sub-Saharan Africa.* Kampala: APCA.

(32) APCA (2010) *Competency Framework for Palliative Care Draft Document.* Kampala: APCA.

(33) Callaway, M., Foley, K., De Lima, L., et al. (2007) Funding for palliative care programs in developing countries. *Journal of Pain and Symptom Management,* **33** (5), 509–13.

(34) Harding, R., Powell, R.A., Downing, J., et al. (2008) Generating an African palliative care evidence base: The context, need, challenges and strategies. *Journal of Pain and Symptom Management,* **36** (3), 304–9.

Chapter 20

Palliative care in the global context: Understanding policies to support end-of-life care

David Clark

This chapter reviews the progress that has been made in research into global palliative care development during the first decade of the new millennium. It sets out the work that has been done by key non-governmental organizations to promote palliative care internationally, focusing particularly on the years after 2000. It then considers some innovative empirical studies on palliative care development that have provided data to map provision at the national level, sometimes with a focus on world regions. It highlights the scale of the research challenge involved in producing and maintaining an accurate analysis of the global state of palliative care. It then goes on to explore the role of funding agencies and the extent to which palliative care has been 'framed' within international policy discourse. Above all it will emphasize the still-limited progress that has been made in integrating palliative care within the architecture of global, regional, and national policy-making.

Contextual issues and organizational development

Before the year 2000 there was little systematic understanding of how palliative care was developing in the global context. Whilst activists in the field did occasionally comment on international links and initiatives, there was no evidence from research studies to shed systematic light on the state of service development, policy recognition, or the general 'vitality' of palliative care in different settings around the world. Some countries had established national associations for palliative care, occasionally with directories of services, but in the main it remained difficult to access any useful information about resources and infrastructure other than through local contacts. The idea of collaborative endeavours in policy innovation, service development, or research to promote palliative care in the international context was barely recognized. Accordingly, the evidence base for palliative care provision and the notion that it might be rooted in public health approaches were weakly developed and often not considered by palliative care activists to be a high priority (1).

The start of the new millennium, however, was a key time in the development of palliative care globally. A European Association for Palliative Care (EAPC) had been active since 1988 (2). In some western European countries, palliative care was maturing as a discipline (3); in eastern Europe the first signs of growth were appearing and a regional Task Force had been established in 1999 (4). In the United States, hospice programmes had been developing since the 1970s, Medicare funding had been achieved in 1982, and during the 1990s there was considerable growth in the involvement of philanthropic organizations in the wider promotion of palliative care within the health care system and as a field of teaching and research. The United States also provided an administrative home to the International Association of Hospice and Palliative Care (IAHPC), which had grown out of the International Hospice Institute, founded in 1980. In South America, the 1994 Declaration of Florianopolis (5) had drawn attention to the need for better access to opioid medications for cancer and palliative care; in 2000 a Latin American Association of Palliative Care was formed. In south-east Asia no regional association for palliative care yet existed, though considerable development had taken place in Australia and Japan, with several other countries making progress, but in 2000 India and China faced enormous challenges with only meagre palliative care resources and infrastructure. In Africa, as the HIV/AIDS epidemic hit, just a few countries had good models for palliative care delivery and the coordination of an African professional organization was badly needed.

All around the globe palliative care leaders bemoaned the same problems: a lack of public recognition and understanding of their work; professional indifference on the part of many health and social care providers; a lack of third-party funding to set up demonstration projects; poor recognition of palliative care within the architecture of both national and international health policy; weakly developed training programmes with few routes for accreditation and professional recognition; and a limited evidence base about the overall development of palliative care and its efficacy, costs, and benefits.

It was not until 2003 that the first 'summit' on international palliative care development took place, in the Hague. Others followed in Seoul in 2005, Nairobi in 2007, and Vienna in 2009—leading that year to the creation of the Worldwide Palliative Care Alliance. These meetings brought together the existing organizations with international palliative care interests, as well as other 'outward facing' national associations from specific countries, together with funders, activists, and researchers. In 2003 a group of national experts worked with the Council of Europe to produce a set of guidelines on palliative care, which it described as an essential and basic service for the whole population. The recommendations appear to have been used quite actively in some countries with less-developed palliative care systems, particularly in eastern Europe, where they served as a tool for advocacy and lobbying (6). By 2003 the European Society for Medical Oncology was giving greater recognition to palliative care. In 2004 the European Federation of Older Persons also launched a campaign to make palliative care a priority topic on the European health agenda (7). The same year, WHO Europe produced an important document on *Better Palliative Care for Older People*, aiming to 'incorporate palliative care for serious chronic progressive illnesses within ageing policies, and to promote better care towards the end of life'(8). A companion volume, *Palliative Care: The Solid Facts* became a resource for policy-makers in a context where 'the evidence available on palliative care is not complete and . . . there are differences in what can be offered across the European region'(9).

Crucially, the remaining world regions also formed associations for palliative care in the early part of the decade: Asia Pacific in 2001 (10) and Africa in 2004. In the UK in 2002, Help the Hospices re-launched an international Hospice Information service, in partnership with St Christopher's Hospice. In 2000, the Open Society Institute (OSI) launched its International Palliative Care Initiative (IPCI). In 2005 activists in the 'summit' meetings worked together to create the first World Hospice and Palliative Care Day, which ran annually thereafter. The Venice Declaration of 2006, brought forward by IAHPC and EAPC, called for strategies and resources to support research activity on palliative care in developing countries (11). In 2007, a set of 'commitments' for palliative care improvement was entered into by palliative care associations at the Budapest congress of the EAPC (12). In the same year, in collaboration with 25 other organizations, the IAHPC developed a list of essential medicines for palliative care in response to a request from the Cancer Control Program of the World Health Organization (WHO) (13). During this period debates also began to emerge in which access to palliative care was constructed as a human right (14), and access to palliative medication was incorporated into a resolution of the United Nations Commission on Human Rights (15) reflecting a growing interest in the relationship between palliative care services and their accessibility to the populations of individual countries.

As the first decade of the twenty-first century closed, the palliative care community appeared organized as never before, with growing levels of commitment to international development issues, but major challenges still in prospect. In addition a range of studies was emerging which could underpin development with the beginnings of an evidence base. These studies were limited by the methodological and practical challenges of research on an international scale, but began to describe the key issues and to map an agenda for scientific collaboration in a rapidly developing field.

Key studies

Early projects

The first research study to explore the development of palliative care in a comparative manner across jurisdictions focused on seven western European countries (16). It showed two forms of variation in the delivery of palliative care (17). First, palliative care services were found in a variety of settings: domiciliary, quasi-domiciliary and institutional. Second, these forms were not prioritized equally in each country. Allowing for population differences, there were great variations in the numbers of palliative care services across countries, and the number of specialist palliative care beds per head of population varied from 1:c18,000 persons in the UK to 1:c1.9m in Italy.

This work led directly to another study which successfully mapped the development of palliative care across 28 former communist countries in eastern Europe and Central Asia (18). Only Poland and Russia had more than 50 palliative care services and 5 countries had no identified palliative care services. Home care was the form of service most commonly found, followed by inpatient provision. There was a great absence of hospital mobile teams, as well as services in nursing homes and day care provision. Only 48 paediatric palliative care services were identified, covering just 9 of the 28 countries.

Using a related approach, a team at the University of Giessen carried out a study covering 16 countries across eastern and western Europe and incorporating a comprehensive analysis of demographics, the history of hospice and palliative care, the number of current services, funding, education and training of professional staff, and the role of volunteers, with an in-depth case portrayal of particular services (19).

Under the present author's leadership, in the period 2003–9, the International Observatory on End of Life Care became the key source of palliative care mapping studies around the world, constructing national reports for over 60 countries (20). In particular it carried out major reviews of palliative care development in Africa (26 countries) (21), the Middle East (six countries) (22), and south-east Asia (three countries (23)), as well as a study covering the whole of India (24). These reviews had several key features in common. They established the number and character of palliative care services existing in a given country, they described the associated funding arrangements, the level of policy support and the specific context of opioid availability. They also contained rich narratives of experience, based on interview accounts from local activists in palliative care.

Global comparison of palliative care development

Emerging from the IOELC studies was a first attempt to map the level of palliative care development for every country in the world, using a four-part typology first developed in the African study (25). The number of countries in each category were: 1) no identified activity 78 (33%); 2) capacity building, but with no operational services 41 (18%); 3) localized provision, without extensive coverage 80 (34%); 4) development approaching integration with the wider health care system 35 (15%). The typology differentiated levels of palliative care development in both hemispheres and in rich and poor settings. It showed that only half of the world's countries had some form of designated palliative care service.

By presenting a 'world map' of hospice–palliative care provision, the authors aimed to contribute to the debate about the growth and recognition of services and in particular whether or not the four-part typology reflects *sequential* levels of palliative care development.

European rankings

The EAPC Task Force on the Development of Palliative Care in Europe reported on an assessment of the state of palliative care development in 47 countries (26) and initially used the simple expedient of ranking countries by services per million in the population (27). In 2008 this was extended in a collaborative study, which built on and updated the data from 2005 and specifically focused on the 27 members states of the European Union (28). This study was important in moving beyond a descriptive comparison of the data, to sketch out the beginnings of a more detailed method for ranking the 27 countries by the level of their palliative care development. Two types of indicator were used for each country: 1) numbers of palliative care services per million population; 2) a measure of the 'vitality'

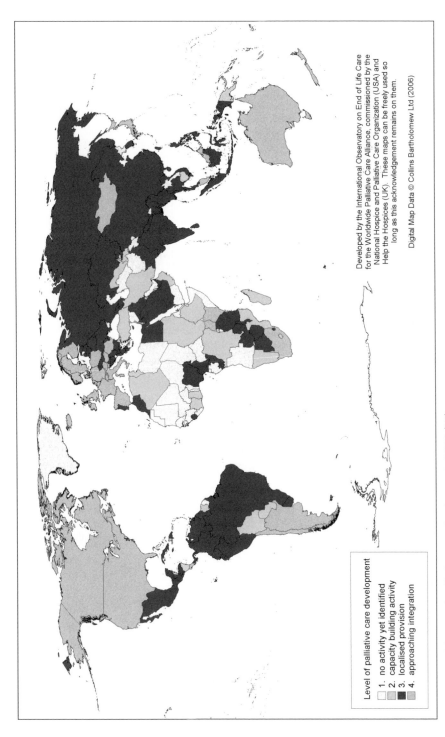

Developed by the International Observatory on End of Life Care for the Worldwide Palliative Care Alliance, commissioned by the National Hospice and Palliative Care Organization (USA) and Help the Hospices (UK). These maps can be freely used so long as this acknowledgement remains on them.

Digital Map Data © Collins Bartholomew Ltd (2006)

Level of palliative care development

1. no activity yet identified
2. capacity building activity
3. localised provision
4. approaching integration

Fig. 20.1 The 'world map' of palliative care development, 2008 (25).

of palliative care based on such factors as the existence of a national association, directory of services, physician accreditation, numbers attending EAPC congresses, publications on palliative care development. In the ranking, 75% of the score was given to the number of services and 25% to 'vitality'. The UK was ranked first with a score of 100% and all other countries were then placed in relation to it. The main weaknesses of the method however were: a lack of confidence in the comparability and accuracy of the inputted data and the use of a *relative* ranking, based on the UK as the highest performer, rather than an *absolute* scale.

Global Quality of Death Index

Building on this work a study commissioned by the Lien Foundation in Singapore and carried out by the Economist Intelligence Unit was published in 2010 (29). This too attempted a ranking of palliative care development in 40 countries of the world, with a more complex set of indicators. The Quality of Death Index scored on 24 indicators in 4 categories, each with a separate weighting: 1) basic end-of-life health care environment (20%); 2) availability of end-of-life care (25%); 3) cost of end-of-life care (15%); 4) quality of end-of-life (40%). The study again ranked the UK with the best quality of death, owing to its advanced hospice care network and long history of state involvement in end-of-life care. Some advanced nations rank poorly on the Index, however—for instance Finland at 28 and South Korea at 32. The report noted the high position of Hungary (11th) and Poland (15th). The USA, however, with the largest spending on health care in the world, ranked just 9th in the Index, principally due to limited public funding for end-of-life care, the costs to the patient and the restriction of government-funded reimbursements through Medicare only to patients who give up curative treatments.

The report noted that across the world, public healthcare funding often prioritizes conventional treatment and provides only partial support for end-of-life care services, meaning such care must rely on philanthropy and community help. It took the view that a widespread cultural belief in affluent countries that governments should provide and pay for healthcare services has hampered private sector provision of end-of-life care services. At the other end of the scale are developing countries such as China and India, where state funding levels for end-of-life care are very low, provision is patchy and localized and most people pay for everything themselves.

Strengths and weaknesses of the studies

There is no doubt that these studies faced a number of challenges and were only partially successful in overcoming them. Certainly, they demonstrated that by working in partnership with local service providers, activists and policy makers, it was possible to build up an evidence-based picture of palliative care development in the international context. But at the same time they struggled to attain comparability between settings and to generate accurate data about specific services and activities. Some of this can be attributed to language problems and difficulties of communication across cultures and settings and to variations that exist between health care systems, which make for difficulties in comparing services.

There were obvious problems too in the standardization and definition of terms such as 'hospice', 'inpatient unit', or 'mobile team', which do not have a universal currency. Similarly, the researchers often faced the problem of determining what is to be counted. Is the unit of analysis an organization, for example a hospice, or is it the number of services that it provides—inpatient, outpatient, domiciliary? Quantitative analysis is further hampered by the absence of accurate registers of palliative care services, making studies dependent on figures generated by local activists, who might incline to under-estimate or over-estimate what exists—or simply not have the wherewithal to obtain accurate data. A further criticism is that the studies have tended to focus on the delivery of what are to varying degrees *specialist* palliative care services, opening up the criticism that palliative care may also be provided by others, for example in primary care or hospital settings. All of these issues will need consideration if the quality of comparative international palliative care studies is to be improved. Certainly the 'second generation' of such studies will have something on which to build and the prospects of higher quality research outcomes are good.

Funders and policy-makers

During the period 2000 to 2010 it became increasingly clear that if palliative care was to make progress with its objectives for international development, two key issues would require attention. In the short run, third party funding would have to be identified to stimulate capacity-building and service development, leading to more interest in the role of national and international donors and ways in which they might be drawn to palliative issues. There was also an increasing awareness that to achieve sustainable programmes of palliative care education and service delivery, it would be necessary to achieve greater recognition within public policy—both at the level of national jurisdictions and internationally.

Funders

Some international palliative care funders are well known and have a relatively high profile, but many are not of this type. The first ever review of such funding from all sectors of philanthropy including private and community foundations, public charities and corporate grant making was conducted in 2007 (30). The study identified 354 national and international donors that support hospice and palliative care activities in five world regions. From this an eight-category typology of donors was developed: 'Multilateral', 'Bilateral', 'Humanitarian', 'Faith-based', 'Business', 'Hospice support', 'Association', 'Other'. Among these, the Humanitarian group was found to be the largest with 124 (35%) organizations, whereas the Multilateral group was the smallest with 9 (3%). An analysis of each group's area of activity showed that the largest number of donor organizations was active in central and eastern Europe and the Commonwealth of Independent States (157; 44%), followed next by Africa (141; 40%). Only 22 (6%) were active in Latin America and the Caribbean and 19 (5%) in the Middle East. The number of donors and their areas of activity indicated that, around the world, many palliative care developments remain dependent on third party funding.

The Global Fund to Fight AIDS, Tuberculosis, and Malaria represents a new type of partnership between governments, civil society, the private sector and affected communities. Established in 2002, it works closely with other multilateral and bilateral organizations and supports their work by the provision of substantially increased funding. Importantly, the Global Fund does not initiate or operate programmes, nor does it determine which policies, activities, or types of care should be implemented; such decisions rest entirely with local organizations. Consequently, some proposals may include palliative care, others not, depending on the locally determined needs and priorities.

In 2004, a major global policy initiative was launched by the United States Agency for International Development (USAID), known as the President's Emergency Plan for AIDS Relief (PEPFAR) (31). Fifteen billion dollars was committed to the project, across 15 countries, and 15% of budget was ear-marked for palliative care. The funding study shows how hospice and palliative care initiatives, particularly in sub-Saharan Africa, have been major beneficiaries of PEPFAR, both for service delivery and organizational capacity-building.

Intergovernmental agencies

A key aspiration within the palliative care community has been to engender interest in and support for palliative care on the part of intergovernmental agencies and particularly those with a major influence on global policy making. The World Health Organization stands out as the first major intergovernmental agency to take an active interest in international palliative care development and its contribution has been well described (32). Undoubtedly, in many resource poor countries the input of the WHO has been significant in promoting cancer pain and palliative care developments. Less clear is the enduring relevance of the WHO approach in the more affluent nations. Of more significance is the question of whether the WHO 'public health model' of palliative care is fully adequate to tackle the barriers to development that exist. The 'foundation measures' for example, are persuasive in their descriptive power, but do not seem to offer an adequate model for action and change. Meanwhile, other organizations have inserted 'symbolic language' about palliative care into their policies, for example the World Health Assembly statement on cancer prevention and control, 2005 and the action plan on ageing of the United Nations Programme on Ageing, 2002 (updated 2008). But the effect of such endeavours is difficult to judge, other than in relation to general awareness-raising.

Prospects for global improvement

Taken together, across the world, there is a growing nexus of funders, intergovernmental organizations, philanthropic bodies, and non-profit organizations that are devoting some or all of their interest to palliative care development. The decade after 2000 saw a great burst of international activity from within the palliative care community. New associations came into being, interchange and information flow between key players increased, and high-level declarations resonated from palliative care congresses, intent on raising the profile of end of life issues. For the first time in its short history, palliative care became the focus of international and comparative research studies and an evidence based picture emerged of palliative care provision around the world. Greater interest in palliative care was also seen on the part of philanthropic and intergovernmental donors. It was a decade of considerable achievement. But at the same time it exposed some specific problems.

Palliative care remained limited by an inward-looking culture. This manifested itself in several ways. Major conferences rarely featured key figures from outside the specialty (the International Congress on Palliative Care, held bi-annually in Montreal, being an exception to this). Research collaborations were similarly constrained. There was a striking absence of senior figures from oncology, old age medicine, psychiatry, and primary care working towards the development of palliative care and making appropriate connections. Even public health showed little engagement, despite the efforts of some palliative care leaders to champion their work within a public health model. Such observations, it might be argued, could seem consistent with the emergence of a new field. By 2010 only 17 countries had recognized palliative medicine as a separate area for specialization (33). There was much to do in order to build up internal critical mass—in service provision, in education, and in research programmes. Yet the field also appeared pre-occupied with questions of definition (a major backlash resulted when the new definition of palliative care produced by WHO in 2002 labelled it 'an approach') and there was much argument about differences between 'hospice', 'palliative', 'supportive', and 'end-of-life' care. The huge appetite for these debates within the palliative care world seemed incommensurate with the interest of external colleagues. Indeed, when others did look in from the outside they were prone to ask some simple but challenging questions: what is palliative care doing for people with HIV disease; how is it responding to the growing needs of ageing populations with high levels of co-morbidity at the end of life; what can it teach primary care and the specialties of hospital medicine; how can it be 'mainstreamed' into general health and social care and what is the evidence for its cost effectiveness? Certainly, there were achievements in all of these areas, but the 'scaling up' of activity in education, research, and service delivery continued to challenge the resources of the palliative care community.

Beyond this, it must be asked whether the global infrastructure for palliative care development is fit for purpose. How integrated are the programmes of the various regional associations? How effective are the relationships between the growing numbers of organizations that claim a mandate to support the global improvement of palliative care? Above all, how effective are these groups in engaging with the major challenges that remain? In particular this includes the need to create better articulation between the interests of palliative care and the architecture of global policy.

The years after 2000 gave birth to the twin ideas that palliative care is both a public health and a human rights issue. Both are contentious. The first assumes the insertion of palliative care into the public health system, thereby positioning it within a discourse of 'need', 'supply', and 'resource allocation'. But there is another version of palliative care as a public health issue which focuses on a 'health promoting' dimension, sees the main source of end of life care as families and communities (not specialists and services), and which argues for a societal reappraisal of death, dying and bereavement (34). The goal in this version is to achieve a greater measure of compassion and dignity in all aspects of dying and death in whichever aspect of society they are manifested, and certainly not within the health care system alone. The second assertion—that palliative care is a human rights issue—may prove challenging to progress. Recognition of palliative care as a human right (35) has been developing and access to palliative medication has been incorporated into a resolution of the United Nations Commission on Human Rights (36), but the goals of such work are difficult to define and the likelihood of reaching them is highly unpredictable. A number of 'public health' palliative care demonstration projects are said to have gained traction—in Africa and India, as well as in the wealthier nations. But demonstration projects with weak evidence surrounding them and rights-based arguments as a spur to policy change seem likely to attract only limited interest in an increasingly constrained fiscal environment.

For such reasons, palliative care remains poorly framed within evidence-based global policy-making. It is clear that the discourse surrounding the global development of palliative care is still weakly articulated and relatively sparse. Within the palliative care field, especially among clinical academics and researchers, there is an understandable and strong focus on demonstrating the efficacy of palliative care interventions. This concentrates efforts in characterizing different syndromes and clusters of pain and other symptoms and on measuring the relative impact of differing therapeutic regimes on 'outcomes' of care. A smaller group is focused on the economic costs and benefits of good palliative care— for the health care system as well as for patients and families. Far less effort is expended on understanding how palliative care is positioned within the language of global policy-making. Palliative care is not one of the Millennium Development Goals. It is hard to find in the priorities of the United Nations, UNESCO and other global organizations. It has only the most tentative recognition in the frameworks of the World Bank, the Global Fund, and in the concerns of the world's largest philanthropic donors and foundations. Much more needs to be done to demonstrate the links between primary care and palliative care, to explore the role of palliative care in poverty reduction and community cohesion, and to examine how palliative care can reduce social, economic, and gender inequalities (37).

By 2010, the global palliative care community could claim some significant successes. With a growing global infrastructure for advocacy, fund-raising, and collaboration, the next decade will be crucial in breaking through to a higher level of policy recognition. Such recognition is vital if the world's palliative care needs are to be met in an equitable and culturally sensitive manner and a true public health orientation to end-of-life care is to be achieved.

References

(1) Stjernsward, J, and Clark, D (2003) Palliative care—a global perspective. In G Hanks, D Doyle, C Calman, and N Cherny (eds), *Oxford Textbook of Palliative Medicine*, 3rd edn. Oxford: Oxford University Press.

(2) Blumhuber, H, Kaasa, S, and de Conno, F (2002) The European Association for Palliative Care. *Journal of Pain and Symptom Management*, **24** (2): 124–7.

(3) ten Have, H, and Clark, D (eds) (2002) *The Ethics of Palliative Care: European Perspectives.* Buckingham: Open University Press.

(4) Luczak, J, and Kluziak, M (2001) The formation of ECEPT (Eastern and Central Europe Palliative Task Force): a Polish initiative. *Palliative Medicine*, **15**: 259–60.

(5) Stjernswärd, J, Bruera, E, Joranson, D, et al. (1995) Opioid availability in Latin America: The Declaration of Florianopolis. *Journal of Pain and Symptom Management*, **10** (3): 233–6.

(6) Cherny, NI, Catane, R, and Kosmidis, P (2003) ESMO takes a stand on supportive and palliative care. *Annals of Oncology*, **14** (9): 1335–7.

(7) See: http://www.eurag-europe.org/palliativ-en.htm.

(8) Davies, E, and Higginson, IJ (eds) (2004a) *Better Palliative Care for Older People*. Copenhagen: World Health Organization.

(9) Davies, E, and Higginson, IJ (eds) (2004b) *Palliative Care: The Solid Facts*. Copenhagen: World Health Organization.

(10) Goh, CR (2002) The Asia Pacific Hospice Palliative Care Network: A network for individuals and organisations. *Journal of Pain and Symptom Management*, **24** (2): 128–33.

(11) The Declaration of Venice. Palliative Care Research in Developing Countries. www.hospicecare. com/dv/english.html_.

(12) Radbruch, L Foley, De Lima, L, Praill, D, and Fürst, CJ (2007) The Budapest Commitments: Setting the goals A joint initiative by the European Association for Palliative Care, the International Association for Hospice and Palliative Care and Help the Hospices. *Palliative Medicine*, **21** (4): 269–71.

(13) http://www.hospicecare.com/resources/pdf-docs/iahpc-em-summary.pdf, accessed 4 August 2010.

(14) Harding, R. Palliative care: a basic human right. id21 Insights Health, 8 Feb. 2006: 1–2. http://www.id21.org/zinter/id21zinter.exe?a=9&i=InsightsHealth8Editorial&u=458167f2.

(15) Commission on Human Rights Resolution 2004/26: Item 7c calls on states 'to promote effective access to such preventive, curative or palliative pharmaceutical products or medical technologies.' Available via http://www.ohchr.org/english/; accessed June 2007.

(16) ten Have, H, and Janssens, R (eds) (2001) *Palliative Care in Europe*. Amsterdam: IOS Press; ten Have, H, and Clark, D (eds) (2002) *The Ethics of Palliative Care: European Perspectives*. Buckingham: Open University Press.

(17) Clark, D, ten Have, H, and Janssens, R (2000) Common threads? palliative care service developments in seven European countries, *Palliative Medicine* **14** (6): 479–90.

(18) Clark, D, and Wright, M (2003) *Transitions in End of Life Care: Hospice and Related Developments in Eastern Europe and Central Asia*. Buckingham: Open University Press.

(19) Gronemeyer, R, Fink, M, Globisch, M, and Schuman, F (2005) *Helping People at the End of their Loves: Hospice and Palliative Care in Europe*. Berlin: Lit Verlag.

(20) Clark, D, and Wright, M (2007) The International Observatory on End of Life Care: A global view of palliative care development. *Journal of Pain and Symptom Management* **33** (5): 542–6.

(21) Wright, M, and Clark, D (2006) *Hospice and Palliative Care Development in Africa. A Review of Developments and Challenges*. Oxford: Oxford University Press.

(22) Bingley, A, and Clark, D (2009) A comparative review of palliative care development in six countries represented by the Middle East Cancer Consortium (MECC). *Journal of Pain and Symptom Management*, **37** (3): 287–96.

(23) Wright, M (2010) *Hospice and Palliative Care in South East Asia*. Oxford: Oxford University Press.

(24) McDermott, E, Selman, L, Wright, M, and Clark, D (2008) Hospice and palliative care development in India: A multi-method review of services and experiences. *Journal of Pain and Symptom Management*, **35** (6): 583–93.

(25) Wright, M, Wood, J, Lynch, T, and Clark, D (2008) Mapping levels of palliative care development: A global view. *Journal of Pain and Symptom Management*, **35** (5): 469–85.

(26) Centeno, C, Clark, D, Lynch, T, Rocafort, J, Greenwood, A, Flores, LA, De Lima, L, Giordano, A, Brasch, S, and Praill, D (2007) *EAPC Atlas of Palliative Care in Europe*. Houston: IAHPC Press.

(27) Clark, D, and Centeno, C (2006) Palliative care in Europe: An emerging approach to comparative analysis. *Clinical Medicine*, **6** (2): 197–201.

(28) Martin-Moreno, J, Harris, M, Gorgojo, L, Clark, D, Normand, C, and Centeno, C. *Palliative Care in the European Union*. European Parliament Economic and Scientific Policy Department 2008. IP/A/ENVI/ST/2007-22. PE404.899 [online], http://www.europarl.europa.eu/activities/committees/studies/download.do?file=21421, accessed March 2010.

(29) http://www.lifebeforedeath.com/qualityofdeath/index.shtml, accessed March 2011.

(30) Wright, M, Lynch, T, and Clark, D (2008) *A Review of Donor Organisations that support Palliative Care Development in Five World Regions*. Lancaster: International Observatory on End of Life Care. http://www.eolc-observatory.net/pdf/Final_Donor_Report.pdf, accessed March 2011.

(31) http://www.pepfar.gov/, accessed November 2007.

(32) Stjernsward, J, and Clark, D (2003) Palliative medicine—A global perspective. In D Doyle, GWC Hanks, N Cherny, and KC Calman (eds), *Oxford Textbook of Palliative Medicine*, 3rd edn. Oxford: Oxford University Press, 1199–224.

(33) Clark, D (2010) International progress in creating palliative medicine as a specialized discipline. In G Hanks et al. (eds), *Oxford Textbook of Palliative Medicine*, 4th edn. Oxford: Oxford University Press, 9–16.

(34) Kellehear, A (2005) *Compassionate Cities: Public Health and End-of-Life Care*. London: Routledge; Kellehear, A (2003) *Public Health Challenges in the Care of the Dying*. In P. Liamputtong and H. Gardner (eds), *Health, Social Change & Communities*. Melbourne: Oxford University Press, 88–99.

(35) Harding, R. Palliative care: a basic human right. id21 Insights Health, 8 Feb 2006: 1–2. http://www.id21.org/zinter/id21zinter.exe?a=9&i=InsightsHealth8Editorial&u=458167f2.

(36) Commission on Human Rights Resolution 2004/26: Item 7c calls on states 'to promote effective access to such preventive, curative or palliative pharmaceutical products or medical technologies.' available via http://www.ohchr.org/english/, accessed June 2007.

(37) Clark, J (2010) Terminally neglected? The marginal place of palliative care within global discourses on health. Unpublished MA thesis. Sheffield: University of Sheffield.

Chapter 21

The importance of family carers in end-of-life care: A public health approach

Allan Kellehear

Introduction

The family care of a dying loved one has been at the centre of all end-of-life care throughout human history. Both among hunter–gather economies and pastoral communities family care has toiled at the tasks of feeding, toileting, and cleaning as well as attending to the physical torments of the dying person. In all societies that care has also included liaison with religious authorities and with the healers of their time. In modern affluent contexts these tasks remain important but are often less recognized, eclipsed as they often are by recent academic, professional and cultural obsessions about 'health services' for end-of-life care. Nevertheless, family care of the dying remains crucial to any holistic consideration of end-of-life care everywhere.

This chapter will review the key social and cultural dimensions that influence family carers, also noting how less recognized influences, such as hidden relationships, might be important influences on family care behaviour. The chapter will argue for a public health response to family care that goes beyond direct service provision. I will argue that health promotion, community development, and service partnerships are crucial to enhancing and supporting family carers.

Family care is frequently an arduous set of tasks that can sometimes minimally involve basic cooking, cleaning, bathing, and toileting but can and often expands to include semi-nursing or medical tasks such as wound care, body repositioning and lifting of patients, preparations of medicines and massage. Furthermore it is common for carers to be go-betweens for patients and their medical and allied staff both at home and in hospital or hospice situations. This does not begin to describe the further roles of emotional care and support, the roles of spokesperson, advocate, or proxy decision-maker (see (1,2) for a thorough review of the empirical research on these many tasks). In all these myriad of practical tasks a number of social dimensions complicate and compound these family duties. I review these below.

Social dimensions of family end-of-life care

Gender issues

Women have traditionally assumed much of the brunt of family care. Furthermore, because women tend to outlive their male partners in modern industrial contexts two other consequences reinforce this gender inequality at the end of life. Women tend to be the main carers of their male partners because more women frequently outlive them and secondly, more of these widows tend to be institutionalized at the end of life because there is no one to look after them in their own homes when they begin to age and die (3).

Finally, some studies have indicated that more women than men report higher levels of perceived stress during their caring (4–6). Some of this burden of stress during care may in part be attributable to the micro-politics of gender relations during care, that is, to the possibility that men will make more demands on a female spouse than women might make on their male spouse carers. Alternatively, more women than men may feel/perceive/receive less actual support than is offered to male carers because male carers might more widely be viewed as vulnerable or unskilled in matters to do with domestic care more generally.

Financial issues

Several studies have noted the important impact that a lack of financial resources can play in the nature and level of family carer stress (7–9). Hudson (10), for example, reported that a quarter of his sample of 106 caregivers had stopped work or taken part-time work in order to care for dying family members at home. Although resigning from full-time work enables individuals to fully concentrate their attention on major round-the-clock care tasks, for a family member at home, it can also have important negative consequences.

These problems include increasing the possibility of social isolation, reducing overall financial capacity at home, and narrowing the number of psychological and social respite breaks during the course of care. Soothill and colleagues (11) in their survey of nearly 200 carers noted that 44% were retired leaving this group, at least in principle, vulnerable to additional financial pressures and risks directly relating to caring. Furthermore, retiring or retiring early to care for dying family members can reduce capacity to deal with costs associated with long-term care. In these ways, most carers are prone to the costs of additional equipment, medications, travel costs, or home care costs on their incomes whether they are retired, working part-time, or working full-time with a significant mortgage (9).

Social isolation

Social isolation is one of the most widely self-reported problems associated with family caregiving. Some of this may be attributed to the need to reduce paid employment. Other influences include the need to reduce social outings and recreational networks as the tasks of care become increasingly more complex and involving for the carer. Even a carer's own poor health has been implicated in increasing isolation as a carer's own illness or carer-related fatigue and injury reduce social contact outside the household.

Soothill and colleagues (11) make the most pertinent observation in this literature on social isolation when they note that although the majority of people have friends and relatives who live nearby only a minority of these people ever offer supportive services. Clearly one of several assumptions are being made by the majority of people in communities that surround carers of dying people at home.

Perhaps people do not know what to offer other family carers or perhaps they believe that any offer would be time-consuming for them. Some may believe that offers of care would only increase a family carer's stress by having people near who are willing to help but may be less skilled. Other people might believe that family care of the dying is too private and intimate or perhaps too difficult or dreadful for distant family or friends to help.

Some people may also believe that formal services are adequate or indeed that some carers do not wish to accept help or support. Whatever the 'real' reason/s behind the lack of community support it is clear that an important key to relieving carer stress and burden, as well as promoting a seamless continuity of care is the challenge of developing community capacity for this challenge. This challenge is, in turn, further complicated by the fact that carer's views of caring are not necessarily those of the dying person.

Dying person's views vs carer's views

Although it has long been recognized among Western people that most people wish to die at home surrounded by friends and family the carer reality of delivering this wish at home is entirely another matter. Some of the social dimensions already mentioned provide a picture of caring that is fraught with financial, interpersonal, and technical problems and one that is frequently coloured by common scenes of fatigue, loneliness and feelings of personal inadequacy. There have been conflicting complaints among research respondents that professional services and information are inadequate to many carers needs or that broader community or family fail to support them.

Some people have traced their unmet needs to conventional care from hospitals or long-term care rather than palliative care services (12) although others mainly expressed satisfaction with these services compared to managing the daily personal tasks of care and life in general (11;13). Although positive experiences are beginning to be reported in the literature (14) including the strengthening of relationships and improved levels of coping and confidence, for medical and other social reasons dying at home may not be appropriate for both carer and dying person.

In fact, Stajduhar (9) reports that some caregivers feel 'pressured' to provide home care as part of a dying person's wish to die at home as well as a growing view that dying at home 'is best'. Such views about dying at home are increasingly being enshrined in recent policy changes that encourage the dying persons to receive the majority of their care at home (4). But there are other social dimensions to differing views between dying and their carers.

Serious illness and dying often alter one's usual roles and relationships in important and sometimes disturbing ways. Adult children who are ill or dying may experience unwelcome role reversals from parents, their children or spouses. Fluctuating states of health or illness can be ignored by an overall assumption of inadequacy in dying people by their carers. Valued roles or tasks may be prematurely given up–or taken away from dying people (3). For fear of being viewed as ungrateful, few dying people may voice protest or criticism. From the same motives and disadvantaged position the common overwhelming attention of friends and family who visit frequently can be a welcome source of support for carers but an added source of stress for the dying person (15). Although research comparing carers and cancer patient views exist in the literature (13) research into carers experience of the social care of dying are yet to adopt this serious comparative dimension to see which parts of these worlds overlap and which parts may collide.

Disenfranchised carers

Although much of the literature on caring attempts to scrutinize needs and satisfaction with professional support and information, or gauge how adequate or otherwise the support is for carers, there have been few attempts to explore the problem of disenfranchised caring. The problem of disenfranchised grief has been openly acknowledged for some time now (16)—the unrecognized grief over lost animal companions, covert sexual relationships or ignored social experiences. However, the same recognition of this common problem for carers is yet to occur in the family carers literature in any significant way. There has been some research recognition about how the disenfranchised care that adults living with HIV/AIDS often receive from parents sometimes excludes or limits the care that former or current lovers can provide. Nevertheless, this problem of unrecognized same-sex relationships also includes past or current heterosexual and bisexual relations.

Furthermore, there is little recognition that *dying people commonly also see themselves as carers* [see (17) for an excellent discussion of this issue]. In other words, in the matter of providing psychological and social support it is important to recognize that *both* 'formal' professional and family carers AND the patient are commonly engaged in what all parties view as 'caring for one another'.

Therefore hidden relationships, and the most obvious one before carers—the dying person—are frequently unrecognized relationships of care that we know little about either because we have not adequately explored these populations in the care literature or because the dying person is always stereotypically cast as a receiver of care only and not as a population that also provide caring roles. The inadequacy of this research state of affairs notwithstanding, disenfranchised carers of the dying from their former and currently unrecognized relationships, and care from dying persons towards their carers, remain an important potential dimension of care to recognize in our professional practices.

Cultural and international dimensions of family end-of-life care

Home vs institutional care: symbols of family care?

With some historical exceptions, home care for dying people has been a longstanding desire and custom for people in the Western world for many years (18). However, both the desire and the custom of caring for dying family at home are not cross-cultural and this is an important cultural difference of care to consider. For some Chinese families, for example, a death at home may bring 'bad luck' or ill fortune on a household—something both families and the dying person wish to avoid if at all possible (19). For many Japanese families, dying at home may suggest to neighbours that a family caring for their dying relative does not have the financial resources for 'better' care in a hospital—or worse—that this care is not being offered for selfish reasons.

These observations highlight the need to thoroughly investigate the preferences of all carers but especially those who may not share common preferences for care in some locations or may do so but for different reasons. In this way, the reasons are as important to

establish as the preferences themselves. But in this context there are even further complications worth identifying.

International and mixed family carers

Most countries nowadays are experiencing a global form of multi-culturalism either welcomed or forced upon them in a post-colonial, high-migrating world situation. What this
means for end-of-life care in general, and families in particular, is that assumptions about
care are now diverse, contingent, and uncertain. Definitions about what constitutes 'care'
may differ even within families as migrant spouses or parents diverge over the 'right'
place to die, the 'right' people to perform intimate tasks of care, or the complex problem
of privacy in small ethnic communities who rely on interpreters. Families that were once
large, extended and may have included servants are now small, dislocated and may now
be commonly confronted with significant communication challenges to even articulate
their needs to others.

Some international communities within a country may be quite small with their usual
internal social or religious divisions unable to ignore each other. Such divisions might be
ignored in the larger populations of the home country but may act as sources of embar-
rassment, inadequacy or resentment in dislocated contexts in a new country. Small but
diverse international communities can mean that small precious items important to the
comfort of the elderly, seriously ill, or dying may be difficult or impossible to obtain. For
example, steamed rice and some kinds of sweet jellies are important to Japanese people
in illness, most especially the elderly who have very specific beliefs about the health
properties of their rice. But that medium-grain Japanese-style rice is absent from most
supermarkets in the UK where it is usually only obtainable from large metropolitan
centres such as London. Family care in these kinds of cultural contexts can be fraught
with culture-specific complexities and difficulties and immeasurably add to the stress of
that care.

Family care in developing nations

Although tuberculosis, malaria and other infectious diseases still dog the poor nations of
the world, HIV is quickly establishing itself as the most important cause of death in these
global contexts. There are currently over 40 million people worldwide infected with this
virus (20), with 5 million new infections annually (21). Most of these people who have
reliable access to antivirals can expect some 10 years life expectancy from diagnosis but
without these antivirals future prospects are considerably less (22). HIV/AIDS is now the
fourth biggest killer in the world today (23).

Irrespective of attempts to stop the spread of HIV, some 25 million people have already
died and many millions more will suffer the same fate. For regions such as Africa, where
prevalence can be between 30 to 50% of the population (24), end-of-life care must depend
heavily on family because health services are meagre, non-existent or a causal part of the
HIV epidemic itself (25). Historically, one might expect traditional customs and supports
to play an important role in this care. Unfortunately, this is seldom the case because the

virus itself is highly stigmatized and feared. Shame is frequently associated with the virus because various folk theories often attribute death to some moral wrong-doing or witchcraft from others (26). Furthermore, family often experience this shame, stigma, and social rejection by association leaving both dying people and their families without traditional supports (27).

In Eastern Europe, since the collapse of the former Soviet Union, villages were emptied from their working age men and women as poverty spread and the able bodied looked for work in foreign countries. Often this desperate search for work takes these populations to far flung countries in western Europe as illegal workers, refugees, or unfortunate subjects of human trafficking. This leaves a major gap in the ability of families to care for their aging and dying as villages in eastern Europe see a preponderance of young children and old people. The customary care provided by adult children, and especially women, is seriously compromised in these kinds of national context (28;29).

Public health support for family care at the end of life

The various social and cultural dimensions of care outlined above strongly suggest the need to think outside of direct service supports for family carers. This is because professional support services, support groups, respite care, and educational interventions, although important to improving the lot of family carers (12), do not address the everyday world of work, school, or recreational contexts of living and dying. Professional supports occupy only a slim body of time and interaction compared to the far more numerous relationships and time that people spend with their usual social contacts and supports. This means that it is to these 'usual' and wider social supports and contexts that we must look to strengthen. This strengthening of wider supports can enhance seamless before-, during-, and after-care relationships with professional services. Furthermore, for economically poor and service-impoverished areas in developing nations, recognition of these non-professional supports may be a simultaneous recognition that these are the *only* supports available.

Furthermore, many of the social problems of family care—of isolation, lack of respite care, of stigma and disenfranchisement, or cultural fragmentation, may be addressed by wider public health approaches that target misinformation, ignorance and or community-wide fears and prejudice. For example, the importance of sex education, improved access to effective contraception and non-family supports, as well as anti-discrimination legislation and information have greatly improved the health and safety of heterosexual teenagers as well as the gay community. These health promotion improvements have complemented health service provision by ensuring that the problem of sexually transmitted diseases, unwanted pregnancies or the stigma of sexual deviance is not simply addressed by services alone. Communities are active participants in this form of health care and support—schools, workplaces, social clubs, and churches but also by mainstream media outlets such as newspapers or television, and information and education notices strategically placed in locations as different as dance venues, toilets and community noticeboards.

A public health approach not only recognizes the importance of people as users of health services but equally the importance of building health and preventing illness or disease in the social settings of the everyday life of the communities they serve.

Community development initiatives—helping communities identify and address their own health and social care needs—are valuable strategies to enhance the community capacity to support families that are supporting their dying parents, spouses, children, or friends. Furthermore, in international contexts where poverty, war, or meagre health services preclude a major health services response to dying and their family carers, broader models of health care may need to be called forth. A public health approach to end-of-life care that incorporates health promoting palliative care, community development and service partnerships will be crucial to the support of families in all these diverse arrangements and limitations. What are the principles of a public health approach to end-of-life care that can enhance family care of the dying?

Principle ideas driving a public health approach

Because family carers may be subject to discrimination, poor social support, or personal isolation, direct support services such as counselling, respite care, or other direct professional services can be practically helpful and of genuine value to carers. However, supports such as respite care are not designed for *prevention and harm reduction* efforts that would reduce the stress and lack of support at the centre of the problem itself. For example, the personal experience of bereavement may be worsened by the common belief that the bereaved should 'get over it' after a few weeks. Counselling may help the bereaved person understand unhelpful community attitudes and to deal with the personal pain of being a victim of them but it does not prevent the problem itself.

Identifying information that will combat ignorance about grief in the wider community— or ignorance about caring—relies heavily on *community participation*. In facilitating any change, identifying the barriers and incentives to that change is crucial—and few people know better what these barriers and incentives might be than the communities them- selves found in schools, workplaces, churches, or families. Inside every community in schools or workplaces, for example, are people who have had direct experience of the problems of caring for the chronically ill, the aged, or the dying. Encouraging commu- nities to explore and exploit that social experience and wisdom among themselves is a crucial step in raising consciousness about a social issue that effects everyone. In these processes the personal experiences, once identified and observed as a re-occurring expe- rience affecting many people, soon become identified as a wider social concern to be addressed as a social task for all. Community participation then, is of paramount impor- tance to the identification, design AND success of any community education and support programme.

Inside this community development approach to health promotion *education and the development of supports* occur by building on existing skills and wisdom of individuals AND within the communities that might support those individuals. By encouraging groups and communities such as families, schools or workplaces to address their own perceived needs and develop strategies for dealing with them community initiatives create 'ownership'—and therefore sustainability—of personal AND public programmes.

Public health approaches to palliative care have been in existence for some time in Australia where these are known as 'health promoting palliative care' (HPPC) programmes (30;31). Health promoting palliative care programmes are programmes designed and developed to promote the idea that care in matters to do with death and loss is everyone's responsibility—not just from professional staff to patients and their families but also staff to staff, staff to patients and their families, community to families and health service professionals. The goals of HPPC (30) consist of:

- Providing education and information for health, dying and death
- Providing social supports—both personal and community
- Encouraging interpersonal reorientation
- Encouraging reorientation of palliative care services
- Combating death-denying health policies and attitudes.

In this context, palliative care services think about what community partnerships, activities and roles they might play in developing their own and the wider community's capacity to cope with death, loss, and care.

Examples of public health approaches from Australian palliative care services are presented in Box 21.1.

Conclusion

The social history of dying indicates that human beings have always cared for their dying—and their families—*as a whole community* (18). Hunter–gather communities have shared the task of care for the seriously ill and have supported families involved more directly in that care. This is also true for peasant societies. The development of urban societies has promoted economic specialization and social diversity, and those developments have been hallmark characteristics of modernity itself.

All these developments have witnessed the rise of cross-cultural forms of reliance and dependency on professionals and their services. In the last 100 years this has made dying people more dependent on health services at the same time as isolating families from wider community supports as folk understandings of 'care' gradually transformed themselves into notions of 'expertise'. We are now seeing a major rethinking of these changes.

The recognition of the importance of family and community care is on the ascendant and this volume is testimony to this fact. The facts of family care and its common consequences—social inequalities, isolation, role ambiguities, financial strains, and many other stresses—suggest the need for a wider public health approach to family care. The idea that we can prevent or reduce the harms for carers through service partnerships and community development are prompting new health service experiments in several countries, such as the ones described here for Australia. There is a greater willingness to entertain new ideas, a greater curiosity to explore the limits to public health in the context of end-of-life care. Such initiatives and desire augur well for public health developments in end-of-life care and they must surely bode well for family carers everywhere.

Box 21.1 Two public health examples from Australian palliative care services

1. In Newcastle city in the Australian state of New South Wales, the regional palliative care service for that city covers some 350,000 residents. For some years now the palliative care service has been actively engaged in relationships with local media, schools, and the community in general to promote awareness—not simply about palliative care—but how to live and live well with death, dying, loss and care.

Staff at this service have been involved with radio programmes as well as active contributors to the local newspapers so they are able to promote community discussion of experiences about death, dying, loss, and care by relating experiences from their workaday world of professional care. Also inside these stories are other stories about family and community care. More directly the Newcastle (Hunter Region) team have been involved in what is commonly termed a 'café conversation' or 'World Café'. In these social activities, a real local café is hired or freely participates in a community invitation to discuss an important life-issue such as mortality.

Local education authorities have been contacted and schools visited by palliative care staff to facilitate their own 'needs assessment'. Key among the priorities for teachers is what to say and how to be helpful to students who have parents who are living with life-threatening illness or who die. Communication issues about what to say to people affected by death or heavy care responsibilities are particularly important to teachers. The development of resources to help students and staff with these communication issues is developed.

Sometimes, the need for grief education is subsequently identified and experts invited to conduct workshops for students or staff. Often simply reflective sessions or the combing through of institutional memory can help both staff and students identify what has helped in the past and what has not. Feedback style evaluations have affirmed that these type of efforts in community capacity building for the general public or schools have been practical and helpful in subsequent relationships encountering death-related events.

2. The Hume Regional Palliative Care (HRPC) team in the northern part of the Australian state of Victoria has had similar success with its health promoting palliative care work (32). This team covers some 40,000 square kilometres and consists of 5 specialist palliative care units and 17 local palliative care volunteer groups.

After initial workshops on health promoting palliative care to clinical staff, volunteers and their managers a health promotion resource team was brought together from both volunteers and staff who had attended the earlier in-service education workshops. This team coordinated and supported the work of other staff and volunteers in the development of community activities and partnerships across the region. The Big 7 Checklist (see (31)) was used to assess between possible community activities as ones that might engender a public health mission and those that might not.

Box 21.1 Two public health examples from Australian palliative care services *(continued)*

Some of the practical outcomes of HRPC efforts included: One larger rural town exploring how young people can communicate creatively about the reality of loss and grief in their lives. The partnerships involved developing a performance event that included local youth service workers, a school nurse, community health workers, a church minister, the local palliative care loss and grief coordinator and volunteer service, a music therapist and other community members with creative talents. The event has been linked with other youth funding schemes, which in turn, increased its potential as a sustainable project.

Another project created an older adult day-activity programme that explored how to assist their clients reflect on personal and family resources that have been used throughout their life span. This was done through photos, stories, memory boxes and the commencement of an illustrated journal including each participant's life story as shared. They involved the local primary school, the adult learning centre and the community health centre as partners in the project making it sustainable and accessible to others within their community.

Another programme involved an adult education centre in a small town that ran two courses for carers in their community. The aim was to strengthen their knowledge of available community support, to inform about loss and grief, to provide resources and skills and access to a sustainable self-help network.

One palliative care volunteer service commenced discussion with their local government council to establish a reflective space at the city cemetery to shelter families and carers visiting people who have died on the palliative care programme and who are buried there. A partnership between them and the local cemetery trust, the local hospital and the palliative care service saw a rotunda and garden area built.

There were numerous World Café events across the length and breadth of the region; other projects that involved church groups, palliative care service involvement of information stands at community festivals and horse racing events. Local business houses were asked to support a 'care for the carers' day where businesses were asked to donate products or services that would help carers. Examples included food, massage, gifts or discounts to relaxing venues. Many other projects, too numerous to mention here (see (32)), were also started and continue in this innovative health promotion programme. The preliminary evaluation of these programmes suggest that they were enthusiastically embraced by the community's involved, were practical and helpful, did indeed build capacity to help beyond direct services and improved the relationship between palliative care services, families, and the wider community (33).

References

(1) Stajduhar, K., Cohen, R. (2009) Family caregiving in the home. In P. Hudson & S. Payne (eds), *Family Carers in Palliative Care*. Oxford: Oxford University Press, 149–68.

(2) Ferrell, B., Borneman, T., Thai, C. (2009) Family caregiving in hospitals and palliative care units. In P. Hudson & S. Payne (eds), *Family Carers in Palliative Care*. Oxford: Oxford University Press, 131–47.

(3) Kellehear, A. (1994) The social inequality of dying. In C. Waddell & A.R. Petersen (eds), *Just Health: Inequality in Illness, Care and Prevention*. Melbourne: Churchill Livingstine, 181–89.

(4) Payne, S., Smith, P., Dean, S. (1999) Identifying the concerns of informal carers in palliative care. *Palliative Medicine* **13**, 37–44.

(5) Scott, G., Whyler, N., Grant, G. (2001) A study of family carers of people with a life-threatening illness 1: The carers' needs analysis. *International Journal of Palliative Care* **7** (6), 290–97.

(6) Goldstein, N.E., Concato, J., Fried, T.R., et al. (2004) Factors associated with caregiver burden among caregivers with terminally ill patients with cancer. *Journal of Palliative Care* **20** (1), 38–43.

(7) Neale, B. (1991) Informal palliative care: a review of research on needs, standards and service evaluation. Occasional Papers 3, Trent Palliative Care Centre.

(8) Emmanuel, E.J., Fairclough, D.L., Slutsman, J., and Emanuel, L.L. (2000) Understanding economic and other burdens of terminal illness: The experience of patients and their caregivers. *Ann Intern Med* **132** (6), 451–9.

(9) Stajduhar, K.I. (2003) Examining the perspectives of family members involved in the delivery of palliative care at home. *Journal of Palliative Care* **19** (1), 27–35.

(10) Hudson, P. (2003) Home-based support for palliative care families: Challenges and recommendations. *Medical Journal of Australia* **179** (6), S35–37.

(11) Soothill, K., Morris, S.M., Harman, J.C., et al. (2001) Informal carers of cancer patients: What are their unmet psychosocial needs? *Health and Social Care in the Community* **9** (6), 464–75.

(12) Harding, R., Higginson, I. (2003) What is the best way to help caregivers in cancer and palliative care? A systematic literature review of interventions and their effectiveness. *Palliative Medicine* **17**, 63–74.

(13) Thomas, C., Morris, S.M., and Hardman, J.C. (2002) Companions through cancer: The care given by informal carers in cancer contexts. *Soc Sci Med* **54** (4), 529–44.

(14) Hudson, P. (2004) Positive aspects and challenges associated with caring for a dying relative at home. *International Journal of Palliative Care* **10** (20), 58–64.

(15) Kellehear, A. (1990) Dying of cancer: The final year of life. Switzerland: Harwood Academic Publishers.

(16) Doka, K. (ed.) (1989) *Disenfranchised Grief*. Lexington, MA: Lexington Books.

(17) Vafiadis, P. (2001) *Mutual Care in Palliative Medicine: A Story of Doctors and Patients*. Sydney: McGraw-Hill.

(18) Kellehear, A. (2007) *A Social History of Dying*. Cambrige: Cambridge University Press.

(19) Chan, C.L.W. & Chow, A.Y.M. (eds) (2006) *Death, Dying and Bereavement: A Hong Kong Chinese Experience*. Hong Kong: Hong Kong University Press.

(20) World Health Organisation (2005) *AIDS Epidemic Update 2005*. Geneva: UNAIDS.

(21) Economic and Social Commission for Asia and the Pacific (2003) HIV/AIDS in the Asian and Pacific Region. New York: United Nations.

(22) Fleming, P.L. (2004) The epidemiology of HIV and AIDS. In G.P. Wormser (ed.), *AIDS and Other Manifestations of HIV Infection*. San Diego: Elsevier, 3–29.

(23) Healey, J. (ed.) (2003) *HIV/AIDS*. Sydney: Spinney Press.

(24) Ferrante, P., Delbue., Mancuso, R. (2005) The manifestation of AIDS in Africa: An epidemiological overview. *Journal of Neurovirology* **1**, 50–7.

(25) Volkow, P., del Rio, C. (2005) Paid donation and plasma trade: Unrecognised forces that drive the Aids epidemic in developing countries. *International Journal of STDs and AIDS* **6**, 5–8.

(26) Liddell, C., Barrett, L., Bydawell, M. (2005) Indigenous representations of illness and AIDS in Sub-Sahara Africa. *Social Science & Medicine* **60**, 691–700.

(27) Songwathana, P., Manderson, L. (2001) Stigma and rejection: Living with AIDS in Southern Thailand. *Medical Anthropology* **20** (1), 1–23.

(28) Wright, M., Clark, D. (eds) (2006) *Hospice and Palliative Care in Africa: A Review of Developments and Challenges.* Oxford: Oxford University Press.

(29) Bingley, A., McDermott, E. (2007) Resilience in resource-poor settings. In B. Monroe & D. Oliviere (eds), *Resilience in Palliative Care: Achievement in Adversity.* Oxford: Oxford University Press, 261–79.

(30) Kellehear, A. (1999) *Health Promoting Palliative Care.* Melbourne: Oxford University Press.

(31) Kellehear, A. (2005) *Compassionate Cities: Public Health and End of Life Care.* London: Routledge.

(32) Kellehear, A., Young, B. (2007) Resilient Communities. In B. Monroe and D. Oliviere (eds), *Resilience in Palliative Care: Achievements in Adversity.* Oxford: Oxford University Press, 223–38.

(33) Rumbold, B., & Gear, R. (2004) *Evaluation of Health Promotion Resource Team: Hume Regional Palliative Care Caring Communities Project 'Building Rural Community Capacity Through Volunteering'.* Melbourne: La Trobe University Palliative Care Unit.

Part VII

Conclusion

Chapter 22

Conclusions: Palliative care—the need for a public health approach

Luc Deliens and Joachim Cohen

Introduction

Until recently, little attention has been given to the development of a public health approach to palliative care at the end of life. With this book we hope to have shown the challenges and potential of a public health approach which is focused on populations rather than on individual patients and their families. This book provides a wide range of information about public health at the end of life and it shows evidence that it is unlikely that good dying for all will be attained by limiting our societal efforts to the improvement of palliative medicine or palliative nursing. There is no doubt that both clinical disciplines still need to be improved, but this in itself will be insufficient to bring about good end-of-life care in all nations and for all patients in need. This book includes an overview of the clinical and social context of death and dying, the provision, access and characteristics of end-of-life care, the differences between care settings, inequalities at the end of life, and the identification of under-served groups within society, and, in the last part, end-of-life care strategies and policies.

We hope that this book, with its valuable contributions from many internationally recognized authors from many countries and several continents, will support the development of a complementary public health policy for palliative care, and that clinicians, public health professionals, and researchers will reach out to and reinforce each other in the effort to develop palliative care across all nations and continents.

Palliative care and public health

According to the World Health Organization, palliative care is an approach that improves the quality of life of patients and their families facing the problems associated with life-threatening illness, through the prevention and relief of suffering by means of early identification and impeccable assessment and treatment of pain and other problems, physical, psychosocial, and spiritual. In addition to attending to physical needs, palliative care explicitly includes the addressing of psychosocial and spiritual needs. Such holistic care is complex and frequently multidisciplinary and is ideally initiated at the time of diagnosis of serious or life-threatening illness, independently of prognosis, and is delivered in concert with curative or life-prolonging therapies provided these are beneficial to the patient. Furthermore this complex care needs to be coordinated by a key caregiver; in some countries or health care systems this is often a general practitioner, in others a nursing home or palliative care physician, a district nurse or a palliative nurse. Hence, good palliative care requires a wide multidisciplinary clinical approach and coordinated caregiving at the end of life. While in most parts of the world this kind of high quality end-of-life care is not yet available, there is also not one country in the world where high quality palliative care is accessible for all in need, independent of their disease, age, gender, socio-economic or ethnic background. There are pervasive cultural, attitudinal, structural and financial barriers to the optimal accessibility of palliative or end-of-life care, and public health researchers must study and identify these barriers and come up with solutions to overcome them. In order to take into account culturally and socially sensitive aspects of health service delivery at the end of life, adapted research designs must be developed and implemented.

Whatever are the best palliative services available in any country, in order to know which patients and people have access to them, societies must monitor not only the quality of palliative care provision but also its accessibility. This book demonstrates clearly that the accessibility of end of life or palliative care varies substantially according to differences in age, disease, culture and social characteristics and conditions. In order to achieve proper end-of-life care for all, we need a population perspective, and this perspective must take into account different disease trajectories (not just the cancer trajectories), different age groups, and different cultures, while policy-making must be multisectoral: public health at the end of life integrates demographics, sociology, and epidemiology with policy-making, organizational and economic skills, together with the skills and knowledge of clinical palliative care. In order to achieve good end-of-life care for all, it is not sufficient to have good nurses and good physicians; we must also have good monitoring systems in a context of advanced policies with a population approach.

As editors of this book, we have found it a pleasure to go through the chapters and learn so much about the cultural, social, and policy aspects of end-of-life care and public health. In this last chapter, we are glad to share these insights with you.

Cultural context

The cultural context in which death takes place has been mentioned by several authors as important in developing sensitive end-of-life care. In general in many Western cultures, attitudes toward disease and death are barriers to the optimal employment of palliative care services (Chapter 11). Current 'consumer society' culture celebrates activity, accomplishment, and youth and denies death; it appears to consider not only health but also immortality as products to which people are entitled. Advances in public health and the technologies of medicine feed this death-denying culture, and patients, families, and physicians may pursue questionably effective, burdensome therapies rather than confront the fact that a life may be coming to its end. Partly for these reasons, palliative care consultation is often deferred until the final days or hours of life.

People with serious illnesses are often in unknown territory (Chapter 8). Not only have they not experienced such illness before nor faced their imminent mortality but, in present-day Western culture, many may not have witnessed another person's death. They may feel disorientated and unsure of what is important and what is not, so providing someone with a clear diagnosis and prognosis so that they can use the knowledge in a way that gives them purpose requires honesty and sensitive communication skills from clinicians. Moreover, the patient's wishes, values, and norms are at the real centre of palliative care and in order to benefit fully the patient must have the right to be fully informed.

Another deeply concerning cultural aspect of death and dying is the existence of a selective attitude towards older people. Ageism is described as the presence of a belief, held by a health care provider, that conditions such as depression, pain, and other disorders are a normal part of aging and that the older individual will not benefit from treatment (Chapter 13). This attitude can discriminate against or otherwise disadvantage an older adult in the nature of the care provided. Among health care professionals, ageism can manifest itself in the belief that poor health is an inevitable consequence of aging. Health care professionals can make assumptions about older patients based on age rather than functional status. As in other forms of prejudice and discrimination, ageism is a product of culture, an attitude or belief that is endemic in society and that may manifest itself in the delivery of health care. The evidence suggests that older adults are less likely to be given proven medical interventions, often leading to inappropriate or incomplete treatment. Research also reveals that older adults may be ignored by physicians or may suffer inappropriate aggressive treatment. Both extremes reveal a lack of understanding of how to manage and treat the complex health needs of the older adult. This selective attitude is totally inappropriate in palliative care.

In some cultures however, older people's perceptions may also have a positive effect on end-of-life care. Interesting findings on the effect of cultural sensitivity and meaning on place of death are clearly described in Chapter 2. The greater likelihood of *elderly, compared with younger, cancer patients dying at home* in some countries such as Italy or Taiwan *may be due to cultural considerations.* Taiwanese culture values *shou zhong zheng qin* (dying naturally of old age at home in one's bed) as the most glorious and fortunate way of dying. Taiwanese people are highly motivated to fulfil an older family member's wish for *shou zhong zheng qin* as an aspect of filial piety.

Of course delivering end-of-life care will be different in different cultures. Models of palliative service delivery in Western countries will not necessarily work well in developing countries and the needs for palliative care will be different. However, a public health end-of-life care approach for Africa needs also to take into account the differences in resources and available services across the continent, and policy will differ from region to region or country to country. The African continent has diverse characteristics, populations, languages, cultures, health care systems, policies, resources, and levels of access to medications. The differences between sub-Saharan and other parts of Africa are great, though we have only been able here to focus on palliative care in countries in sub-Saharan Africa (Chapter 19). There is an overwhelming need for quality palliative care services across sub-Saharan Africa. Centres of excellence exist and enormous advocacy gains have been made. Lessons have been learnt in terms of coverage, lobbying and advocacy, and innovative low-cost palliative care that can be useful for other regions of the world. However, palliative care remains a public health priority within the region and practitioners must continue to be innovative, adapting and developing appropriate models of care to meet the public health needs of all.

Social and demographic issues

Although it is difficult to estimate what the appropriate level of palliative care provision in a population should be, this book demonstrates clearly that provision of palliative care varies considerably between countries (Chapter 6 and Chapter 7). Many patients across the world have little or no access to palliative care due to lack of provision while within nations with good provision there is considerable local variation in both provision and access (Chapter 16). Patients differ in their access to palliative care on the basis of diagnosis, age, gender, socio-economic status, ethnic background, and the availability of a family carer.

Populations are aging, and increasing numbers of people are reaching the end of life. The overall picture of the circumstances of death and dying is one of common complex and multiple symptoms, emotional, spiritual, and social concerns, with more similarities than differences in the experience of patients with different conditions (Chapter 3). There are often gaps in the provision of services providing support and symptom relief, but equally examples of inappropriate or over-treatment, mainly in hospitals. Family members and caregivers often carry a great burden and their own health suffers. Older people, those from low socio-economic groups and black and minority ethnic groups often experience disadvantage in access to services despite similar levels of problems. Making palliative care for all more of a public health priority would create more opportunities for equal access to all patients.

The issues of gender and the differences between male and female deaths are illustrated in several chapters. Women have traditionally borne much of the brunt of family care (Chapter 21) and tend to outlive their male partners, leading to two other consequences which reinforce gender inequality at the end of life: they tend to be the main carers of their male partners and then to be institutionalized themselves at the end of their own life. Their children may have moved away, particularly from rural communities (Chapter 16) and there is no one left to look after them; their health, and wealth, are likely to have been undermined by having cared for their male partner (Chapter 5), and because they live longer they are more likely to face the prejudices against the very old, including those which affect the likelihood of end-of-life decisions with a potential or certain life shortening effect (Chapter 4).

Under-served patient groups need selective policies

It is clear that continued support of palliative care integration into acute and chronic care models, as well as the implementation of end-of-life practice guidelines based on culturally sensitive quality indicators, should become public health policy priorities (Chapter 6).

Given the demographic transition and the shift in developed societies of place of death towards care home and nursing home, the organization of a care home or a nursing home and the quality of its care have significant influence on end-of-life care (Chapter 10).

Because in Dutch nursing homes physicians are on-site, they serve as 'gatekeepers' and tend not to hospitalize patients with, for instance, dementia. On-staff physicians provide continuity of care, similar to that provided by the family physician, which reduces the rate of hospitalization of older people with ambulatory care-sensitive conditions. In the US, with less physician presence in nursing homes, this continuity role may be served by an on-site nurse practitioner who can also lower hospitalization rates in dementia patients. Reimbursement practices also influence end-of-life care decisions in nursing homes, such as financial payment for feeding tubes in the US, so their use is not discouraged. The effect is evident in that feeding tubes are used more frequently in for-profit nursing homes.

Despite the need to develop good end-of-life care in long-term care settings, a large majority wants to stay at home and wants to extent or prevent a transfer to a long term setting if possible. This means that developing palliative care services in primary care remain an important public health challenge, with many common challenges across different countries with different health care systems (Chapter 9).

An aging population will contribute to increases in long-term conditions, and hence an increasing number of people will die after an illness trajectory of frailty or dementia. This means that the fact that those with non-malignant conditions remain under-served in palliative care is problematic. Several reasons for this disadvantage are discussed in Chapter 12, one of them that understanding the transition from actively curing disease to accepting an approaching death is often more difficult for non-cancer patients. Planning end-of-life care and palliative care services for those with non-malignant conditions will therefore be one of the public health challenges.

Children are another under-served group. Although childhood death in developed countries is an infrequent event, the provision of paediatric health care before death, specifically or more generally in the setting of a grave life threatening illness, is also a public health issue (Chapter 14) which demands not only an individualized plan of clinical care but also a population-level approach. Chapter 14 on paediatric palliative care outlines a public health framework for paediatric palliative and hospice care to facilitate the focus on key public health concerns and to better understand how to apply them in the context of paediatric palliative and hospice care.

People with intellectual disabilities are among the most vulnerable in society. The lack of use and access to end-of-life care for people with intellectual disabilities is becoming an issue of increasing concern and adjustments to palliative care provisions and access are urgently needed (Chapter 15). Such adjustments include the need to modify communication, allowing extra time, the inclusion of family and other carers as partners in care, finding creative ways to meet individual needs, and liaising with other service providers. This alone is not enough: there also needs to be a commitment at regional and national level to providing policies and guidelines for services around inclusion of people with intellectual disabilities, and to supporting training initiatives.

Many rural/remote populations and some urban sub-populations also have inequalities that disadvantage them when ill, with end-of-life inequalities being particularly concerning (Chapter 16). Chapter 17 appraises evidence, principally from the UK and the USA, to determine in which ways the socially excluded—the poor, black, and minority ethnic groups, asylum seekers and refugees, the homeless, those within the penal system, and drug users—fare with respect to accessing palliative care and related services during advanced disease and at the end of life. It is important for researchers to increase our understanding of these inequalities, so that services for terminally ill people and their families better meet the needs of these under-served populations.

Public health at the end of life needs clear policy and vision on how end-of-life care should be developed and organized. This vision can best be developed and promoted within an international framework like the World Health Organization (WHO).

Palliative care as a human right: a call for an international policy agenda

Palliative care remains poorly framed within evidence-based global policy-making (Chapter 20). It is clear that the discourse surrounding the global development of palliative care is still weakly articulated and relatively sparse. Until now limited efforts have been focused on understanding how palliative care is positioned within the language of global policy-making. Palliative care is not one of the Millennium Development Goals; it is hard to find in the priorities of the United Nations, UNESCO and other global organizations. In 2011, the global palliative care community can claim some significant successes but with a growing global infrastructure for advocacy, fund-raising, and collaboration, the next decades will be crucial in breaking through to a higher level of policy recognition. Such recognition is vital if the world's palliative care needs are to be met in an equitable and culturally sensitive manner and a true public health orientation towards end-of-life care is to be achieved.

The most powerful tool for promoting and improving palliative care provision and access for all nations and all patient groups, independent of nation, race, religion, gender, age, or disease, could be the international positioning and implementation of palliative care as a human right. This would imply the moral and political call for international assistance and cooperation for access to all essential palliative or end-of-life care services and medicines. Access to essential medicines is a critical problem that plagues many developing countries (Chapter 19) With a daunting number of domestic constraints—technological, economic, and otherwise—developing countries are faced with a steep uphill battle to meet the human rights obligation of providing essential medicines. To meet these challenges, the international human rights obligations of international assistance and cooperation can play a key role in helping developing countries fulfil the need for access to essential medicines and essential end-of-life services.

This book has identified a number of under-served groups in end-of-life care, and an international coordinated action by, e.g., the WHO could establish a human rights agenda for '*equal access to end-of-life care for all*' (Chapter 18). Parallel to its promotion of prevention through the '*health for all*' strategy of the twentieth century, the WHO can establish an international agenda promoting palliative or end-of-life care for all in the twenty-first century. This would focus the efforts of the different nationally developed end-of-life care strategies towards more coordinated international action and promote not only improvements in palliative medicine and palliative nursing, but also promote and coordinate different intersectoral efforts to improve end-of-life care. It is not only the clinical sector which must promote end-of-life care concepts and infrastructure but also schools, universities, social and cultural organizations and even private companies. Hence, end-of-life care strategies have to develop a societal and population approach, alongside a clinical and individual patient one. The WHO could set an agenda with very concrete targets and deadlines and invite all governments to fit their end-of-life care strategies and policies into this framework. The palliative care community across the world could collaborate in this and start developing a policy based on the premise that palliative care is a human right and hence all people have equal rights to access it. To be successful in this the international palliative care community needs to expand the current understanding of end-of-life care from a clinical to a public health perspective.

Editing this book has been a pleasure and we have learned a great deal because the material in it presents an entirely different perspective on palliative and end-of-life care from that of traditional textbooks. We hope you too enjoyed reading it.

Index

DATE DUE

			PRINTED IN U.S.A.